ENVIRONMENTAL HEALTH ETHICS

Environmental Health Ethics illuminates the conflicts between protecting the environment and promoting human health. In this study, David B. Resnik develops a method for making ethical decisions on environmental health issues. He applies this method to various issues, including pesticide use, antibiotic resistance, nutrition policy, vegetarianism, urban development, occupational safety, disaster preparedness, and global climate change. Resnik provides readers with the scientific and technical background necessary to understand these issues. He explains that environmental health controversies cannot simply be reduced to humanity versus environment, and he explores the ways in which human values and concerns – health, economic development, rights, and justice – interact with environmental protection.

David B. Resnik, JD, PhD, is Bioethicist at the National Institute of Environmental Health Sciences, National Institutes of Health. Dr. Resnik additionally holds the positions of Adjunct Professor of Philosophy at North Carolina State University and Associate Editor of *Accountability in Research*. He has written eight books and numerous articles on ethical, philosophical, and legal issues in science, medicine, and technology. He is also Chair of the NIEHS Institutional Review Board, which oversees and reviews research projects that include human participants.

ENVIRONMENTAL HEALTH ETHICS

DAVID B. RESNIK

National Institute of Environmental Health Sciences

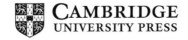

CAMBRIDGE
UNIVERSITY PRESS

CAMBRIDGE UNIVERSITY PRESS
Cambridge, New York, Melbourne, Madrid, Cape Town,
Singapore, São Paulo, Delhi, Mexico City

Cambridge University Press
32 Avenue of the Americas, New York, NY 10013-2473, USA

www.cambridge.org
Information on this title: www.cambridge.org/9781107617896

First published 2012

Printed in the United States of America

A catalog record for this publication is available from the British Library.

Library of Congress Cataloging in Publication data
Resnik, David B.
Environmental health ethics / David B. Resnik.
p. ; cm.
Includes bibliographical references and index.
ISBN 978-1-107-02395-6 (hardback) – ISBN 978-1-107-61789-6 (pbk.)
I. Title.
[DNLM: 1. Environmental Health – ethics.   2. Environmental Medicine – ethics.
3. Environmental Policy.   4. Environmental Pollution – ethics, WA 30.5]
613′.1–dc23   2011052380

ISBN 978-1-107-02395-6 Hardback
ISBN 978-1-107-61789-6 Paperback

This book is dedicated to Rachel Carson.

CONTENTS

FIGURES AND TABLES

ACKNOWLEDGMENTS

I would like to thank for following individuals for helpful comments and critiques: Bruce Androphy, Lisa DeRoo, Michael Fessler, Andrew Jameton, Paul Jung, Freya Kamel, Matt Longnecker, Zubin Master, Liam O'Fallon, Walter Rogan, Bill Schrader, William Suk, and Dan Vallero. This book is the work product of an employee or group of employees of the National Institute of Environmental Health Sciences (NIEHS), National Institutes of Health (NIH); however, the statements, opinions, and conclusions contained herein do not necessarily represent the statements, opinions, or conclusions of NIEHS, NIH, or the U.S. government.

ABBREVIATIONS

AIDS	Acquired Immune Deficiency Syndrome
ANWR	Alaska National Wildlife Refuge
ASU	Arizona State University
BPA	Bisphenol A
CAA	Clean Air Act
CBPR	Community-based participatory research
CDC	Centers for Disease Control and Prevention
CFC	Chlorofluorocarbon
CLIA	Clinical Laboratory Improvement Amendments
CPR	Cardiopulmonary resuscitation
DDT	Dichlorodiphenyltrichloroethane
DEET	N,N-diethyl-3-methylbenzamide
EPA	Environmental Protection Agency
ESA	Endangered Species Act
FDA	Food and Drug Administration
FEMA	Federal Emergency Management Administration
FFDCA	Federal Food, Drug, and Cosmetic Act
FIFRA	Federal Insecticide, Fungicide, and Rodenticide Act
FQPA	Food Quality Protection Act
FWS	Fish and Wildlife Service
GM	Genetically modified
GMO	Genetically modified organism
HDL	High density lipoprotein
HIV	Human immunodeficiency virus
IOM	Institute of Medicine
IPCC	Intergovernmental Panel on Climate Change
IPM	Integrated pest management
IRB	Institutional Review Board
KGOE	Kilograms of oil equivalent
KKI	Kennedy Krieger Institute

LD	Lethal dose
LD$_{50}$	Lethal dose 50 percent
LDL	Low density lipoprotein
LSD	Lysergic acid diethylamide
MRSA	Methicillin-resistant *Staphylococcus aureus*
MTD	Maximum tolerable dose
NAS	National Academy of Sciences
NHLBI	National Heart, Lung, and Blood Institute
NIEHS	National Institute of Environmental Health Sciences
NIH	National Institutes of Health
NIMBY	"Not in my backyard"
NIOSH	National Institute for Occupational Safety and Health
NOAA	National Oceanic and Atmospheric Administration
NOAEL	No observed adverse effect level
NRC	National Research Council
NTP	National Toxicology Program
OSHA	Occupational Health and Safety Administration
PCB	Polychlorinated biphenyl
PD	Parkinson's disease
PM	Particulate matter
POP	Persistent organic pollutant
PP	Precautionary principle
PTSD	Post-traumatic stress disorder
RCT	Randomized controlled trial
RfD	Reference dose
SDWA	Safe Drinking Water Act
TB	Tuberculosis
TSCA	Toxic Substances Control Act
UN	United Nations
UNICEF	United Nations Children's Fund
USDA	United States Department of Agriculture
VOCs	Volatile organic compounds
WHO	World Health Organization

I

INTRODUCTION

Over an increasingly large area of the United States, spring now comes unheralded by the return of birds, and the early mornings are strangely silent where once they were filled with the beauty of bird song.

Rachel Carson (1962: 97)

Rachel Carson launched the modern environmental movement in 1962 when she published *Silent Spring*, a book that documented the harmful effects of pesticides on birds and other nonhuman species. The book was serialized in the *New Yorker* prior to its full publication and was widely read after it was placed in the Book of the Month Club and became a best seller on the *New York Times* list. Carson had been aware of the potential hazards of pesticide use since the 1940s, but she became especially concerned when one of her friends had published a letter reporting the deaths of numerous birds on her property after aerial dichlorodiphenyltrichloroethane (DDT) spraying. In *Silent Spring*, Carson argued that DDT can cause reproductive problems, such as sterility, weak eggs shells, and embryo death in a variety of bird species, which leads to population decline (Carson 1962). She warned that, one day, the world would have a silent spring (i.e., no birdsongs) if steps were not taken to restrict the use of DDT and other pesticides. Carson discussed several examples of how pesticides can harm human beings, including a case in which farm workers had suffered toxic reactions from pesticide exposures. She also claimed that the chemical industry had spread false or misleading information about pesticide safety and that government agencies had not carefully examined industry claims.

Carson was a scientist, writer, and devoted lover of nature. She was born on May 27, 1907 in Springdale, Pennsylvania. In 1929, she graduated from Pennsylvania College for Women (now known as Chatham College), majoring in science. She then studied at the Woods Hole Marine Biological Laboratory in Massachusetts. In 1932, Carson received a master's degree in zoology from Johns Hopkins University. She worked for the U.S. Bureau of Fisheries in the 1930s and became editor-in-chief of U.S. Fish and Wildlife Service publications. While working for the federal government, Carson wrote pamphlets on conservation of natural resources and edited scientific articles. She also wrote articles on nature for newspapers and magazines. In 1952, she quit her government position to devote more time to writing. She published a highly acclaimed book, *The Sea Around Us* in 1952, followed by *The Edge of the Sea* in 1955. As a result of these books and other publications, Carson became a well-known popular science writer. She was inducted into the American Academy of Arts and Letters and won a National Audubon Society Medal. In 1964, Carson published an essay, "The Sense of Wonder," about the importance of nurturing a child's sense of wonder about the natural world. Carson had a radical mastectomy in 1960, and died of breast cancer four years later on April 14, 1964 at age 56 (Lear 2009).

Silent Spring generated tremendous controversy as soon as it was published. Industry representatives and some scientists branded Carson as a subversive, hysterical woman, who lacked the qualifications to investigate the complex issues related to pesticide use. She received personal attacks and threats of legal action. Other scientists and members of the public shared her concerns and called for new efforts to protect the environment from hazardous chemicals and pollution (Lytle 2007). In June 1963, Carson gave testimony about the dangers of pesticides to the U.S. Senate Subcommittee on Government Operations. President John F. Kennedy also ordered the Science Advisory Committee to conduct an independent review of Carson's research. The Science Advisory Committee concluded that Carson's assertions about the potential dangers of pesticides were well-founded, a finding that promoted a strengthening of U.S. pesticide regulations (Lytle 2007). As a result of growing concerns about DDT's potential effects on human beings and the environment, Sweden banned DDT in 1970, and the U.S. Environmental Protection Agency (EPA) banned the use of DDT except for specific public health purposes in 1972 (Robson et al. 2010). In the United States, the EPA regulates the sale, distribution, and use of pesticides and other chemicals.

DDT was first synthesized by Austrian chemists in 1873, but the compound did not generate much interest until Swiss chemist Paul Müller patented it in 1940 and explored its uses as a pesticide. Müller won the Nobel Prize in Physiology and Medicine in 1948 for his work demonstrating that DDT can kill a variety of insect pests, including mosquitoes, lice, and houseflies (Nobelprize.org 2010). Research conducted since the 1960s has yielded vital information about how DDT can cause harm to wildlife and humans. DDT is a persistent organic pollutant (POP), which can accumulate in organisms higher up the food chain and slowly degrades in the environment (Longnecker et al. 1997). Inside an organism, DDT may break down into DDE or DDD, which may be metabolized into other forms. DDT is stored in fatty tissues. Predatory birds, such as eagles, falcons, and pelicans, are particularly susceptible to the effects of DDT. It is also highly toxic to cats, crayfish, shrimp, and some species of fish (Agency for Toxic Substances and Diseases Registry 2002), and has been classified by the National Toxicology Program (NTP) as moderately toxic to humans. DDT exposure has been linked to premature birth, low birth weight, and developmental problems, and is associated with an increased risk of some types of cancer. DDT has been classified by the NTP as reasonably anticipated to be a human carcinogen (Agency for Toxic Substances and Diseases Registry 2002; National Toxicology Program 2009). There is some evidence that DDT causes genetic damage and disrupts human reproductive and endocrine functions even

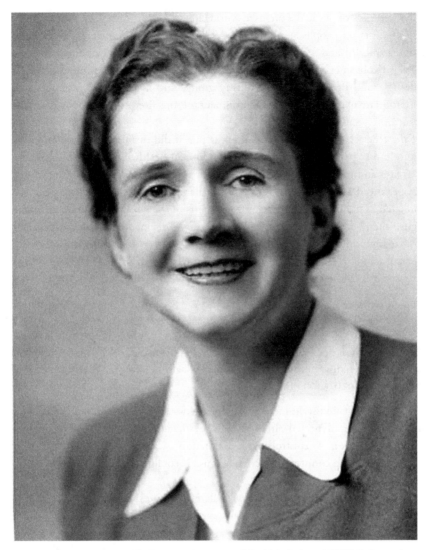

Figure 1.1. Rachel Carson (courtesy of the U.S. Fish and Wildlife Service).

in low doses (Longnecker et al. 1997). In 2001, more than 150 countries signed the Stockholm Convention on Persistent Organic Pollutants, which calls for the elimination of DDT and ten other POPs (Robson et al. 2010). See Figure 1.1 for photo of Rachel Carson.

Silent Spring initiated an ethical and political debate concerning the proper use of pesticides that continues today. A pesticide is a substance used to destroy, control, repel, or mitigate a species considered to be a pest, such as some types of insects, ticks, rodents, fungi, plants, microbes, worms, and even fish and birds (Environmental Protection Agency 2010a). People have been using chemicals to control pests since the nineteenth century.

Over 5 billion pounds of pesticides are used worldwide each year. Although pesticides can have harmful effects on people, nonhuman species, and the environment, they can also promote human health and well-being by preventing the spread of disease and improving crop yields (Robson et al. 2010). Though many environmental groups oppose the use of pesticides (Beyond Pesticides 2010), industry groups and many scientists endorse the safe and appropriate use of pesticides (Environmental Protection Agency 2009a; Croplife America 2010).

One of the chief criticisms of Carson's book is that it did not pay sufficient attention to the vital role that pesticides play in promoting human health. DDT had been widely used in the 1940s and 1950s to control disease-carrying mosquito populations in the United States, Europe, and the South Pacific. As a result, malaria and typhoid fever have been virtually eliminated as public health threats in many parts of the world (Robson et al. 2010). Critics argued then – and continue to claim now – that Carson's book is an antipesticide manifesto that undermines human health (Lytle 2007; Murray 2007). But this criticism misrepresents Carson's views about pesticides. Carson recognized the importance of using effective measures, including pesticides, to prevent insect-borne diseases:

All this is not to say there is no insect problem and no need of control. I am saying, rather, that control must be geared to realities, not to mythical situations, and that the methods employed must be such that they do not destroy us along with the insects.... It is not my contention that chemical insecticides must never be used. I do contend that we have put poisonous and biologically potent chemicals indiscriminately into the hands of persons largely or wholly ignorant of their potentials for harm. (Carson 1962: 20, 22)

Carson argued that the indiscriminate use of pesticides should be eliminated in favor of responsible use. She advocated alternatives to pesticides, such as the use of natural predators and sterilization, to control insect populations. Carson also warned that overuse of pesticides could be counterproductive because it could lead to pesticide resistance (Carson 1962).

The use of DDT to prevent the spread of malaria illustrates vividly some of the ethical dilemmas concerning pesticide use (Resnik 2009). Although malaria is no longer a significant problem in most of the world's developed nations, many developing nations still suffer under the burdens of this disease. Malaria is a parasite carried by females of the genus *Anopheles*. It produces fever, chills, headaches, and muscle pains, and can cause anemia, impaired consciousness, convulsions, kidney failure, and death. Approximately 350 million–500 million people contract malaria each year, mostly in nations in sub-Saharan Africa and the tropics (Centers for Disease Control and Prevention 2007). More than three million people die each year from malaria, most of them young children. Every thirty seconds a child dies from malaria (Kapp 2004). While there are medications that can treat malaria, prevention is the preferred method for reducing the impact of the disease on the human population, especially in countries that lack adequate health care resources. Methods of preventing infection include wearing protective clothing, using mosquito nets and repellants, as well as controlling the malaria vector (World Health Organization 2010). Vector control includes methods that disrupt the life cycle of mosquitoes, such as eliminating sources of stagnant water that serve as breeding grounds for mosquitoes, and the application of pesticides to kill mosquitoes in their adult or larval forms. In 2006, the World Health Organization (WHO) announced it would support limited use of DDT, such as spraying the chemical on interior walls or mosquito netting, to control malaria (World Health Organization 2006). Infectious disease specialists, public health advocates, and others have also supported limited use of DDT to control malaria (Roberts et al. 2000; Kapp 2004). Many sub-Saharan countries, including South Africa, Uganda, Zambia, Zimbabwe, and Kenya currently use DDT to fight malaria (Hecht 2004).

The WHO's endorsement of the limited use of DDT for malaria control has generated considerable controversy. Opponents of DDT use argue that because the chemical persists in ecosystems for many years and accumulates in species higher up in the food chain, it poses a risk to nonhuman species, including some species of birds and fish. DDT also poses risks to human health, which are not well understood at present, such as interference with reproductive and endocrine functions and neurological development. Moreover, some mosquito populations have become resistant to DDT as a result of overuse, and continued use may increase resistance. DDT may also disrupt ecosystems by altering the balance of different species in the food web, such as predatory birds. Disruption of ecosystems can have broad-ranging effects on human and nonhuman populations (Wilcox and Jessop 2010). Other strategies for controlling the spread of malaria, including medication, protective clothing and nets, and even the limited use of pesticides other than DDT, are preferable to limited DDT spraying, according to many (Berenbaum 2005; Pesticide Action Network of North America 2007).

The question of whether to use DDT to control malaria raises complex scientific and ethical issues:

- What are the hazards to human health and the environment posed by the limited use of DDT? Can these hazards be mitigated or controlled?
- Will limited use of DDT increase DDT resistance? Can DDT resistance be prevented?
- What are the alternatives to DDT use? How safe and effective are these alternatives?
- How should we weigh the uncertain long-term risks to human health posed by DDT use, such as endocrine disruption or cancer, against the near certain short-term benefits, such as malaria prevention?
- How should we balance human health against risks to nonhuman species and the environment posed by DDT use?
- Because children are more likely to die from malaria than adults, should public health measures emphasize short-term benefits to children over possible long-term risks to adults?
- What is the extent of a government's moral authority to regulate chemicals, such as pesticides, that can save lives but may also cause harm?

These and other issues related to DDT used to control malaria exemplify some of the themes that are the focus of this book. Dilemmas, problems, and questions concerning the relationship between human health and the environment have come to occupy center stage in a number of different areas of public concern, such as genetically modified (GM) crops, antibiotic resistance, air and water pollution, hazardous waste disposal, food safety and nutrition, meat eating, urban planning, housing, occupational safety, disaster preparedness, nanotechnology, climate change, and population control. Many authors have written about these topics from various disciplinary perspectives including ecology, public health, medicine, toxicology, economics, law, sociology, theology, philosophy, and political science. I have chosen to add my voice to this conversation in order to offer a unique viewpoint that incorporates insights from ethical theory, environmental science, and public health. The title of my book – *Environmental Health Ethics* – signifies this perspective.

Because many of the issues are complex, timely, and nuanced, this book should be regarded as a starting point that prompts further debate by scholars, scientists, students, and others, not as a definitive analysis of every topic under consideration. Indeed, because the latest scientific and legal developments have an important bearing on most of these issues, some of the conclusions drawn in this book may be out-of-date in a few years. That concern need not worry us here because my aims are to introduce specialists and lay readers to unfamiliar issues; explore relationships among ethics, the environment, and human health; and incorporate insights from diverse fields of study. The net result of this endeavor will, I hope, open up new areas of inquiry and offer fresh perspectives on old problems.

One of the central themes of the book is that most of the difficult environmental health questions we face involve conflicts among fundamental values, such as human rights, economic development, public health, justice, and environmental protection. To think clearly about resolving these conflicts it is important to develop a conceptual framework that distinguishes among these different values and includes a method for resolving conflicts

Traditional ethical theories lack the tools to deal with environmental health issues, because they tend to be human centered, focusing on human rights, duties, and values, with scant attention to other species or the environment. In the last two decades, philosophers and theologians have developed theories that extend the scope of ethical concern beyond the human realm to consider the value of other species and the environment. Most of these new theories, however, deal with human interests in general terms and do not distinguish between human health and other values, such as economic development and social justice. However, it is important to think about how all of these different values interact and potentially conflict to deal with environmental health issues (Resnik 2009).

For example, water pollution, which is often a by-product of economic development, can threaten nonhuman species and ecosystems. It is tempting to think of clean water policy debates as boiling down to economic development versus the environment. However, the issues are not that simple. Water pollution also negatively impacts human health and has implications for social justice because it may affect people differently, depending on where they live. However, economic development can have positive effects on human health and social justice by creating jobs, income, housing, and wealth. Poverty and unemployment contribute to poor health (Marmot and Wilkinson 2005). Government policies dealing with water pollution therefore need to take into account not only environmental protection but also economic development, human health, and social justice.

Many commentators and organizations tend to view promoting human health and protecting the environment as complementary objectives. For example, the mission of the Environmental Protection Agency (EPA) is to protect human health and the environment (Environmental Protection Agency 2011a). Though environmental protection and public health promotion often go hand-in-hand, they are still distinct values that may sometimes conflict, as illustrated by the dilemma mentioned earlier concerning the use of DDT to control malaria. Environmental protection may also conflict with public health when a community is deciding whether to build a dam on a river to provide enough water for its population. Having an ample supply of clean water is essential for public health, but damming the river could have adverse impacts on species and the ecosystem (Ford 2010).

A key question explored in this book, therefore, is how best to balance competing values in environmental health decision making. In Chapter 4, I will describe a method for ethical decision making that aims to achieve a fair and reasonable balance between competing values and moral principles. It is important to consider environmental and public health concerns, as well as economic and social ones. My balancing approach stems from recognition that ethical and policy decisions often involve difficult choices between competing interests and values, and that practical answers usually reflect compromises among opposing viewpoints (Rawls 2005). Decision-making methods with a particular ideological, economic, or religious slant are likely to alienate opponents, instead of inviting them to engage in a serious discussion about what to do. Compromises may not be palatable to those who maintain unwavering allegiance to particular principles or ideals, but they are often the best way to involve different stakeholders, such as environmentalists, public health advocates, and leaders from business, industry, and government in working toward effective solutions to difficult problems (Brand 2009; Master and Crozier 2011).

Another theme of the book is that interactions between human health and the environment put a new twist on some of the traditional questions of ethics. For example, the conflict between individual rights and the common good is a perennial issue for ethics, political philosophy, and legal theory. In the environmental health arena, questions about the moral basis for government restrictions on property rights play a critical role in policy debates about urban sprawl, a pattern of uncontrolled development around the edge of a city. In the United States, communities have taken various measures, such as prohibitions on new housing construction on rural land and zoning laws that mandate high-density, mixed-use development, which are intended to counteract urban sprawl. Public health advocates and environmentalists have championed these measures as a way to reduce the impact of diseases associated with urban sprawl, such as obesity, diabetes, heart disease, and asthma, and to protect the environment from further damage (Heaton et al. 2010). Property owners and developers have argued, however, that these policies are an unjustified restriction on their rights, and they have succeeded in forestalling antisprawl policies in many locations (Resnik 2010).

Justice is another traditional ethical concern that appears in a different light when considered in the context of human health and the environment. For many years, debates about justice have focused on social institutions and relationships among human beings. For example, questions about the distribution of income and wealth in society have to do with the structure of social institutions (Rawls 1971). As we shall see in this book, however, questions about justice also arise when one considers the health impacts of pollution, urban development, waste disposal, climate change, energy production, and other environmental issues. It is important to address questions concerning the distribution of health in the environment, and processes for making decisions related to environmental policies (Shrader-Frechette 2002, 2007a). Various chapters in this book will highlight these issues, and an entire chapter will be dedicated to environmental justice.

The plan for the book is as follows. Chapters 2 to 4 will examine the fundamental issues related to environmental health ethics, including an overview of environmental health (Chapter 2) and ethics (Chapter 3); and development of a principle-based approach to ethical decision making related to environmental health (Chapter 4). Chapter 4 will articulate principles for decision making, including respect for human rights, promotion of social utility, justice, protection of animal welfare, stewardship of natural resources, sustainability, and precaution. Ethical decision making concerning environmental health issues should strive to achieve a fair and reasonable balance among these different principles. Decisions and policies should also be consistent and based on evidence and arguments open to public criticism. Chapters 5 to 11 will apply the conceptual framework developed in the first part of the book to practical problems related to environmental health, such as GM crops, pesticide use, pollution, food safety and nutrition, nanotechnology, housing, urban planning, occupational health, population control, climate change, and research with human subjects. Chapter 12 will summarize the major findings and conclusions of the book.

AN OVERVIEW OF ENVIRONMENTAL HEALTH

There are a number of different ways of defining environmental health. Some describe it as a scientific field of study similar to biology or chemistry, while others refer to it as an applied discipline similar to medicine or public health, and still others include both characterizations (Fromkin 2010; World Health Organization 2010b). The National Institute of Environmental Health Sciences (NIEHS), a branch of the National Institutes of Health (NIH), describes environmental health as both a scientific field of study that attempts to understand "the complex relationship between environmental risk factors and human biology within affected individuals and populations" and as an applied discipline that "uses this knowledge to prevent illness, reduce disease, and promote health" (National Institute of Environmental Health Sciences 2006: 5).

Many different scientific disciplines develop knowledge related to environmental health, including: ecology, toxicology, epidemiology, exposure biology, environmental medicine, genetics and genomics, cell and reproductive biology, endocrinology, neurology, microbiology, environmental economics, climatology, and meteorology (Frumkin 2010a). Applied environmental health disciplines implement practices and policies that promote environmental health. These include: occupational health, industrial hygiene, solid and hazardous waste management, water management, public health, forestry management, urban planning, agriculture, environmental engineering, ergonomics, and environmental law and ethics (Frumkin 2010a). (See Table 2.1.)

To clarify the definition of environmental health, it is important to distinguish between different environmental risk factors. Biological factors include the various organisms and species in our environment, such as bacteria, fungi, food crops, trees, birds, insects, cattle, rodents, as well as larger units of biological organization, such as ecological communities, ecosystems, and the biosphere (Frumkin 2010). Chemical factors include water, oxygen, carbon dioxide, nitrogen, phosphates, pesticides, food preservatives, industrial waste, heavy metals, and other substances that have an impact on health (Frumkin 2010). Physical factors include the physical aspects of our environment, such as geology, weather, gravity, heat, and electromagnetic radiation (Frumkin 2010). Social factors include characteristics

Table 2.1. *Environmental Health Disciplines*

Scientific Disciplines	Applied Disciplines
Ecology	Solid and hazardous waste management
Toxicology	Hydrology and water management
Exposure biology	Occupational health and industrial hygiene
Epidemiology	Public health
Environmental medicine	Urban planning
Genetics/genomics	Civil engineering
Cellular and reproductive biology	Environmental engineering
Endocrinology	Environmental consulting
Neurology	Agriculture
Microbiology	Pest management
Meteorology and climatology	Forestry management
Environmental economics	Environmental law and ethics

of human societies that can affect health, such as warfare, racism, poverty, religion, buildings, infrastructure, social institutions, and occupations (Marmot and Wilkinson 2005; Barr 2008). Additionally, many human diseases result from gene-environment interactions (Olden 2006). For example, Type II (insulin-resistant) diabetes results from genetic predispositions in combination with excessive caloric intake and insufficient exercise (American Diabetes Association 2010).

Although the definition of environmental health should be broad, it is prudent to focus research on environmental factors that we are able to control or mitigate. For example, we have no control of the amount or type of solar radiation that reaches the Earth from the Sun. We do, however, have an ability to affect the protective ozone (O_3) layer in the atmosphere, which blocks harmful ultraviolet radiation. In the 1970s, scientists discovered that a variety of compounds, such as chlorofluorocarbons (CFCs), cause ozone depletion when released into the atmosphere. Recognizing the dangers of ozone depletion, countries around the world have reached international agreements and adopted domestic laws that regulate CFSs and other ozone depleting substances (Environmental Protection Agency 2010b). While the study of the Sun's energy production should be left to astrophysicists, environmental scientists can study the formation of the ozone layer, how different compounds affect it, and how ozone depletion can cause diseases, such as skin cancer.

Focusing on aspects of the environment that we can control or mitigate does not mean we should take a stoic attitude toward the environment, accepting whatever fate may befall us, because our ability to affect or respond to the environment changes with advances in science and technology. For example, at one time it was not possible to accurately predict natural disasters such as hurricanes, tornadoes, tsunamis, floods, and volcanoes. Advances in meteorology, geology, and oceanography have made it possible to forecast, prepare for, and respond to natural disasters. Advances in engineering, architecture, building construction, and other sciences have allowed us to create structures that are able to withstand high winds, earthquakes, and floods. One day we may even be able to prevent asteroids or comets from causing cataclysmic destruction to human civilization and the entire biosphere (Science Daily 2009).

It is also prudent to focus environmental practice and policy efforts on factors that are not totally dependent on divisive politics in order to avoid wasting valuable time, energy, and public support in intractable debates that are beyond the expertise of environmental scientists and practitioners. Warfare has profound implications for human health and disease. Over 100,000 civilians have been killed in the Iraq War that began with the U.S. led invasion in the spring of 2003, and many hundreds of thousands have been injured (Iraq Body Count 2010). The war has also decimated the country's public health infrastructure and other resources necessary for health, such as agriculture, roads, water and sewer systems, and electric power, which has led to an increase in maternal and childhood mortality, starvation, and infectious diseases (World Health Organization 2007). While it is important for environmental scientists to understand and mitigate the human toll of war and to advocate for peaceful means of settling conflicts, direct involvement in antiwar efforts, such as lobbying and letter-writing campaigns, could detract from environmental scientists' primary mission, which is health oriented. Environmental health is primarily a scientific discipline and an applied practice, not a political party or movement.

Though it is important to avoid overly politicizing environmental health, environmental health is not purely apolitical. Political, economic, and moral values often influence decision making related to the science of environmental health. Politics often comes into play when the government is deciding how to allocate public funding for science projects (Resnik 2009b). If a government agency decides to increase the amount of funding for research on climate change, then it has made a decision that this research is politically or morally important. Economic interests have a direct bearing on funding decisions made by private companies (Resnik 2007). If a pesticide company decides to sponsor research on the safety of one of its products, then it has made this decision because it believes that the research will contribute to the company's profit margin.

Political and economic values often influence the interpretation of data produced by scientific research (Resnik 2007). For example, politics and economics have played a major role in the debate about climate change. Since the 1980s, scientists have gathered considerable evidence that the Earth is becoming warmer as a result of the increasing atmospheric levels of greenhouse gases such as carbon dioxide and methane produced by human activity. The administration of President George W. Bush took a skeptical view about climate change and resisted national and international efforts to minimize or mitigate global climate change such as restrictions on hydrocarbon emissions. The Bush administration's policies were largely influenced by business interests, especially the oil industry, which opposed any restrictions on carbon emissions (Resnik 2009b). Although the vast majority of scientists accept the hypothesis that human activities are causing global warming, many politicians and some scientists continue to doubt this hypothesis and oppose measures to prevent or reduce global warming (Revkin 2009, Rosenthal 2010).

Political, economic, and moral values also have a major impact on the formation of policies related to environmental health, such as government rules, regulations, and guidelines. For example, the Clean Air Act, which was passed by the U.S. Congress in 1963 and amended in 1970 and 1990, authorizes the EPA to enact and enforce regulations to protect the public from airborne contaminants that are hazardous to human health (Clean Air Act 1963). Congress passed that act because it determined that protecting the public from air pollution was an important goal. Politics also has entered into decisions related to enforcement of the act. Under the Bush administration the EPA did not apply the Clean Air Act to carbon dioxide emissions (CO_2), because it did not view CO_2 as a hazardous airborne contaminant. Under the administration of President Barack Obama, who was elected with strong support from environmentalist groups, the EPA has begun to take measures, such as mandatory reporting of greenhouse gases, which may lead the agency to regulate these substances in the future (Environmental Protection Agency 2010c). (Climate change will be discussed in greater detail in Chapter 9.)

Values play a central role in scientific and practical decisions related to most of the topics discussed in this book. I will discuss and explore these different values in Chapters 3 and 4 and at other appropriate places. For now, I will simply note that while choices related to environmental health science and practice should reflect a careful consideration of the different values at stake, this does not mean that environmental health is a purely political or humanistic enterprise. At its core, environmental health is a scientific discipline and an applied practice that seeks to promote health and prevent disease. Though environmental health incorporates human values into decision making, it is also based on evidence from well-designed experiments and observational studies (Shrader-Frechette 1994, 2007; Elliott 2011).

Questions about the role of human values in environmental health also play an important role in understanding what we mean by "health." The World Health Organization (2010c) defines health as: "a state of complete physical, mental, and social well-being and not merely the absence of disease or infirmity." While this definition has some intuitive appeal, it has been criticized as too broad, because it includes more than absence of disease but also complete social well-being (Boorse 2004). Taken literally, this implies that health includes many different factors essential to social well-being, such as a living wage, education, community, happiness, and freedom from discrimination or political or religious persecution. Such a broad definition of health medicalizes social and political problems and would entail that environmental health should be concerned with human rights, poverty, warfare, discrimination, justice, and so on. The WHO definition would overly politicize environmental health and obligate environmental health researchers and practitioners to tackle social and political problems well beyond their domain of expertise or authority.

Boorse (1977, 2004) has developed a narrower, more scientific definition of health. According to Boorse, a healthy organism is one that functions normally, and a disease is deviation from normal functioning. Normal functions are traits that have been designed by natural selection to perform specific tasks that contribute to reproduction or survival.

(Natural selection is discussed in more depth later in this chapter.) For example, one of the normal functions of the liver is to detoxify the blood. The liver has this function because blood detoxification contributed to the reproduction and survival of animals that possessed this trait. A liver that does not detoxify blood properly is diseased, and animals that cannot detoxify blood die from a buildup of toxins. Normal functions include not only biological traits but also behavioral and psychological ones, according to Boorse (2004). A person who has Alzheimer's disease has abnormal brain functioning, characterized by the formation of amyloid plaques in brain tissue, and exhibits abnormal behaviors, such as dementia, difficulties in communicating, and emotional disturbances (National Institute on Aging 2010).

Though I think Boorse offers a clear and convincing account of health and disease, his views have some flaws. One of the main criticisms of Boorse' view is that it is too scientific and does not give sufficient attention to the role that social values play in defining and recognizing diseases (Kovács 1998). For example, some loss of sexual function is a normal part of the aging process for men and women, but most people in the United States and other developed countries consider age-related loss of sexual function to be a medical condition requiring treatment. Even though some loss of sexual function during aging is biologically normal, we regard sexual dysfunction as a disease because people value sexual pleasure and intimacy. Social values play a significant role in the decision to treat other conditions that are typical of our species as diseases, such as tooth decay, overbite, wisdom teeth, baldness, slight nearsightedness or farsightedness, and hyperactivity in children. Though most conditions are classified as diseases because they are biologically abnormal, some conditions are classified as diseases because they interfere with achieving socially valued goals (Richman 2004). Health and disease are, at their core, scientific concepts, but they are not purely value-free.

A BRIEF HISTORY OF ENVIRONMENTAL HEALTH

Human beings have recognized the relationship between environmental factors and health and disease throughout history. Ancient people knew the importance of having access to clean water, as there is evidence that the Greek, Roman, Egyptian, Indian, and South American civilizations had water and sewer systems. The Romans built extensive systems of pipes, aqueducts, pumps, baths, and fountains. Ancient people also understood the importance of preserving food and not eating spoiled food. The Jewish prohibition on eating pork came from recognition that eating this type of meat can cause disease (Fromkin 2010). During the Black Death, an outbreak of the bubonic plague that decimated European populations in 1300s, people thought that something in the environment was causing the disease, but they did not have a good understanding of the source. The plague was carried by fleas on rats, but many Europeans mistakenly thought the plague was carried by cats, which they regarded as agents of the devil. Many people killed domestic house cats, which only made the problem worse because cats eat rats. The practice of killing cats stopped when it became apparent that people who kept their cats were protected from the plague (Abee 2008).

Environmental health as a scientific study began in the 1700s, with the growing recognition of the health problems associated with rapidly growing cities, such as air pollution from coal-burning factories, horse manure, and sewage. Epidemiology started to emerge as a scientific discipline in the seventeenth and eighteenth centuries as researchers, such as John Graunt (1620–1674), Willima Farr (1807–1883), and Edwin Chadwick (1800–1890) compiled and analyzed demographic and health-related data on various populations. Chadwick was asked by the British government to investigate a possible relationship between sanitation practices and outbreaks of typhoid fever and influenza. Chadwick's report argued that overcrowded homes, impure water, unsanitary living conditions, and other environmental factors contributed to many different health problems. Chadwick's report led to the formation of the Central Board of Health in 1848, which appointed local boards to oversee trash collection, sanitation, sewage disposal, and clean water. Chadwick advocated for toilets in every home and removal of sewage from the city to the farmland where it could be used as fertilizer (Frumkin 2010a). The English physician John Snow (1813–1858) investigated the cholera outbreak in London in 1854. Snow observed that people who drank from the Broad Street pump had a much higher incidence of cholera than people who did not drink from the pump. Snow hypothesized that contaminated water from the Broad Street pump was the source of the outbreak, and he convinced the local authorities to deactivate the pump, which led to an abatement of the disease (Frumkin 2010a).

During the Industrial Revolution, working conditions in factories, mines, and mills produced many occupational fatalities and injuries (Frumkin 2010a). In England, Charles Turner Thackrach (1795–1833) published a book that raised greater awareness of work-related hazards and led to the passage of the Factory Act (1833) and the Mines Act (1842). The novels of Charles Dickens, such as *Oliver Twist* (1838), called attention to the plight of the urban poor and the social conditions they faced. In the United States, Alice Hamilton (1869–1970) made important contributions to occupational health by documenting links between toxic exposures and illnesses among factory workers and miners and through her service as the director of Illinois's Occupational Disease Commission. As a professor at Harvard University, Hamilton published books on health hazards in the workplace (Frumkin 2010a). The organized labor movement in the first half of the twentieth century in the United States led to safer working conditions for factory workers, mill workers, and miners.

The publication of *Silent Spring* in 1962, discussed in Chapter 1, helped to launch the modern environmental health movement. Inspired by Carson's book, other scientists began paying greater attention to chemical hazards in the environment. Irving Selikoff (1915–1992) demonstrated that workers exposed to asbestos developed various lung diseases, including cancer and mesothelioma. Other scientists also studied cancers related to exposures to other chemicals in the workplace, such as bis-chloromethyl ether, vinyl chloride, and polychlorinated biphenyls (PCBs). Herbert Needleman, a pediatrician and child psychiatrist at the University of Pittsburgh, conducted research in the 1970s and 1980s demonstrating the detrimental effects of lead on cognitive development. His work supported bans on lead in gasoline and interior paints as well as efforts to remove lead paint from older homes (Goodman 1997; Frumkin 2010a).

Since the 1970s, environmental health has expanded beyond its traditional concerns with occupational health, exposures to hazardous substances, and hygiene to address socio-economic factors that influence health and global concerns. In the 1980s, scientists, leaders of minority groups, and public health advocates recognized that unequal exposures to environmental risks raises issues of civil rights and social justice, which led to the birth of the environmental justice movement (Bullard 1994), which will be discussed in greater depth in Chapter 10. Researchers also explored how other socioeconomic factors such as race/ethnicity, poverty, discrimination, and education, can adversely impact health, which initiated a research program known as the social determinants of health (Marmot and Wilkinson 2005). Environmental health researchers have focused more on global environmental issues since the 1980s, such as the health impacts of global climate change, overpopulation, and economic development. Ecologically sustainable development has been a major focus of environmental health since the United Nations (U.N.) formed the World Commission on Environment and Development in 1983 (Frumkin 2010a). (These topics will be discussed in greater depth in Chapter 9.)

ENVIRONMENTAL HEALTH DISCIPLINES

As noted earlier, many different scientific disciplines have a bearing on environmental health. I will not give an overview of all of these disciplines in this book but will discuss several that play a key role in environmental health. I will assume that readers already have some basic knowledge of biology and chemistry.

ECOLOGY

Ecology is the study of how organisms interact with their environment, including biological factors or conditions, such as other organisms, as well as nonbiological ones, such as water, air, soil, and solar radiation. Ecologists are especially concerned with how different natural systems interact and function. Levels of biological organization studied by ecologists, from smallest to largest include: genes, organisms, populations, species, biological communities, ecosystems, biomes, and the biosphere. A population is a group of organisms that belong to the same species living in a particular location, such as a forest or mountain range. A species is an interbreeding population of organisms. An ecosystem is a complex set of interactions between different species living in a common environment, a web of life. Some examples of ecosystems include lakes, rivers, forests, wetlands, caves, city parks, and coral reefs. Biomes are collections of ecosystems, such as deserts, tropical forests, temperate forests, arctic tundra, and grassy plains. The biosphere consists of all of the ecosystems and organisms in the world. Ecology, at the level of the biosphere, is concerned with understanding how all living things depend on other living things to live and prosper (Stebbins 1982; Wilcox and Jessop 2010).

Ecosystems are organized into different levels based on energy production and consumption. At the bottom of the ecosystem's food chain are autotrophs, or primary producers, which make their own food. Terrestrial autotrophs include plants, algae, lichens, and bacteria, which use the energy provided by sunlight to produce organic materials, such as carbohydrates, lipids, and proteins. Above the autotrophs are primary consumers, which feed upon the primary producers. In a North American forest ecosystem, primary consumers include herbivores, such as deer, elk, rabbits, mice, beavers, moles, and various species of birds, reptiles, amphibians, worms, and insects. At the top of the ecosystem are secondary consumers, which feed on primary consumers. In a North American ecosystem these include coyotes, wolves, foxes, mountain lions, bears, predatory birds, spiders, and some species of insects, reptiles, and amphibians. Energy is lost as heat as it moves up the different levels of the food chain, which explains why the amount of biomass decreases by an order of magnitude as one moves up the food chain. If the amount of biomass found in primary producers is x, then the ecosystem can support a biomass of primary consumers of $1/10x$ and a biomass of secondary consumers of $1/100x$. All of the different roles in the ecosystem – primary producers, primary consumers, and secondary consumers – are necessary for the proper functioning of the ecosystem as a whole. If secondary consumers become endangered or extinct, for example, primary consumers will overfeed on primary producers, which will put a stress on those populations. If primary consumers decline in population, due to hunting or fishing, for example, then secondary consumers will lose a food source (Wilcox and Jessop 2010).

The science of ecology emerged in the 1800s from the study of natural history. The English natural historian, Charles Darwin (1809–1882), proposed a theory of evolution by natural selection, which has shaped the development of all of the life sciences, especially ecology. In his *On the Origin of Species by Means of Natural Selection* (1859), Darwin argued that species are not static entities but change over time in response to environmental conditions. Existing species can die out and new ones can emerge. Natural selection, according to modern evolutionists, occurs when there are heritable, random variations among members of a population that confer adaptive advantage (i.e., fitness) in a common environment and members that are better adapted out-survive and out-reproduce those that are less adapted. Over time, the genetic and phenotypic composition of the population changes as a result of differential reproduction and survival among members of the population (Stebbins 1982). A new animal or plant species emerges when interbreeding populations become reproductively isolated, so that they can no longer interbreed. Isolation can result from genetic differences between populations or phenotypic ones, such as mating behavior or anatomy (Stebbins 1982).

Natural selection is important for understanding how populations, species, biological communities, and ecosystems can change over time, and how they can affect each other. For example, flowering plants have developed traits that encourage pollination by bees and seed dispersal by birds; herbivores have developed traits that help them to feed on plants and hide or flee from carnivores; mammals have evolved an immune system to defend against microbial infections; insects have developed resistance to pesticides. An entire ecosystem can change over time as a result of changes among species living in the ecosystem. For example, a significant decline in annual precipitation over many years in a geographic area can lead to changes in the ecosystem because plants that are better adapted to low precipitation conditions are likely to be more successful than plants that require more precipitation. These changes are likely to affect herbivores that eat the plants, which may affect the carnivores that eat the herbivores (Mayr 2001).

Natural selection is also important for understanding how human activities affect populations, species, communities, and ecosystems. A common example of human-induced evolution is pesticide resistance. When farmers spray a crop with an insecticide, some of the insects may have a genotype that produces resistance to the pesticide, and they can transmit this genotype to the next generation. Over time, the genotype will increase in frequency in the population, decreasing the effectiveness of the insecticide. A variety of insect species have become resistant to malathion, for example (ffrench-Constant 2007). As predicted by Carson (1962), many populations of malaria-carrying mosquitoes have become resistant to DDT (van den Berg 2009). Antibiotic resistance follows a similar pattern. In many developed countries, methicillin-resistant *Staphylococcus aureus* (MRSA) is becoming a major public health concern, due to overuse of antibiotics. MRSA causes dangerous skin infections, infection in the bloodstream, pneumonia, and death. MRSA infections are the leading cause of death from infectious agents in the United States (DeLeo and Chambers, 2009).

Biodiversity is an important concept in ecology and evolution because genetic and phenotypic diversity are essential conditions for the occurrence of natural selection. Diversity gives species the ability to change over time in response to environmental conditions. Species that lack diversity may become extinct when the environment changes. Lack of biodiversity has been a significant problem for some plants used in commercial agriculture. After years of selective breeding, some species of plants, such as corn, wheat, cotton, and bananas, have lost considerable genetic diversity. As a result, these populations are susceptible to diseases because they contain fewer members that have disease-resistant genes. Lack of diversity between and among species in the ecosystem can also impact the ability of the ecosystem (as a whole) to adapt to changing environmental conditions and stresses, such as changing weather patterns, invasive species, and pollution (Wilcox and Jessop 2010). Human activities, such as farming and urban development, can reduce biodiversity by changing or destroying the habitats of species living in a geographic area, which can result in loss or decline of species (Wilson 1984).

Ecosystem functioning is another important concept in ecology. Ecosystems are able to perform a variety of functions vital for human and nonhuman life. One of the most important functions is circulating and recycling biologically important compounds and elements, such as water, oxygen, nitrogen, phosphorus, and carbon. Microorganisms are the major driving force behind these cycles and constitute most of the Earth's biomass (Wilcox and

Jessop 2010). For example, wetlands are able to filter and purify water that has been contaminated with sewage, pathogens, heavy metals, and hazardous chemicals. Various species in the wetlands remove and metabolize contaminants in the water. When human beings drain wetlands for development, they reduce the ability of the ecosystem to filter and purify water, thereby having a negative impact on all of the species that are affected by contaminants in the water. Saltwater marshes provide barriers to the inflow of saltwater into areas of freshwater. The marshes trap salt water and provide defense against storm surges, thereby protecting the aquatic species that live in freshwater. When saltwater marshes are destroyed, freshwater zones are compromised, which negatively impacts aquatic life (Wilcox and Jessop 2010).

Some elements and compounds concentrate at higher levels in the food chain in a process known as bioaccumulation. For example, mercury exists in the natural environment and is emitted from coal-burning power plants, incinerators that burn medical waste, paper mills, and chemical plants. Bacteria convert the mercury into an organic form (methyl mercury). Aquatic plants take in methyl mercury from the water and soil. Fish at the lower end of the food chain consume plants and do not eliminate the mercury, but store it in their muscle tissues. These fish are eaten by other fish, which are eaten by other fish, and so on. Because mercury is stored in muscle tissue, fish at the highest part of the food chain, such as Albacore tuna, grouper, sea bass, shark, and King mackerel, have higher concentrations of mercury. People who eat fish at the higher levels of the food chain can receive dangerous amounts of mercury if they do not take appropriate steps to minimize their mercury exposure (McSwane 2010). POPs, such as DDT (discussed in Chapter 1), and polychlorinated biphenyls (PCBs) can also bioaccumulate (Wilcox and Jessop 2010).

Ecosystems also regulate weather and climate. At a local level, forests can stabilize air temperatures and regulate extremes of hot or cold. During urban development, forests are removed and replaced with materials that retain heat, such as concrete and asphalt, which create a heat island effect. In the summer, a city is typically several degrees hotter than a surrounding forest because it retains heat more than the forest does (Wilcox and Jessop 2010). Forests can help to mitigate global warming. Forests remove CO_2 from the atmosphere and convert it into biomass, a process known as carbon sequestration. Forests cover 30 percent of the land but contain 45 percent of terrestrial carbon. Tropical forests are especially good at drawing CO_2 from the atmosphere and contain 25 percent of terrestrial carbon. The destruction of forests, especially tropical forests, reduces the ability of the biosphere to sequester carbon, which can contribute to global warming (Bonan 2008). Climate change can also have a variety of negative impacts on human and nonhuman species, which will be discussed in more depth in Chapter 9.

Ecosystems also help to control zoonotic (animal to human) infectious diseases. In a well-functioning ecosystem, species that serve as reservoirs for pathogens that can infect humans are kept in balance. When the ecosystem is damaged, the balance of species is disrupted, which can have an adverse impact on human populations (Wilcox and Jessop 2010). In North America, Lyme disease is transmitted to humans by the black-legged tick (*Ixodidae scapularis*) that carries *Borrelia burgdorferi*, a spirochete bacterium. The white-footed mouse

(*Peromyscus leucopus*) and white-tailed deer (*Odocoileus virginianus*) are reservoirs for *B. burgdorferi*: Larval forms of the ticks that feed on the mouse and deer become infected with *B. burgdorferi* and can transmit it to other species, including humans. The ticks can also feed on other species that are not good reservoirs for *B. burgdorferi,* including other species of rodents, birds, marsupials, and reptiles. When larval forms of the ticks feed primarily on the white-footed mouse or white-tailed deer, the prevalence of Lyme disease in the tick population is higher than when they feed on other species. Some species, such as opossums and squirrels, even function as ecological traps for black-legged ticks in that they kill the larval forms of the tick that attach to them. Thus, loss of species diversity in the ecosystem, as a result of destruction or fragmentation of habitats or other causes, can increase the prevalence of Lyme disease in the tick population, which increases the risk of human infection (LoGiudice et al. 2003; Keesing et al. 2009).

Carrying capacity is another important concept in ecology. Population ecologists study changes in population size and composition (i.e., genetics) over time. Population size is a function of several factors including birth rate, death rate, migration, age of reproduction, and longevity. Populations tend to increase at an exponential rate if not kept in check by predation, disease, starvation, or other causes of population decline. For example, the human population has grown from a few hundred million people around 1600 to an estimated 7 billion people in 2011 (Population Reference Bureau 2009). In his *Essay on the Principle of Population* (1798), Thomas Malthus (1766–1834) wrote about the problems of overpopulation in England. Malthus hypothesized that the human population was growing faster than the food supply. When population growth exceeds the food supply, starvation would occur, which keeps the population in check. Other scientists who expanded upon Malthus' ideas developed the concept of carrying capacity, which is the population size that can be supported within a particular area, given resource constraints, such as food, water, and habitat (Wilcox and Jessop 2010). Since the 1960s, scientists and political leaders have recognized that many environmental, economic, medical, and political problems are a direct result of the Earth's burgeoning human population. Some believe that human population is fast approaching the Earth's carrying capacity (Cohen 1995).

Carrying capacity is closely related to the concept of sustainability. Sustainability is the capacity of a system to endure over time. There are different concepts of sustainability, including ecological sustainability, economic sustainability, and political sustainability. In ecology, sustainability is the capacity for a biological system, such as a population, species, or ecosystem, to endure over time. As noted earlier, biodiversity is important for ecological sustainability because this allows an ecosystem to withstand and adapt to changing conditions. Sustainability can also be understood as the ability of human populations to prosper over time. For this to happen, people need to practice good stewardship of the Earth's resources so that future generations will have enough resources to prosper (World Commission on Environment and Development 1987). According to many scientists and scholars, current rates of population growth and resource use are placing tremendous stresses on the environment and are not sustainable over time (Rockström 2009). Population growth and resource use must be kept in check so that future generations will have the resources they need (World Commission on Environment and Development 1987). Because sustainability of the human population involves policies related to economic development and population control, the sustainability of the human population includes economic and political, not just ecological dimensions. These issues will be discussed in more depth in Chapter 9.

TOXICOLOGY

Toxicology is an interdisciplinary field that investigates the adverse effects of chemicals on organisms (Richardson and Miller 2010). Toxicologists study the effects of chemicals on many different organisms, including plants, insects, laboratory mice, and human beings. Chemicals can produce a variety of signs and symptoms that indicate toxicity in animals and human beings, ranging from minor adverse effects, such as skin irritation, headache, nausea, dizziness, and mucosal inflammation, to significant adverse effects, such as kidney failure, liver failure, cardiac arrhythmia, stroke, and permanent disability or death. Toxicology plays an important role in risk assessment of a variety of chemicals, including new drugs, industrial chemicals, and pesticides. Toxicologists may work for private companies, such as pharmaceutical manufacturers or pesticide companies, universities, or government agencies, such as the FDA, EPA, NTP, Centers for Disease Control and Prevention (CDC), or National Institute for Occupational Safety and Health (NIOSH) (Richardson and Miller 2010).

One of the central concepts of toxicology is that the dose makes the poison, a principle articulated by the Swiss alchemist Paracelsus (1493–1541) over 500 years ago. The meaning of this fundamental idea is that all chemicals can be toxic at sufficiently high doses and nontoxic at sufficiently low doses. How much of a chemical is needed to produce acute toxicity (i.e., toxicity from a single exposure or multiple exposures in a short time) depends on the properties of the chemical. For example, a lethal dose (LD) of acetaminophen, the active ingredient in Tylenol, is 500 mg/kg for a healthy adult (Richardson and Miller 2010). A 70 kg (154 lb) man could die if he receives a 35 gm dose of acetaminophen. A maximum safe dose is 4000 mg/24 hours. However, doses higher than 4000 mg/24 hours can cause toxic effects, such as nausea, abdominal pain, diarrhea, vomiting, convulsions, and liver damage (Medline Plus 2009a). Some chemicals have LDs that are much higher or lower than acetaminophen's. For example, an LD of saxitoxin (shellfish toxin) is 0.003 mg/kg. One of the most important tasks for toxicology is to establish the dose-response relationship for different chemicals (Richardson and Miller 2010).

The acute toxicity of a chemical also depends on the physiology and metabolism of the organism receiving the dose. Among human beings, toxicity can be affected by a number of different factors, such as age, disease status, drug interactions, and genetics. Many drugs that are safe for adults at a particular dose are not safe for children, because children metabolize drugs differently. Also, some drugs that are safe for young adults at a particular dose are not safe for senior citizens because aging can affect drug metabolism. A drug that is safe for healthy adults at a particular dose may not be safe in people who have diseases that cause liver damage, such as hepatitis or alcoholism, because the liver plays a major role in drug metabolism. Likewise, diseases that cause kidney damage, such as diabetes and some types of cancer, can also have an impact on safe drug dosing, because the kidneys also help to eliminate drugs from the body. A variety of medications interact in potentially dangerous ways, which can impact dosing (Physicians' Desk Reference 2010). For example, a class of antidepressant drugs known as selective serotonin reuptake inhibitors can interact with other drug classes, such as opioids, monoamine oxidase inhibitors, antimigraine agents, antiemitics, and some types of antibiotics to produce serotonin syndrome, a life-threatening condition resulting from too much serotonin in the nervous system (Dvir and Smallwood 2008).

A number of studies have shown that genetic factors can affect toxicity. For example, the cytochrome P450 system is a family of enzymes that plays a key role in drug metabolism carried out by the liver and other tissues. Variations in the genes that code for these enzymes can affect the metabolism of a number of different drugs, including antidepressants, beta-blockers, opioids, chemotherapy agents, and others. Due to variations in cytochrome P450 genes, the speed of drug metabolism can vary among people. Because people with particular cytochrome P450 variants may metabolize drugs at different rates, a dose of a drug that is safe and effective for one person may be toxic for another with a particular variant, and nontoxic and noneffective for another person with a different variant (Lynch and Price 2007). Variations in cytochrome P450 genes can also affect susceptibility to some types of cancer, because some people produce carcinogenic metabolites (Richardson and Miller 2010). Variations in cytochrome P450 genes and other genetic factors can also affect a person's susceptibility to developing dangerous drug interactions, such as serotonin syndrome, mentioned earlier (Dvir and Smallwood 2008).

Acute toxicity also varies across species and phyla, due to differences in metabolism, protein synthesis, and other functions. For example, theobromine, a chemical in chocolate, can cause toxic reactions in dogs at 130mg/kg. Theobromine content varies with the darkness of chocolate. Milk chocolate has about 4 mg/gm of theobromine, but semisweet chocolate has as much as 16 mg/gm. 1300 mg of theobromine would be toxic to a 10 kg (22 lb) dog. This would be equivalent to eating 81.25 gm (2.87 ounces) of dark chocolate. Signs and symptoms of theobromine toxicity in dogs include: irritability, rapid heart rate, increased urination, muscle tremors, vomiting, and diarrhea (Vetrica 2004). The same amount of chocolate might make a human being feel full of chocolate but not sick. Theobromine is more dangerous for dogs than humans because dogs do not metabolize this chemical as quickly as humans. Glyphosate, a chemical contained in the herbicide Roundup, is extremely toxic to many plant species. As little as 10 micrograms of glyphosate can kill a single plant in the wild, and aerial spraying of Roundup may kill plants up to 100 meters away from the targeted area (Greenpeace 1996). Glyphosate is not very toxic to most animal species and humans. Glyphosate's LD for humans is about 5,600 mg/kg (Richardson and Miller 2010). Glyphosate inhibits the shikimic acid pathway, a chemical reaction that actively growing plants use to synthesize several amino acids. Glyphosate is not very dangerous to animals, because they do not have the shikimic acid pathway (Greenpeace 1996; Richardson and Miller 2010).

Many chemicals that do not produce acute toxicity at a particular dose may still produce toxicity after many years of exposure (chronic toxicity) (Richardson and Miller 2010). For example, tobacco smoke contains over fifty known carcinogens, but lung cancer typically develops only after several decades of smoking (Lubin and Caporaso 2006). Some chemicals cause acute and chronic toxicity. Ethyl alcohol, a chemical in wine, beer, whiskey, and other alcoholic beverages, can produce vomiting, seizures, reduced respiration, seizures, hypothermia, and death. The LD for alcohol is a function of the percentage of alcohol in the bloodstream, which depends on a number of factors, including the person's weight, how many alcoholic drinks they have consumed in a period of time, the percentage of alcohol in those drinks, other drugs they have been taking, metabolism, and alcohol tolerance. Many years of excessive drinking can lead to liver cirrhosis, which can cause nausea, vomiting, abdominal pain, jaundice, bleeding of the gums, weight loss, and, if not treated, death (Medline Plus 2009b). Toxicologists tend to focus on acute toxicity, while other researchers, such as epidemiologists, focus on chronic toxicity.

One of the most important questions for toxicology is whether there is a threshold dose below which no adverse effects will occur. In animal dosing experiments, the concept of a no observed adverse effect level (NOAEL) is important for making regulatory decisions. An NOAEL for a chemical is the highest dose at which no adverse effects are observed (Richardson and Miller 2010). If a chemical produces no adverse effects at a particular dose, it is considered "safe" at that dose. In making regulatory decisions concerning safe human pesticide exposures, the EPA uses three uncertainty factors of ten. It divides the NOAEL dose in laboratory animals by a factor of ten to take into account differences between humans and animals, then by another factor of ten to account for variations among humans, and then by another factor of ten to provide extra protection for children. So, the safe dose or reference dose (RfD) for a pesticide in humans is 1/1000 the NOAEL dose in animals, under EPA rules.

Though most chemicals have a threshold effect, some carcinogens, such as dioxin, are not considered safe at any dose. Additionally, research has shown that some chemicals have a nonlinear dose-response curve. Some chemicals activate a particular biochemical pathway at a low dose and inhibit the same pathway at a high dose. Chemicals that have these properties can be dangerous at low and high doses. For example, endocrine disruptors are chemicals that alter the function of the body's endocrine (hormone) system (National Institute of Environmental Health Sciences 2010a). Many of these chemicals mimic the properties of hormones in the body by activating hormone receptors or preventing hormones from activating these receptors. Bisphenol A (BPA), a chemical that activates estrogen receptors, exhibits adverse effects even at low doses (vom Saal and Hughes 2005). Other endocrine disruptors include DDT, PCBs, phthalates, dioxin, and arsenic. Because not all chemicals follow a linear dose-response curve, determining what constitutes a "safe" dose for a chemical can be a challenging task for scientists and regulators (Richardson and Miller 2010; Elliott 2011).

To understand dose-response relationships, it is important to have information about the amount of the chemical that an organism is exposed to as well as the route of exposure. In mammals, the main types of environmental exposure are through the skin (dermal), lungs (inhalation), and by the digestive system (ingestion). In medicine, chemicals also may be administered through the vein (intravenous) or through the muscle (intramuscular). The route of exposure can make a tremendous difference concerning the effects of the chemical on the body, such as toxicity. For example, chlorpyrifos is ten times more toxic when exposure occurs through the digestive system rather than the skin (Richardson and Miller 2010).

Chemicals enter the body through a process known as absorption. All of the different routes of exposure have barriers that block the entry of chemicals or pathogens. Some chemicals are betters at crossing these different barriers than others. For example, the digestive system has a large surface area that is designed to absorb many different types of chemicals and deliver them to the bloodstream, including water-soluble and fat-soluble compounds. The skin has been designed to protect the body from invasion. However, some chemicals, such as fat-soluble compounds, can easily penetrate the skin and enter the bloodstream. The lungs contain a large surface area designed to promote gas exchange and block entry from pathogens and airborne particles. However, water-soluble compounds, fat-soluble gases, small particles, and aerosols can enter the bloodstream through the lung alveoli (Richardson and Miller 2010).

Once a chemical enters the bloodstream, it can travel around the body in a process known as distribution. Chemicals will tend to move from areas of high concentration (such as the point of entry) to areas of low concentration (such as other areas in the body). Ingested chemicals may go directly to the liver via the portal vein. Chemicals can go anywhere in the body once they enter the bloodstream, but they may not be able to cross the blood-brain or blood-testes barriers, which block large molecules, pathogens, and hydrophilic compounds (Richardson and Miller 2010).

Metabolism begins as soon as a chemical enters the bloodstream. Though almost all cells in the body have some capacity to metabolize exogenous chemicals, most metabolic reactions occur in the liver, under the control of various enzymes. Many of these metabolic reactions convert chemicals into compounds that are more soluble in water, so they can be more easily excreted. Metabolism generally has two phases. Phase I reactions increase the polarity of chemicals (thus making them more soluble in water) and decrease toxicity. Oxidation is the most common Phase I reaction. In oxidation reactions, compounds gain positive charge by the addition of oxygen or the removal of hydrogen. The most important oxidation reactions are carried out by the cytochrome P450 system (discussed earlier). In Phase II reactions, toxins are combined with organic molecules to produce compounds that are less toxic and more polar.

Most of the time, metabolism converts toxic compounds into chemicals that are less toxic. For example, benzene, which is highly toxic, becomes phenol, which is not. However, sometimes metabolic reactions produce toxic metabolites. For example, methanol, which is not very toxic, becomes formaldehyde and formic acid, both of which are highly toxic. Some metabolic reactions yield carcinogenic products. For example, vinyl chloride is metabolized into a highly reactive compound that causes cancer. Variations in the cytochrome P450 enzyme system can also produce carcinogenic metabolites (Richardson and Miller 2010).

If an enzyme system becomes saturated, a different system may take over. However, sometimes a toxin will persist in the body and produce adverse effects, if it is not metabolized by the preferred chemical pathway. Saturation can occur following a large dose of a particular toxin, or doses of different toxins that are metabolized by the same enzyme system. Drug overdoses can occur when people combine different medications that are safe when taken separately but dangerous when taken together because they saturate an enzyme system (Richardson and Miller 2010).

Excretion follows metabolism. Most toxins and metabolites are excreted through the kidneys, which filter the blood. Filtration occurs in units of the kidney called nephrons. In the nephrons, capillaries known as glomeruli are surrounded by the end of a tubule known as the Bowman's capsule, which collects urine. The urine then flows down the tubule and eventually into the bladder. Blood pressure forces fluid and waste to exit the glomeruli and enter the Bowman's capsule. Compounds that are too large to move through the pores in the glomeruli, such as chemicals that are bound to proteins, may be secreted into the tubules via active transport, in which the body uses energy to move compounds across electrochemical gradients. Chemicals that are useful to the body may be reabsorbed after they enter the tubule. The liver is the other major organ involved in excretion. Excretion by the liver is similar to the kidneys: Wastes cross a barrier through filtration or active transport and become part of the bile, which enters the digestive system through a bile duct. Compounds that are not reabsorbed in the intestines exit the body through the feces (Richardson and Miller 2010).

Toxins can exert different effects on different parts of the body. Because the liver and kidneys handle most the toxins that enter the body, liver or kidney damage is a frequent consequence of toxicity. Toxins can also have a pronounced impact on the heart and lungs because they receive a high blood volume. Toxins can also impact the site at which they enter the body. For example, chlorine gas combines with water in the lungs, airways, nose, mouth, and eyes to form hydrochloric and hypochlorous acids, which cause irritation, swelling, tissue damage, and pain (Richardson and Miller 2010).

Some toxins exert systemic effects. For example, carbon monoxide combines with hemoglobin in red bloods cells, rendering them ineffective at delivering oxygen to the body. Carbon monoxide poisoning is the most common form of acute toxicity due to breathing polluted air (Blumental 2001). Chemicals and biological products (such as proteins, pollen, food, skin, or hair) can also affect the immune system in various ways. Some, such as asbestos and dioxin, suppress the immune response; while others, such as formaldehyde and nickel, can trigger dangerous immune reactions, such as inflammation, difficulty breathing, and shock (Luster and Rosenthal 1993).

Toxicologists use several different systems for classifying toxins. One way of classifying toxins is according to chemical class, such as acids, alcohols, heavy metals, oxidants, and solvents. Another way is by source of the toxin, such air pollutants, food additives, industrial wastes, and water pollutants. A third way is to classify toxins by how they affect the body: Nephrotoxins affect the kidney; hepatotoxins – the liver; cardiotoxins – the heart; neurotoxins – the nervous system; immunotoxins – the immune system; mutagens – the genome (Richardson and Miller 2010).

Animal experiments play an important role in toxicity testing. Government agencies, such as the EPA and FDA, require extensive data from animal studies before making regulatory decisions. A common test is the LD_{50} test, an experiment in which dosing is increased until 50 percent of the animals die from an acute toxic exposure (Richardson and Miller 2010). Another common test strategy involves administration of doses to animals for a longer period of time (several months) to determine whether a chemical increases the risk of cancer. Animals are divided into experimental and control groups, and compared at the end of the trial. Scientists euthanize the animals and perform pathology studies to detect the presence of cancerous or precancerous tumors and other evidence of carcinogenesis.

While animal experiments can yield important information about toxicity, there are some methodological problems with applying the results of animal research to human beings. First, there are significant metabolic and physiologic differences between animals and humans. When choosing an animal for a toxicology experiment on a particular chemical, it is important to use a species that has metabolic pathways similar to those found in human beings. Second, some relevant signs and symptoms that appear in human beings may be difficult to model in animals, due to neurological, behavioral, or other differences between animals and humans. For example, human beings may experience confusion, irritability, dizziness, and other psychological or behavioral effects due to chemical toxicity, which are difficult to reproduce in animals (LaFollette and Shanks 1997). Third, animal studies usually involve administration of extremely high doses of chemicals (mega-doses) over a relatively short period of time, which is not a good model of toxicity in human beings, because people typically are exposed to smaller doses of chemicals over a longer period of time. To overcome this problem and develop better models of human toxicity, some scientists are exploring strategies for administering lower doses to test subjects for longer periods of time. These studies may not produce the definitive outcomes one would see in an LD_{50} test, but they may yield important information about how chemicals affect mammalian metabolism and physiology (Meyer 2003; Gerde 2005). (The ethics of animal toxicology experiments will not be examined in this book. For further discussion, see LaFollette and Shanks 1997; Shamoo and Resnik 2009.)

Other methods of investigation in toxicology include desktop analysis and in vitro testing. In desktop analysis, toxicologists draw inferences from quantitative structure-activity relationships among molecules. For example, if a chemical with a particular structure is known to produce certain toxic effects, a toxicologist may infer that a chemical with similar structure will produce similar effects, under the guiding assumption that similar structures produce similar effects. In in vitro testing, toxicologists expose cultured animal, human, or other cells to a potential toxin to observe cellular responses, such as metabolic reactions and genetic mutations (Richardson and Miller 2010). Advances in stem cell science have made it possible to develop various human tissues types (liver, heart, nerve, and so on) from adult and embryonic stem cells for toxicity testing, an important advance in *in vitro* research (Davila et al. 2004).

EPIDEMIOLOGY

Epidemiology studies the distribution of health in society and the environmental and genetic factors that contribute to disease. Epidemiologists investigate population trends, such as the relationship between exercise, caloric intake, and diabetes, as well as local disease epidemics, such as an outbreak of food-borne illnesses at a local restaurant or a high incidence of cancer near a toxic waste site. Epidemiologists may study populations at a local, regional, national, or global level (Steenland and Moe 2010).

Epidemiologists distinguish between two different ways of describing disease frequencies in a population. The prevalence of a disease is the percentage of people in the population with the disease at a particular time. The incidence of a disease is the percentage of new cases in the population in a time period, a year, for example. A chronic, incurable disease such as type II diabetes, could have a high prevalence but a low incidence, because cases could accumulate in the population at a slow, but steady rate. Acute, short-term diseases, such as the common cold, could have a high incidence but a low prevalence, because while many people will get the cold each year, far fewer will have it at any one time (Le and Boen 1995).

There are different types of study designs in epidemiology. The most basic division is between observational studies, which gather data on human subjects in their natural environment without manipulating the conditions; and experimental studies, which gather data on human subjects under controlled conditions. Common types of observational studies are: case reports, descriptive studies, ecological studies, prospective cohort studies, retrospective case-control studies, and cross-sectional studies. Common types of experimental studies are: clinical trials and exposure studies (Resnik 2008a). These different studies have advantages and disadvantages and are useful for achieving different sorts of scientific goals.

Descriptive studies are preliminary investigators of disease prevalence in a population. Descriptive studies gather information on the prevalence of different diseases as well as demographic factors, such as age, race, sex, income, location, and so on. Descriptive studies do not attempt to test hypotheses concerning disease factors or trends, but they provide useful information for designing more rigorous investigations (Steenland and Moe 2010).

Ecological studies investigate correlations between disease rates and environmental or other factors at the population group level. Ecological studies do not gather data on specific individuals but compare different groups, such as Japanese versus Americans, residents of Nevada versus residents of Utah, and so on (Steenland and Moe 2010). For example, Lee (1976) compared colon cancer mortality rates among people living in Japan, the United States, and

Wales to that of Japanese Americans. The study gathered data on sex, race, age of death, and other variables, and noted that colon cancer mortality rates had risen dramatically in Japan since World War II. The study speculated that differences in mortality rates were due to environmental factors (such as diet) rather than genetic factors (Lee 1976). One methodological weakness of this study is that it gathered data from populations, not individuals. Thus, at best the study can provide information about general trends rather than individual risk factors. Ecological studies, like descriptive studies, are useful in generating hypotheses concerning disease risk and environmental conditions, but not in testing hypotheses (Steenland and Moe 2010).

Prospective cohort studies are designed to test specific hypotheses concerning diseases and environmental or other factors. These studies include two groups: the cohort and a control group. Individuals in the cohort have a common characteristic of interest, such as a particular occupation or environmental exposure. Individuals in the control group do not have this characteristic. The two groups are matched with respect to relevant demographic and other factors, such as age, race, sex, education, and so on. The two groups are followed over a long time period (often ten years or more), and data are collected at various intervals concerning diseases and health status. At the end of the study, researchers can compare disease rates among the two groups, and statistical inferences may be drawn concerning environmental and other risk factors for diseases (Steenland and Moe 2010).

One of the most important prospective cohort studies is the Framingham Heart Study, a joint project of the National Heart, Lung, and Blood Institute (NHLBI) and Boston University. Begun in 1948, the Framingham study has followed a cohort of people living in Framingham, MA, with the goal of identifying environment risk factors for heart disease. Framingham investigators have collected information about health status of the participants, environmental risks factors, such as smoking, diet, occupation, medications, exercise, and demographic information. Framingham investigators have also collected blood samples from the participants and analyzed genetic factors related to health and disease. The study originally enrolled 5,209 men and women between ages 30 and 62. In 1971, the study enrolled 5,124 adult children and spouses of the original participants; in 1994, the study enrolled an additional 506 participants to increase the diversity of the population and later expanded this enrollment with an additional 410 members. In 2002, the study enrolled grandchildren of the original participants. The Framingham study, which has generated hundreds of publications, has shown that cigarette smoking, high blood pressure, high blood cholesterol levels, obesity, and menopause increase the risk of heart disease, and that high levels of high density lipoprotein (HDL) cholesterol and exercise decrease the risk of heart disease (Framingham Heart Study 2010).

Although prospective cohort studies can provide useful information that can be used to test hypotheses, they have methodological problems that must be addressed. Because prospective studies follow a large group of individuals for a long time (twenty years or more) they can be expensive to conduct and can suffer from high attrition rates, because people decide to drop out of the study or cannot be recontacted (Steenland and Moe 2010). If attrition rates are high, this can bias the results, because the people who stay in the study may be different from those who do not.

Selection bias and confounding can impact prospective cohort studies. Selection bias occurs when the cohort or control groups do not represent the general population. For example, if there are social, cultural, or ethnic differences between people living in Framingham, MA, and other places in the United States, this could bias the study. Confounding occurs when there are variables that affect relationships between disease outcomes and risks factors that have not been included or adequately controlled in the study. For example, if a study examines the relationship between welding and lung cancer but does not control for smoking as a risk factor, then smoking status could confound the study, because smoking, and not welding, might be the most significant risk factor for lung cancer (Steenland and Moe 2010).

Case-control studies include people with a disease of interest (cases) and a group of nondiseased people matched to the cases (controls). In these studies, investigators look back into the past to determine risk factors for the disease in question, such as environmental exposures, demographics, and so on. For example, Elbaz et al. (2009) conducted a case-control study on Parkinson's disease (PD) and occupational exposures to pesticides. The study included 224 PD cases and 557 controls without PD from a group of French agricultural workers. The investigators asked the subjects about occupational exposures to different types of pesticides and other risk factors, such as smoking, well-water drinking, and family history. They found that the PD was positively associated with professional pesticide use and that the risk of PD increased with the number of years of exposure to pesticides. They also found that organochlorine insecticides pose a greater risk than other types of pesticides.

Case-control studies face some of the same methodological hurdles that can affect the other research designs. Because these studies ask individuals about what happened to them in the past, they face potential problems related to human memory (recall bias). People may not remember what happened to them, or they may remember incorrectly. Recall bias can sometimes be addressed by supplementing human memory with objective data, such as medical records, birth records, and employment records. Case-control studies also are subject to selection bias, because the cases and controls may not represent the general population (Steenland and Moe 2010).

Cross-sectional studies provide a snapshot of a population in time. They measure disease prevalence as well as other relevant variables, such as environmental exposures, demographics, and so on. Cross-sectional studies may also include data from interviews or surveys (Steenland and Moe 2010). Because cross-sectional studies focus on a single point in time, they do not provide evidence of causality, which occurs over time, but they can suggest relationships between different variables, which can be investigated by other types of studies. Cross-sectional studies also provide useful background information for other study designs. For example, before conducting a case-control study of a particular disease in a population, it is important to have information about the prevalence of the disease in the population, as well as other information from cross-sectional studies because this information can help an investigator to select cases and controls that are representative of the population.

Clinical trials investigate the safety and efficacy of a health intervention, such as a test or treatment. Though most people associate clinical trials with tests of new medications, clinical trials are used to investigate many different therapies other than drugs, including biologics, medical devices, psychotherapy, public health interventions, and environmental health interventions. The "gold-standard" for clinical research is the randomized controlled trial (RCT), which involves random assignment of subjects to one of two or more different treatment groups, including an experimental group and a control group. Subjects in the control group may receive a standard treatment or a placebo. Usually placebo controls are not used if a standard treatment is available. If a placebo group is not used, the experimental treatment will be compared to a standard therapy. Randomization helps to reduce the potential for bias in the assignment of subjects to different groups, and placebos compensate for therapeutic improvements resulting from the placebo effect (Resnik 2008b).

There are four different phases of clinical trials. Phase I trials are small studies (50–100 subjects) lasting several months whose main goal is to assess the safety of a new treatment. Phase I studies are conducted after animal studies have demonstrated that a new therapy is safe enough to attempt in human beings. Phase I studies are usually conducted on healthy volunteers, though some Phase I studies are conducted on patients with terminal diseases who have few alternatives for treatment other than experimental therapies. One of the goals of a Phase I drug study is to determine the maximum tolerable dose (MTD) for a new therapy. Doses are increased until subjects experience intolerable symptoms, such as severe nausea, vomiting, or headaches, or physiological problems indicative of toxicity. Phase I drug studies also investigate drug uptake, distribution, metabolism, and excretion (Shamoo and Resnik 2006).

Phase II studies may begin if Phase I testing shows that a new treatment is safe enough to attempt in patients. Phase II studies are larger than Phase I studies (about 300 subjects) and last longer (one to two years). Phase II studies gather dose-range data related to the efficacy and safety of a new treatment. Phase III may begin if Phase II studies show that a new therapy is safe and effective. Phase III studies are larger than Phase II studies (1,000–3,000 subjects) and may last many years. Phase III studies gather additional efficacy and safety data at the anticipated therapeutic dose. If a new therapy completes Phase III testing successfully, then it may be approved for marketing and distribution by a regulatory agency, such as the FDA, if regulatory approval is required. Phase IV studies may be conducted once a new therapy is on the market. The purpose of Phase IV studies is to gather additional efficacy and safety data, especially data pertaining to populations that were not included in Phase II or III testing (Resnik 2008b).

Though RCTs are excellent methods for studying the safety and efficacy of therapies, they raise a number of ethical and policy issues, which have been the subject of debate (Resnik 2009c). Ethical issues related to environmental interventions will be discussed in Chapter 11.

Exposure studies are controlled experiments in which subjects are exposed to an environmental agent, such as ozone or automobile exhaust, to gain a better understanding of how the agent induces adverse effects, such as toxicity. The exposure is carefully controlled and subjects are monitored closely. Biological samples such as urine, blood, and tissue may be collected. The main reason for using human beings as test subjects in these experiments is that other research methods have significant limitations (Resnik 2006). Animal studies can tell us how a substance interacts with mammalian bodies, but it is important to have specific information about how a substance interacts with the human body. Human exposure studies can yield information about absorption, distribution, metabolism, and excretion. Observational studies on human subjects, such as prospective cohort studies or retrospective case-control studies, usually involve exposure to environmental agents that are not well-controlled. Observational studies also may not collect the kind of information that is needed to gain a clear understanding of exposures. In most cases, useful information can be gained from exposure levels that are very low and do not pose significant risks to the subjects. However, environmental exposure studies do raise some ethical concerns, which will be discussed in Chapter 11.

It is also important to mention that meta-analysis is an important research method in epidemiology. Meta-analysis is a statistical technique for combining and analyzing data or results from different studies that address the same or related questions using common measures of effects. Meta-analysis is used typically to combine the results of case-control studies or clinical trials. For example, a class of commonly prescribed drugs known as statins can lower low-density lipoprotein (LDL) cholesterol levels in the blood and reduce the risk of cardiovascular problems. However, studies have reported conflicting results about whether statins increase the risk of Type II (adult) diabetes. To resolve this issue, Sattar et al. (2010) combined the results of thirteen RCTs with a similar design that reported diabetes as an outcome, and they used meta-regression to analyze the results. A total of 91,140 subjects were in the different trials. The investigators found that statins slightly increase the risk of diabetes, with a more pronounced effect among older patients, but that the benefits of statin therapy outweigh the risks.

Like any research tool, meta-analysis has strengths and weaknesses. Statistical power is one of the strengths of meta-analysis because the combined set of data/results is much larger than any of the separate sets of data/results. Because a meta-analysis has greater statistical power than the studies it incorporates it may be able to detect effects that have not been detected previously. A meta-analysis also provides greater generalizability than the smaller studies it incorporates because it includes data/results from many different populations. Meta-analysis has some problems, however. First, to conduct a valid meta-analysis, the different studies in the combined set must define the measured effects in the same way and must have similar study design. These assumptions may not always be met due to differences in research planning and execution. Second, a meta-analysis is only as good as the studies that compose it. If the studies in the combined set have methodological flaws, these will weaken and perhaps invalidate the meta-analysis (Bailar 1997).

Two areas of epidemiology especially important for environmental health are environmental epidemiology and occupational epidemiology. Environmental epidemiology studies involuntary exposures to environmental agents, that is, agents that are not associated with a person's medical condition or lifestyle, such as microorganisms, air pollutants, water pollutants, pesticides, toxic chemicals, radon, lead, mercury, and allergens. Environmental epidemiology usually does not focus on exposures to alcohol, medications, illegal drugs, and various foods. Environmental epidemiologists study exposure to secondhand smoke, not firsthand smoke, because smoking is a lifestyle choice. Although the distinction between voluntary and involuntary exposures is somewhat arbitrary, it is useful for focusing research questions and funding priorities. Moreover, environmental epidemiologists do not ignore voluntary exposures because they must gather data on these exposures to control for possible confounders. An example of an environmental epidemiology study is the Sister Study, a prospective cohort study of 50,000 women in the United States and Puerto Rico, who have not had breast cancer but whose biological sisters have been diagnosed with the disease. The Sister Study collects data on the medical history, demography, and various environmental exposures in order to determine the role of environmental and genetic factors in breast cancer. The women in the study will be followed for ten years (Sister Study 2010).

Environmental epidemiologists study not only endemic diseases, such as cancer, diabetes, or hypertension, but also disease epidemics, such as outbreaks of disease in particular places or populations. A disease outbreak occurs when there is a dramatic rise in the incidence of a disease. Environmental epidemiologists study the causes of the outbreak. For example, in the 1970s, African doctors observed an increase in people who had diseases such as Kaposi's Sarcoma (tumors caused by a type of herpes virus) and Candidiasis (a type of yeast infection), which were associated with a weakened immune system. These patients also had fatigue and dramatic weight loss. In the early 1980s, doctors in the United States observed patients with similar clinical presentations among gay men, intravenous drug abusers, and hemophiliacs, and in 1982 the CDC introduced the name Acquired Immune Deficiency Syndrome (AIDS) to describe this disease. By 1983, there were 3000 known AIDS cases in the United States and 1,000 deaths. In 1984, Robert Gallo and Luc Montagnier identified the pathogen responsible for AIDS and named it Human Immunodeficiency Virus (HIV). Researchers also discovered that the disease is transmitted when someone's mucus membranes come in contact with blood or bodily fluids from an infected person, and the disease attacks immune system cells known as T-cells. Preventative measures, such as condom use and needle exchange programs, were instituted. The prevalence of the virus continued to increase dramatically in the human population: There were 38,000 AIDS cases in eighty-five countries by 1986, 8 million cases worldwide by 1990, and 33 million cases by 2008. More than 25 million people have died of AIDS since 1982 (AVERT 2009).

Occupational epidemiology studies health risks associated with workplace conditions and exposures. As mentioned previously, two of the important figures in the history of environmental health, Charles Turner Thackrach and Alice Hamilton, studied the hazardous conditions associated with coal mining and factory work. The workplace often serves as a laboratory for studying environmental exposures, because people in the workplace are in a geographically isolated place in which they sometimes encounter relatively high exposures to environmental agents over a long period of time. Many carcinogens have been identified in the workplace such as arsenic, radon gas, dioxin, diesel fumes, nickel, and various pesticides. Some of these agents are also found outside of the workplace in much lower concentrations.

Once a health risk is identified in the workplace, additional research is needed to show that it is also a risk outside of the workplace, because workplace exposures are typically much higher than exposures outside the workplace (Steenland and Moe 2010). For example, asbestos is a mineral fiber with flame-retardant properties used in making a variety of construction materials. Asbestos exposures in the workplace have been shown to cause mesothelioma, a rare form of lung cancer. The risks of developing mesothelioma increase with the level of exposure to asbestos. Though the hazards of asbestos exposure were initially identified in occupational settings, there is now evidence that people can contract mesothelioma as a result of exposures outside of the workplace (Asbestos.com 2010; Bourdés et al. 2010).

Occupational epidemiologists study not only dangerous environmental agents in the workplace, but also the adverse effects of hazardous working conditions, such as inadequate ventilation that causes difficulty breathing, poorly designed worksites that increase the risk of accidental injuries, on-the-job stress that leads to psychological problems, noise that induces hearing loss, long work shifts that lead to fatigue and accidents, ergonomically unsound seating arrangements that increase the risk of back pain, inadequate sanitation and hygiene that leads to infectious diseases, and repetitive work motions that cause injuries, such as carpal tunnel syndrome (Perry and Hu 2010).

Occupational epidemiologists also make recommendations for improving health and safety. The United States and many other countries have laws pertaining to workplace health and safety. The Occupational Health and Safety Act, enacted in 1970, authorized the Occupational Safety and Health Administration (OSHA) to set and enforce standards for occupational health and safety. OSHA conducts routine and for-cause inspections of worksites and penalizes companies for failing to adhere to health and safety standards. Federal laws allow states to adopt their own occupational health and safety standards, as long as these are as protective as the OSHA standards. The National Institute for Occupational Safety and Health (NIOSH) conducts research on occupational health and site-specific hazards (Perry and Hu 2010). Conducting research in occupational settings poses some ethical challenges for investigators, which will be discussed in Chapter 11.

Environmental and occupational epidemiologists sometimes study disease clusters where there is an elevated incidence of a disease in a particular place and time. Epidemiologists may investigate a cluster after public health authorities or citizens become aware of it. It can be difficult to determine whether the cases in the cluster result from a common cause or are only due to random variations in patterns of disease. It is not always easy to identify a common cause, due to small sample sizes and numerous uncontrolled environmental factors that may have an impact on the situation. Suppose that seven people living in a small neighborhood near a chemical plant develop leukemia within a period of two years. These cases might be due to a common cause, such as proximity to the plant, but they could also be due to many other factors, such as genetics or other environmental exposures.

An example of a successful identification of the cause of a disease cluster occurred in January 1977, when epidemiologists and infectious disease specialists determined that a species of bacteria (*Legionella pneumophila*) was responsible for an outbreak of pneumonia at the American Legion Convention at the Bellevue Stratford Hotel in Philadelphia in July 1976. The disease sickened 182 Legionnaires and killed 29. The investigators also found that the hotel's air conditioning system was the source of the infection. The findings led to increased regulations for climate control systems. Legionnaire's Disease is a very serious infection with a mortality rate of up to 30 percent (Winn 1988; Centers for Disease Control and Prevention 2008a).

The controversy over Gulf War Illness illustrates some of the difficulties with identifying a single cause for a noticeable increase of disease symptoms in a population. Following the 1991 Persian Gulf War, thousands of military personnel complained of a variety of symptoms they believed were related to their service in the conflict, including headaches, mood disorders, shortness of breath, gastrointestinal problems, fatigue, rashes, joint pain, sleep disturbances, forgetfulness, and concentration difficulties. Many veterans blamed their illness on toxic exposures encountered in the war, such as chemical weapons, depleted uranium, burning oil wells, pesticides, and petroleum products. Initial inquiries from the Department of Veteran Affairs concluded there was no single cause of all of these symptoms – that there was no Gulf War "illness." However, the controversy of the health of Gulf War veterans continued, and in 1998 the U.S. Congress passed laws directing the Department of Veteran Affairs to contract with the National Academy of Sciences (NAS) to study a possible link between occupational exposures among military personnel who served in the war and illnesses. The Institute of Medicine (IOM), a division of the NAS, published a series of reports that reviewed and summarized the peer-reviewed literature on the health of Gulf War veterans. The IOM concluded that Gulf War veterans had higher symptom rates than military personnel who were not deployed in Iraq at the time, as well as higher rates of posttraumatic stress disorder (PTSD), chronic fatigue syndrome, and fibromyalgia. However, these differences were not explained by a single cause. The IOM report used statistical methods, such as factor analysis, to try to determine whether the symptoms reported by Gulf War veterans constituted a unique syndrome or medical condition. Though Gulf War veterans have significant health problems that require attention, the IOM determined that there is no Gulf War Illness (Institute of Medicine 2006).

Several methodological difficulties have hampered the investigation of the health problems of Gulf War veterans. First, selection bias may have affected some of these studies because the response rate to most health surveys was mediocre, and veterans who responded to health surveys may have been sicker than those who did not respond. Second, recall bias may have affected the studies because data about environmental exposures were based on veteran's recollections, which may be inaccurate. Veterans may have exaggerated or minimized their exposures. Third, there was no way to objectively determine veterans' exposures because measurements were not taken before, during, and after exposures, and it is difficult to use theoretical models to ascertain what these exposures might have been, due to lack of knowledge about many different factors that could have affected exposures, amount of exposure, timing of exposure, wind direction or speed, wearing of protective gear, and so on (Hotopf and Wessely 2005; Institute of Medicine 2006).

The importance of obtaining accurate information about environmental exposures brings us to another important discipline in environmental health: exposure science.

EXPOSURE BIOLOGY

The goals of exposure biology are to 1) quantify hazardous environment exposures, 2) evaluate the different factors that affect exposures, and 3) develop methods to measure exposure and its effects (Ryan 2010). Exposure assessment plays a crucial role in environmental and occupational epidemiology because to determine whether an environmental agent contributes to disease, a scientist must have an accurate and complete understanding of how people are exposed to that agent. Exposure assessment can take place in the natural environment, such as a workplace or home, or in the laboratory.

Several different variables need to be measured to assess exposure to an environmental agent, including the concentration of the agent (magnitude of exposure), the exposure period (duration of exposure), the effectiveness of transfer of the agent to the body, and the absorption of the agent by the body. Concentration is a measure of how much of the agent is in the part of the environment that transfers the agent to the individual, that is, the media. For example, for exposure to carbon monoxide, air is the media. Other common media include: water, soil, dust, food, plants, and animals. Concentrations may be quantified in units of mass per units of mass, for example, parts per million (ppm) or billion (ppb), or units of mass per units of volume, for example, micrograms per liter (Ryan 2010). Carbon monoxide poisoning can begin when a person is exposed to 70 ppm of this gas for a prolonged period of time, and death can result from exposures at 150–200 ppm (Consumer Products Safety Commission 2010). The EPA has determined that safe drinking water should have no more than 0.01 mg/liter of arsenic or 10 ppb (Environmental Protection Agency 2006). Exposure scientists use a variety of scientific instruments and analytical methods to measure concentrations of environmental agents in different media, such as gas or liquid chromatography, mass spectrometry, gravimetric analysis, and trace metal speciation analysis.

Once the concentration level of an agent in the media is determined, it is important to also ascertain how long the agent will be in contact with the body because exposure to a high concentration of a substance for a short time may be less dangerous than prolonged exposure at a lower concentration. Exposure to 150 ppm of carbon monoxide for 0.5 minutes is not very dangerous, but exposure to the same concentration of this gas for an hour is dangerous. To take the period of exposure into account, exposures are usually multiplied by a unit of time, for example, mg/L (hours). In considering the exposure period, it is also important to know whether there are variations in the concentration of the agent during the period, because higher concentrations during a segment of the exposure period could have adverse impacts. For example, suppose one is measuring ozone exposure over a twenty-four-hour period. It would be important to know whether ozone concentrations wax and wane during this time period and the level of the peak concentration (Ryan 2010).

Several different factors can impact the effectiveness of the transfer of the agent to the body, such as wind speed or direction (for airborne particulates), air temperature, the presence of other environmental agents, and protective clothing. Once these factors are taken into account, a potential dose, or the amount of the agent that enters the body, can be determined. The potential dose depends on the concentration, exposure period, and the rate at which the agent crosses the relevant epithelial barrier (i.e., epidermis, lung alveoli, etc.). For example, suppose that a person is exposed to 100 ug/ m^3 carbon monoxide for one hour and that he breathes 10 m^3 per hour. Let's also assume that carbon monoxide only enters the body through the lungs. The potential dose would be:

$$(100 \text{ ug/ } 10 \text{ m}^3) \ (1 \text{ hour}) \ (10 \text{ m}^3/\text{hour}) = 100 \text{ ug.}$$

Assessment of a potential dose can be more complicated when the agent can enter the body through more than one route. For example, an agricultural worker might be exposed to pesticides through respiration, digestion, and skin contact. A potential dose would need to take all of these different exposure routes into account (Ryan 2010).

The actual dose a person receives would depend on one other variable: the percentage of the agent that is actually absorbed by the body. Most agents are not completely absorbed once they reach an epithelial barrier (Ryan 2010). If the environmental agent is completely absorbed, the actual dose would equal the potential dose.

Exposure scientists use direct and indirect methods to measure exposures. Two important direct methods include environmental monitoring and personal monitoring. For example, air pollution monitoring measures concentrations of pollutants, such as ozone and sulfur oxides, in the atmosphere. Carbon monoxide detectors in the home measure the concentration of this gas in the air and sound an alarm if the concentration goes above a preset level. Personal monitoring involves attaching a device to a person to measure their exposures. For example, people who work with radioactive materials, such as radiographers and nuclear engineers or technicians, wear radiation badges to detect their level of exposure to radiation. If excessive exposures are detected, steps can be taken to correct potential problems and reduce risks to workers (Ryan 2010).

Indirect methods do not measure exposure directly but infer probably exposures from data and assumptions. For example, an indirect method of measuring a person's exposure to pesticides would be to measure the level of pesticides on different types of food the person eats, and ask the person to keep a food diary. Exposures could be inferred from this data as well as assumptions about the person's eating habits and other assumptions. Another way of indirectly measuring exposure would be to infer exposures from a person's activity patterns. For example, one could estimate an agricultural worker's exposures to pesticides by determining exposures for different farm activities, and then asking the worker about which of these activities he has performed and for how long (Ryan 2010).

Because the actual dose that a person receives of an agent depends on many factors that often are not easily controlled or determined, such as magnitude, duration, or absorption, many scientists consider the best way to assess exposures is to measure biological markers of exposure (or biomarkers) that yield information about actual exposures. To measure exposure biomarkers, scientists analyze biological samples (blood, urine, saliva, hair, etc.) to detect the presence of the environmental agent in question, one of its metabolites, or a biological response to the presence of the agent or its metabolites (Ryan 2010). For example, police estimate blood alcohol levels by asking suspected drunk drivers to breathe into a breathalyzer machine, which measures the percentage of ethanol in air exhaled by the person. Health insurers determine whether a person has used tobacco by measuring the amount of cotinine (a nicotine metabolite) in the blood, urine, or saliva. One way to measure long-term exposure to inorganic arsenic is to test for the presence of skin lesions, a biological response to inorganic arsenic (Hughes 2006). Airway inflammation is a biomarker for ozone exposure (Alexis et al. 2008). Biomarkers can also be used to detect predispositions for disease and disease progression. For example, BRCA1 and 2 mutations are biomarkers for a predisposition to breast cancer, and cardiac enzymes in the bloodstream indicate a recent myocardial infarction (Decaprio 1997).

Although biomarkers can offer precise estimates of actual exposures, they have some drawbacks. First, though biomarkers indicate that a chemical has entered the body, they do not provide information about the source of the exposure, the magnitude of the exposure, or the duration of the exposure. Second, for many types of research it may be difficult or impossible to measure biomarkers of exposure because the person has already metabolized and excreted the substance. For example, to be effective, a blood alcohol test must be administered before the person eliminates alcohol from their blood. One problem with the study of Gulf War illnesses, mentioned earlier, was the lack of biomarker evidence. Without this evidence, it is difficult to estimate veterans' exposures to environmental agents. Ideally, an environmental health study should include many different exposure measurements to get a complete picture of the interaction between an environmental agent and the human body.

SUMMARY

Environmental health is a field of scientific study and an area of applied practice. The science of environmental health attempts to understand the biological, chemical, physical, and social factors in the environment that affect human health and disease, and the practice of environmental health applies scientific knowledge to decisions and policies that promote health and reduce or prevent disease. This chapter has given a brief overview of some of the concepts, principles, theories, and methods from four key disciplines in environmental health: ecology, epidemiology, toxicology, and exposure biology. The next chapter will present an overview of ethical theory.

3

ETHICAL THEORY

To understand the ethical issues in environmental health, it is necessary to have a good grasp of environmental health and ethics. Chapter 2 presented an overview of environmental health, and the next two chapters will focus on ethics. This chapter will provide the reader with some background in ethical theory, and Chapter 4 will develop a procedure for ethical decision making.

WHAT IS ETHICS?

Ethics can be defined as: 1) a set of standards (or norms) for distinguishing between right and wrong actions, or 2) the study of ethical standards. Ethical (or moral) concepts include such notions as obligation (or duty), virtue, justice, rights, happiness, value, and goodness. The study of ethics can be divided into four different areas: normative ethics, which examines general concepts and principles of ethics; applied ethics, which investigates ethical decision making in particular domains, such as medicine, science, or law; meta-ethics, which analyzes the meaning and justification of ethical concepts and principles; and empirical ethics, which studies moral reasoning, judgment, behavior, learning, and development. For many years, ethics has been predominantly the domain of humanistic disciplines, such as philosophy and theology, but now many empirical disciplines study ethics, including psychology, sociology, anthropology, economics, and sociobiology (Pojman 2005).

Ethics has much in common with, but is different from, the law. Ethics and the law are similar in that they 1) provide guidance for human conduct; 2) deal with similar concepts, such as obligation, duty, rights, and justice; and 3) use the Socratic method, which involves consideration and analysis of opposing viewpoints. However, these disciplines are different in important ways. First, laws are backed by coercive power of the state. If you break the law, you can face a financial penalty, imprisonment, or in some countries, capital punishment. Though some ethical standards, such as prohibitions against murder, are enforced by the state, many are not. Second, we can appeal to ethical standards to criticize, protest, or defend laws. For example, during the Civil Rights Movement in the United States, many people argued that laws requiring racial segregation were unethical, and many people protested those laws through civil disobedience (Pojman 2005).

Ethics is also similar to, but different from, politics. Ethics and politics are similar in that they both provide guidance for human conduct via the development of rules and standards, and they also use similar concepts, such as rights and justice. These two domains focus on different levels of analysis, however. Ethics focuses on the microlevel and asks questions like, "what should I do?" and "how should I make decisions?," while politics focuses on the macrolevel and asks questions like, "what should we, as a society, do?" and "how should we make decisions?" The differences between ethics and politics are often subtle, and many controversial topics, such as abortion, euthanasia, and capital punishment have ethical and political dimensions (Pojman 2005). Though this book will focus on ethical issues in environmental health, it will also consider political ones.

Finally, ethics is similar to but different from religion. Ethics and religion both provide standards of conduct. They also focus on similar concepts, such as obligation, duty, justice, and virtue. But ethics and religion are different in that widely recognized ethical rules and standards, such as prohibitions against murder, rape, theft, and dishonesty, can be defended and embraced without appealing to any particular religious viewpoint. Further, there is considerable evidence that people from very different religious backgrounds accept some common ethical standards (Pojman 2005). Even though ethics and religion are distinct domains, they often overlap. First, as we shall also see, many theologians and religious thinkers have made important contributions to ethical theory and scholarship. Second, for most people, religious ideas and beliefs play an important role in motivating ethical conduct and guiding ethical decision making.

A BRIEF HISTORY OF ETHICS

Chapter 2 gave a brief history of environmental health. The history of ethics discussed in this chapter will be a bit longer because contemporary ethical theories incorporate historical traditions. Ethical scholarship involves an ongoing dialogue with past thinkers and their ideas.

Before there was an academic study of ethics, leading thinkers in different civilizations had developed moral codes, stories, and sayings to provide guidance for living. The Hebrew Bible, or Old Testament, includes books dating from 1400 BCE to 150 BCE. The Ten Commandments, found in the book of *Exodus*, include religious obligations, as the duty not to worship false idols and to keep the Sabbath holy, as well as moral ones, such as the duty not to murder or steal (*Holy Bible* 2004). The book of *Proverbs* contains practical guidelines for living, such as avoiding excessive drinking, adultery, dishonesty, gossip, laziness, and harsh words. The *Tao Te Ching*, attributed to the Chinese philosopher Lao Tzu (600–300 BCE), contains sayings for living a good life in harmony with nature and achieving enlightenment (Lao Tzu 1984). The *Tao Te Ching* serves as a basis for Chinese Buddhism. Another Chinese philosopher, Confucius (551–479 BCE) provided guidance for living a good life and wise governance, and advocated different moral virtues, such as courage, temperance, moderation, and honor (Confucius 1955). Taoism and Confucianism have played an important role in the development of Chinese culture and philosophy and still have considerable influence today.

Although people have developed and followed moral rules for thousands of years, most scholars trace the academic study of ethics to ancient Greece (MacIntyre 2000). Many of the insights developed by the Greeks still have considerable influence over contemporary ethical thinking. The main moral problem that concerned the Greek philosophers was how to live a good life (Rawls and Herman 2000). Plato (428–348 BCE) published thirty-five dialogues, many of which deal with moral questions, such as the meaning of justice and virtue and reasons for obeying the law. Plato was a student of Socrates (469–399 BCE), the father of philosophy, and many of his dialogues involve conversations between Socrates and various students. In the *Euthyphro*, Socrates argues for a separation between ethics and religion. This was an important conclusion for Greek philosophers to reach because it opened the door to developing secular moral concepts and theories (Cooper and Hutchinson 1997).

Plato deals with the problem of virtue in his most famous dialogue, *The Republic* (380 BCE). In this dialogue, Socrates discusses justice, understood as a moral virtue, with several different students. One of these, Glaucon, argues that justice is not valuable for its own sake, but is valuable only for the benefits it confers on a person, such as a good reputation or freedom from punishment. If people did not fear punishment, they would not act justly or praise justice. To illustrate this point, Glaucon tells the story of the Ring of Gyges, which can make the wearer invisible. Glaucon says that anyone who has the ring would use it to commit unjust acts because he could avoid punishment. Plato's answer to Glaucon's challenge is that justice is valuable for its own sake because a person who lacks justice (virtue) in his soul will be destroyed by his appetites or his emotions (Cooper and Hutchinson 1997).

Plato's student, Aristotle (384–322 BCE), developed an account of what it means to live a good life or to be happy in his *Nichomachean Ethics*. Something is good, according to Aristotle, if it performs its function well: a good flute player plays music well, a good axe chops well, and so on. So, a good human being is someone who performs the human function well. What is the function of man? According to Aristotle, human beings have different biological functions, such as growth, reproduction, movement, and so on. Human beings share many of these biological functions with other living things. The function that is distinctively human is activity in accordance with reason. To live in accordance with reason, according to Aristotle, is to apply reason to your decisions and actions, which entails practicing virtue. A good human being, then, is someone who is good at practicing different virtues, such as courage, moderation, justice, kindness, and honesty (Aristotle 2003).

Human virtues, according to Aristotle, are behavioral traits that we develop through practice. Eventually, virtues become habits and we are disposed to act according to those virtues. For example, someone who continually performs kind acts will become a kind person. As kindness becomes a habit, the person will have a psychological disposition to act kindly. To learn how to become virtuous, we must observe virtues in other people and follow their example. Virtues are appropriately situated between two behavioral extremes. Too little courage is cowardice, which is a vice; but too much courage can lead to foolhardiness, which is a vice. Courage is between the extremes of cowardice and foolhardiness (Aristotle 2003).

After the Greeks, another important figure in the history of ethics is the Jewish prophet Jesus of Nazareth (5 BCE-30 AD). Although Jesus was not a scholar in the traditional sense, his teachings have had a considerable impact on ethical thinking in Western cultures and religions. Christians regard Jesus as the son of God and they follow his teachings. Muslims do not believe Jesus was the son of God, but they regard him as an important prophet and follow his teachings. Jesus communicated his ideas through parables, aphorisms, and sermons. Jesus' most important contribution to ethical thought was his emphasis on compassion for one's enemies and people who are poor, hungry, diseased, or socially ostracized. Though he was not opposed to following moral rules, such as the Ten Commandments, he emphasized an ethics of compassion and love: love for God, self, and neighbor. Jesus also taught people to follow the Golden Rule ("do unto others as you would have them do unto you"), and he stressed the importance of forgiveness and humble service to others (*Holy Bible* 2004).

The Dominican monk and medieval philosopher St. Thomas Aquinas (1225–74 AD) incorporated Aristotelian insights into Christian theology. Aquinas, like Aristotle, held that people should practice moral virtue, though he did not believe that happiness consisted solely of living a life of virtue. To be truly happy, one must contemplate God. Aquinas also held that morality is based on natural law, which reflects God's will for the universe. Human legal systems (humans laws) should conform to the natural law. Some things, like life and health, are naturally good, while others, such as death and disease, are naturally evil. Although taking a human life is inherently evil, Aquinas justified self-defense under a doctrine known as double-effect. According to this idea, actions can have intended and unintended effects. If our conduct produces a bad effect (e.g., killing another person) were are not morally at fault for this effect, provided that we were intending to produce a good effect (e.g., saving our own life), we were not intending the bad effect, the bad effect was not a means to produce the good effect, and the good effect outweighs the bad effect (e.g., saving one's life compensates for taking a life). The natural law tradition has had significant influence over the development of Christian ethics, especially Catholic ethics (Pojman 2005).

During the Renaissance, philosophers were less concerned with developing a theory of moral virtue than they were in examining the structure of a moral society. The English philosopher Thomas Hobbes (1588–1679) articulated a strategy for justifying social rules that has played an important role in moral and political theory. Hobbes proposed a philosophical thought experiment known as the state of nature, a hypothetical time in human history before the advent of civilization. According to Hobbes, people in their natural state are selfish and cruel, and life is fraught with perils: One may die from a bad harvest or be killed for one's food. People in the state of nature eventually recognize the benefits of social cooperation, and they form a civil society, governed by various rules concerning ethical conduct, justice, and political decision making. Morality, according to Hobbes, is ultimately based on enlightened self-interest: People make a rational decision to accept moral rules to derive the benefits of civil society. Hobbes thought that the only way to keep social order is for people to succumb to the rule of a strong dictator, whom he called *Leviathan* (Pojman 2005; Hobbes 2006).

The idea of state of nature has influenced many other moral and political theorists, including the English philosopher John Locke (1632–1704) and the French philosopher Jean Jacques Rousseau (1712–1778). Locke argued that in the state of nature people have equal rights to life, liberty, and property. They are free to exercise and enforce these rights. People agree to form a civil society (or enter a social contact) to protect their natural rights, and the main function of government is to safeguard these rights (Locke 1980). People can acquire property by gift, commercial exchange, or by mixing their labor with a common resource. The only limit on the amount of property one can own is a limit imposed by nature: One can acquire property up to the point of spoilage or destruction. Property acquired beyond this natural boundary should be returned to the commonwealth, so that others may use it.

The English philosopher David Hume (1711–1776) sought to discredit the idea that morality is based on human reason, an assumption that had prevailed since the time of the Greeks. For the Greeks, human reason was the key to developing virtue. For Hobbes, Locke, and Rousseau, the decision to form civil society is a rational choice. According to Hume, morality is based not on reason but on passions and sentiments (or emotions), such as sympathy. Hume's main argument for this thesis stems from his understanding of what reason can do: Reason can demonstrate beliefs based on observation of logical relationships, but it cannot convince us about what our ultimate ends (desires, goals) should be. Reason can influence the human will by providing information about how best to achieve our ultimate ends, but it is not the source of those ends (Hume 1978). Reason can tell me how to save a child from drowning, but it cannot tell me whether I should save the child from drowning. Though reason can influence the human will, it cannot, by itself, convince a person to do anything in the practical realm. A related Humean thesis is that normative statements, that is, statements that say what people ought to do, cannot be logically derived from descriptive statements alone, that is, statements that describe facts about the world (Rawls and Herman 2000). For example, one cannot infer "I should take my umbrella" (a normative statement) from "It is raining" (a descriptive statement), without some other statement that has normative content, such as "I don't want to get wet."

The German philosopher Immanuel Kant (1724–1804) tried to answer Humean skepticism about moral reason and sought to reestablish the rational basis for ethical concepts and norms. Kant recognized that people have passions, emotions, and interests, but he held that people have the capacity to transcend these psychological conditions and make choices that conform to moral rules. This capacity to make decisions based on moral principles – also known as rational agency – is what distinguishes people from animals. It is also what makes us truly free. Freedom (or autonomy), for Kant, consists in making our will conform to moral rules. People who decide to make choices based on moral principles have a good will. Kant argued that the only thing that is unconditionally good is a good will. Someone who has a moral virtue, such as courage, but has a bad will, can do many evil things, as a result of his courage or intelligence. Someone who has a good will is motivated to do his moral duty for the sake of duty, not meet the demands of passions, emotions, desires, or to achieve some particular goal (Kant 1964).

Moral duties are determined by a general principle known as the Categorical Imperative (CI). Kant developed three distinct formulations of the CI. According to the first version, one should perform an action only if it could become a law for all people. This version of the CI, like the Golden Rule, emphasizes the universality of moral rules. If an action cannot become a universal rule, due to internal inconsistency or detrimental social implications, then one should not perform the action. For example, lying in order sell a product does not pass the universality test, because if everybody acted this way, people could not trust each other to tell the truth in commercial transactions, which undermines economic transactions. According to the second version of the CI, one should treat humanity, whether in one's own person or in another person, as an end in itself, not as a mere means. This version of the CI emphasizes the inherent value and moral worth of all human beings. We should not perform actions, such as murder, theft, and lying, which treat people as mere things to be manipulated or used to achieve particular ends. According to the third version of the CI, we should perform an action only if it conforms to a rule that would be chosen by rational beings developing a system of common laws. This version of the CI is similar to social contract idea, mentioned previously. Morality is a set of rules for behavior that we, as rational beings, choose to impose on ourselves (Kant 1964; Rawls and Herman 2000).

The British philosopher and economist John Stuart Mill (1806–1873) developed an ethical theory that stands in sharp contrast to Kant's view. Mill held that all moral rules and virtues are founded on the greatest happiness principle or the principle of utility. According to this idea, actions are right insofar as they promote the happiness of all people in society, and they are wrong insofar as they promote unhappiness. Mill equated happiness with pleasure and distinguished between different types of pleasure. Pleasure consists of the satisfaction of appetitive desires, such as the desire for food or sex, but it also consists of the enjoyment of intellectual activities, such as poetry, philosophy, and art. In contrast to Kant, Mill held that moral rules are justified by reference to the ends or consequences they promote: Moral rules are teleological. Kant held that moral rules are justified on their own, without reference to the ends or consequences they promote: Moral rules are deontological (or duty-based). Mill did not offer a direct justification of the principle of utility, because he believed that it was a first principle (or axiom) that any rational person would accept (Mill 2003).

In one of his most influential essays, *On Liberty*, Mill argued against government restrictions on freedom of thought, expression, and action. Mill articulated an important idea in moral and political philosophy known as the harm principle: The only justification for restricting liberty, according to Mill, is to prevent harm to others. Government restrictions on liberty are not justified to prevent people from harming themselves, unless the person is making a choice based on ignorance or lack of decision-making capacity. The government should not restrict free, well-informed choices of competent adults that do not harm other people. Mill rejected paternalistic restrictions on freedom because they generally produce unhappiness and because individuals, not the government, tend to be the best judges of their own good. Mill's strong stance against government paternalism still has relevance to modern debates about the regulation of nutrition, drug use, pornography, sexuality, gambling, and other private actions (Mill 2003).

In the beginning of the twentieth century, philosophers focused on examining the foundations of ethical beliefs, concepts, and rules. Skepticism about the role of reason in ethical judgment and decision making loomed large in these debates. The English philosopher G.E. Moore (1873–1958) argued that ethical concepts cannot be defined in factual terms, such as utility, happiness, or pleasure. Moore held that the concept of good is the most fundamental ethical idea, and that all other ethical concepts and principles are derived from it. To show that good cannot be defined in factual terms, Moore developed an argument strategy known as the open question test. According to Moore, when someone defines "good" by reference to a natural property, we can still ask, "is that good?" Moore also held that there is a logical gap between ethical statements and factual ones. Moore believed that because good cannot be defined, the only way we can know whether something is good is through intuition, not reason (Moore 1903; Pojman 2005).

Other philosophers, known as logical positivists, claimed that ethical statements do not state facts or logical relationships but are simply expressions of emotion. The logical positivists argued that statements only have meaning if they can be verified by referring to observations or logical relationships. A statement like "Murder is wrong" cannot be verified by observing a property, such as wrongness, associated with murder. It also cannot be verified by analyzing the relationship between the concept of murder and the concept of wrongness. Because "murder is wrong" cannot be verified, it is an expression of emotion, not a statement of fact or logic (Ayer 1946). Many philosophers concluded that because ethical statements are not verifiable, they are merely subjective expressions of emotion or cultural conventions. These attacks on the foundations of ethics deterred many philosophers from analyzing specific moral concepts or normative principles. As a result, the academic study of ethics focused on meta-ethical questions and largely ignored practical questions concerning duties, justice, happiness, and virtue.

A notable exception to this trend was the Scottish philosopher W. D. Ross (1887–1971), who argued that moral statements describe our intuitions of right, wrong, good, bad, and so on. Ross argued that ethical conduct is based on seven fundamental duties: fidelity (keeping promises, telling the truth); reparation (righting wrongs); gratitude (being grateful to people who have helped us); nonmaleficence (not harming others); justice (treating others fairly); beneficence (helping others); and self-improvement (improving one's self). Ross' duties are a mix of teleological obligations (such as beneficence) and deontological ones (such as fidelity). These duties are not absolute rules but *prima facie* obligations that sometimes conflict. When two *prima facie* duties conflict, we must examine the situation carefully, obtain the relevant facts, and decide which duty should have priority in the situation. To prioritize duties, we must form a moral intuition about what to do (Ross 1930).

CONTEMPORARY ETHICS

The contemporary study of ethics began, according to many, when American philosopher John Rawls (1921–2002) published *A Theory of Justice* in 1971. Rawls developed a method of moral reasoning that answered some of the skeptical problems relating to the foundations of ethics. Following in the tradition of social contract theorists, Rawls introduced the idea of the original position to justify ethical and social norms. The original position is not a real time in history, but a hypothetical device used to justify principles of justice and morality. In the original position, people are deciding how they will form a society. They are rational agents armed with knowledge of psychology, biology, economics, and other scientific disciplines. They are also behind a veil of ignorance: They do not know who they will be in this society. They do not know their race, social class, or economic status, for example. Because the social contractors do not know who they will be in this society, they will choose rules that protect the interests of all people, especially the least advantaged members of society, because they might be one of those least advantaged people. In deciding upon these rules, the contactors engage in a process known as reflective equilibrium. They propose rules to codify and explain their considered judgments of rightness, justice, and so on. Considered judgments are moral intuitions that have been appropriately purged of any social, economic, or other biases. Once they develop a set of rules, they test these against their considered judgments, and if the set does not fit, they modify it and test it again. The contractors continue developing and revising the social rules until they reach a point, known as reflective equilibrium, where judgments and rules agree with each other (Rawls 1971).

Rawls held that the social contractors would choose two basic principles for the organization of society. These principles would help determine how primary goods would be distributed. Primary goods are things that any rational person would want: rights, liberties, opportunities, income, wealth, and self-respect (Rawls 1971). Rawls' two principles are: 1) basic rights and liberties shall be distributed equally in society; 2) socioeconomic differences among people are acceptable, provided that these differences benefit the least advantaged members of society and there is fair equality of opportunity in society (Rawls 1971). Rawls also argued that these principles are ordered: The first principle must be satisfied first. Rawls argues that the contractors would choose these principles, because they would not know whether they are one of the least advantaged members of society, and they would therefore want to avoid a situation in which the least advantaged members are treated unfairly. Thus, Rawls defends a social order that may involve some redistribution of income or wealth to ensure that there is fair equality of opportunity in society. For example, taxes can be collected to pay for public education, infrastructure, social services, and so on (Rawls 1971).

Part of the genius of Rawls' method is that it bypasses some of the skeptical problems relating to the foundations of ethics. It does not matter whether ethical statements are factual or merely express emotions or intuitions. What matters is that the social contractors in the original position can deliberate about rules that codify and explain these different statements. This idea reopens the door to careful reflection on moral rules and our judgments concerning rightness, wrongness, justice, and virtue in particular situations.

After Rawls, many scholars abandoned their exclusive focus on meta-ethics and clarified, expanded upon, or criticized traditional ethical theories. One of Rawls' colleagues at Harvard University, Robert Nozick (1938–2002), developed a libertarian political philosophy based on Locke's ideas. Nozick argued that people are entitled to acquire an unlimited amount of wealth, provided it is obtained through a process that protects property rights, avoids fraud and theft, and rewards individual achievement. Taxes should pay for institutions that protect natural rights and should not be used to redistribute wealth. Government should be minimal (Nozick 1974). Alasdair McIntyre updated the Greek idea of moral virtue, arguing that virtues are acquired traits that enable people to cooperate with each other in achieving the goals of a social practice (MacIntyre 1984). Richard Brandt developed a form of utilitarianism, known as rule utilitarianism, to counter some objections to Mill's views. According to Brandt, people should act according to a system of ideal rules that maximize overall social utility (1998). Onora O'Neill (1990) and others expanded upon Kantian notions of freedom, dignity, rationality, and practical decision making.

Other scholars have taken ethical theory in new directions. Feminist scholars have argued that traditional ethical theories are overly legalistic and rule-oriented, and do not adequately represent women's moral experiences. To provide more balance in moral theorizing, masculine ethical concepts, such as rights, rules, and duties, should be supplemented by concepts that speak more to women's moral experiences, such as care, relationships, and trust (Gilligan 1993; Held 2007). Communitarians have argued that contemporary ethical theories place too much emphasis on individual rights and autonomy, and that community concerns and values need greater emphasis. Because individuality is shaped, in part, by social and cultural factors, and the idea of moral agency, as found in the works of Kant or Rawls, is too abstract to be useful in ethics (Sandel 1981; Walzer 1983). Since the 1970s, scholars have written about ethical problems in different practices and disciplines, including biomedicine (Beauchamp and Childress 2008), business (DeGeorge 2005), scientific research (Shamoo and Resnik 2009), sports (Simon 2003), government (Thompson 2004), law (Orlik 2007), and the environment (discussed in more depth in Chapter 4).

Another important trend is the increasing interest in studying moral reasoning, judgment, and norms from an empirical science perspective. Psychologists have proposed that children go through distinct phases of moral development (Kohlberg 1981; Gilligan 1993; and Piaget 1997). Psychologists have also studied the various emotional, cultural, ethnic, gender, and racial factors that affect ethical decision making (Hauser 2006; Haidt 2007; Mikhail 2007; Miller 2008). Neuroscientists have explored how moral judgment and reasoning activate different centers in the brain associated with cognition and emotion, and have hypothesized that emotional centers play a crucial role in ethical decision making (Greene et al. 2001; Miller 2008). Anthropologists have studied moral norms in different cultures, looking for similarities and differences (Benedict 1934; Mead 2001). Philosophers and anthropologists have engaged in a heated debate about whether there are some ethical norms common to all cultures (Pojman 2005). Evolutionary biologists have proposed models for the evolution morality in human societies (Buss 2004; Hauser 2006; de Waal 2009).

While most philosophers acknowledge the importance of the empirical study of morality, there is considerable debate about the implications of this endeavor for normative ethical theory (Rosenberg 2000; Pojman 2005). As noted earlier, philosophers such as Hume and Moore have maintained that there is a logical gap between descriptive statements and normative ones, which would imply that descriptions of human evolution, behavior, cognition, and emotion have no direct bearing on normative claims. Aggression is an evolved human behavior. People express aggression in many different ways, such as warfare, sports, games, and forms of violence (Lorenz 2002). However, from the fact that people are naturally aggressive we cannot infer that people should be aggressive, or that an aggressive act is appropriate in some particular situation. We need to appeal to some type of normative theory that stands outside of human nature to tell us how we ought to control, shape, or channel our natural tendencies.

Even if one cannot deduce moral prescriptions from facts about human nature, the empirical study of morality can lend some insight into normative ethics by placing some limitations on the theories we adopt. An ethical theory should be consistent with our understanding of human reasoning, emotion, behavior, and evolution. The limitations on imposed normative ethics by natural science may be tight enough to rule out some types of theories.

FUNDAMENTAL PROBLEMS IN ETHICAL THEORY

As one can see from my synopsis, there are many different well-known ethical theories and traditions. A great deal of ink has been spilled in philosophy attempting to defend moral theories against various arguments and objections to develop an account that best systematizes and explains all of our moral intuitions and judgments. I will not attempt to undertake that task here. Rather, I shall adopt the view, embraced by many, that there is no single "best" moral theory but that different moral theories focus on different aspects of our moral experience (Clark and Simpson 1989; Beauchamp and Childress 2008). Because human moral experience is complex and diverse, we should not expect that a single theory should be able to completely describe and explain it. This is not to say that moral theory has no bearing on ethical decisions, only that it is often useful to consider more than one approach to a particular dilemma or issue. The following discussion of common problems and tensions in ethical theory illustrate this point.

THE INDIVIDUAL VS. SOCIETY

Many different ethical controversies stem from conflicts between the good of the individual and the good of society. The Trolley Problem is a well-known thought experiment that philosophers have used to examine how different theories and principles settle conflicts between the good of the individual and the good of others (Thomas 1976; Foot 1978; Unger

1996). Imagine there is a runaway trolley heading down the tracks. Five people are stuck on the tracks and cannot move away. There is a lever you can pull that will send the trolley down a different set of tracks. However, there is one person stuck on these tracks. Should you pull the lever to divert the trolley, thereby killing one person and saving five? Different ethical theories answer this question in different ways. According to utilitarians, you should pull the lever because this will produce the greatest balance of good/bad consequences. Kantians would say that you may pull the lever only if the action (killing one person to save five) conforms to the CI. Virtue theorists would hold that you may pull the lever if pulling the lever is what a good person would do in the situation. According to the natural law tradition, you should pull the lever only if the bad effect (death of one person) is an unintended consequence of the good effect (saving five), the bad is not a means to the good, and the good outweighs the bad. Psychologists have asked people to respond to the Trolley Problem. 90 percent in one study said they would pull the lever (Mikhail 2007).

Consider a second variation of the Trolley Problem. Suppose that the trolley is on a path to kill the five people and the only way to save them is to push a large man off a bridge onto the tracks below, which will stop the trolley. Surveys show that 90 percent of people would not push the man onto the tracks (Mikhail 2007). One difference between the first and second variations is that in the second variation you are more actively and personally involved in killing a person (Mikhail 2007). Most of the moral theories we have examined would probably not instruct you to push the large man onto the tracks. According to Kantians, pushing the man onto the tracks would be wrong because it would be using him as a mere means to save the five people. The natural law tradition would say that pushing the man onto the tracks would not be justified because this bad effect (killing someone) was a means to achieving the good effect (saving lives). Virtue theorists could say that pushing the man onto the tracks would be wrong because this would make you a bad person – a murderer. Only utilitarianism would imply that you should push the man onto the tracks because you would still be saving five lives and only losing one.

The Trolley Problem illustrates a fundamental tension in ethical theory between protecting the rights and welfare of individuals and promoting the good of society. One reason why philosophers and others have examined the Trolley Problem is that it provides a simple and clear illustration of some ethical tensions in moral theory. Many real world choices are similar to the Trolley Problem in some respects, but they introduce other complications. For example, in May 2011, the Army Corps of Engineers blasted open a levee in Cairo, Illinois, to prevent flooding from the Missouri River further downstream. This decision sacrificed the welfare of residents (mostly farmers) living near the levee to protect whole towns further downriver from flooding (Smith 2011). The decision to open the levee was not simply a matter of the good of the many vs. the good of the few, however, because it also involved questions concerning property rights and social justice.

The Trolley Problem can be used to illustrate differences between moral theories. Utilitarianism tends to favor the good of society over the good of the individual. Some have objected to utilitarianism on the grounds that it does not give sufficient respect to individual rights and welfare (Barcalow 1994). The theory would seem to recommend killing innocent people to save lives. Some utilitarians, such as Brandt, have modified the theory to try to avoid such implications. According to Brandt, if utilitarianism is understood as requiring us to act according to ideal rules that maximize utility, then it will not have the undesirable implication that we should kill innocent people to promote utility, because a rule that allowed us to do this would not be a part of the ideal system of rules (Brandt 1998). A society that has rules against murder is much better off than one that does not.

Kantianism tends to favor the rights and welfare of the individual over the common good. Some have objected to Kantianism on the grounds that it does not give adequate consideration to producing good consequences for society (Barcalow 1994). Suppose a would-be murder needs some information about the whereabouts of his intended victim. You could tell him the truth or tell him a lie. On some interpretations of Kant's theory, you should not lie to the would-be murder because this would be treating him as a mere means to saving human life. But most people would regard this as absurd: It is ethical to lie to a would-be murder to save a life. Some philosophers have interpreted Kantianism so it does not have these undesirable implications concerning the good of society. A rule for action like "I will lie to a would-be murder to save human life" would be acceptable under Kantianism because it could become a universal law (O'Neill 1990).

The point of this discussion is that some versions of utilitarianism and Kantianism have implications concerning the tradeoffs between the good of the individual and the good of society that philosophers and ordinary people would find unacceptable (Pojman 2005; Mikhail 2007). These theories have been modified and interpreted to avoid these undesirable results, but potential conflicts between individuals and society may still remain. One might argue then, that the conflict between the individual and society is a fundamental problem in normative ethics and that no single theory has the complete answer (Barcalow 1994). As we shall see later in this book, this conflict occurs not just at the level of ethical theory, but also in the context of environmental health practices, policies, and research.

JUSTICE

Deciding what is just or fair is another fundamental problem in normative ethics that different theories address in different ways. There are three main areas of justice: criminal (or retributive) justice, social (or distributive) justice, and procedural justice. The main problem of criminal justice is determining the fairness of punishments; for social justice it is deciding what counts as a fair distribution of socioeconomic goods; and for procedural justice it is choosing fair decision-making processes and rules. The formal principle of justice, articulated by Aristotle and accepted by virtually all theorists today, mandates consistency in the application of justice: Equals should be treated equally (Rawls 1971). The rule implies that two people who commit the same crime with the same mitigating factors should receive the same punishment, and that discrimination based on race, ethnicity, or gender is unjust (Barcalow 1994).

There are three basic approaches to distributive justice: egalitarianism, which holds that socioeconomic goods should be distributed to promote equality; libertarianism, which holds that socioeconomic goods should be distributed according to a process, such as the free market, that respects individual property rights, promotes personal responsibility, and rewards hard work and innovation; and utilitarianism, which holds that socioeconomic goods should be distributed to promote the greatest balance of social benefits/harms (Barcalow 1994). There are also variations on these three approaches. For example, Rawls (1971) holds that socioeconomic goods should be distributed according to the difference principle, which promotes equality of opportunity, not equality of outcomes.

Let us consider how these different theories might approach another common thought experiment in ethics, the lifeboat. Suppose that a ship carrying thirty people is sinking at sea and there is only one lifeboat with food, supplies, and enough space for ten people. There are twenty men, five women, and five children on board. The boat is sinking slowly enough that there is time to decide who can go on the lifeboat. How should we make this decision? The rule of "women and children first" has been observed on many sinking boats. The rule seems to stem from a traditional chivalry, in which adult men were expected to demonstrate their courage and honor by sacrificing themselves for the "weaker" sex. There is evidence that the rule was followed, to some extent, during the sinking of the Titanic on April 14, 1912 (Frey et al. 2010). But is it a just rule? One might argue that the rule is sexist because it treats women as a "weaker" sex in need of rescue. Another problem is that it may be counterproductive. Suppose there is a highly skilled male physician on board who could help people on the lifeboat with medical needs and possibly save their lives, and that there are no female physicians with similar skills. Should the male physician be left to die on the ship?

Utilitarianism would endorse taking the physician on the lifeboat to increase the chances of saving more lives. So should we apply this theory to lifeboat ethics? One reason we should be hesitant to adopt this approach is that it says that we should make the selection based entirely on maximizing the social utility, which would imply that we should select people based on their ability to maximize the lives saved on the lifeboat as well as their potential contribution to society, assuming they are rescued. If there are "important" people on the ship who can provide many benefits to society, such as scientists, engineers, educators, or government leaders, utilitarianism would hold that they should be saved. People who would have little to contribute to society if they were saved, such as unemployed actors, ex-convicts, janitors, senior citizens, and disabled people, should be left on the ship.

Should we decide who lives and who dies based on a person's "social worth"? Many people were outraged that a seven person committee at Swedish Hospital in Seattle in the 1960s used social worth criteria to decide who would have access to a limited number of dialysis machines. The decision makers, who became known as the "God Committee," considered a number of different social worth factors when deciding who should go on dialysis, including the candidate's dependents, occupation, education, income, and future potential. The committee was discontinued when dialysis machines became less scarce in the late 1960s. The committee had a significant impact on organ allocation policies in the

United States, however. Decisions about who will receive a new liver, heart, or kidney are based on medical criteria, such as tissue matching, medical need, prospects of survival, and time spent on a waiting list, not on social worth criteria (Pence 2007).

If we do not want to judge people according to their social worth, perhaps a better rule would be to use a random procedure, such as drawing lots, to decide who can be on the lifeboat. A random procedure would be egalitarian in that each person would have an equal chance of being selected. It would be favored by ethical traditions, such as Kantianism and Christianity, which emphasize the inherent dignity and equality of all people. Organ allocation policies in the United States include a random element, because organs are allocated on a first come, first served basis, after medical criteria are applied.

Randomness also has drawbacks. If the physician is not selected in the random drawing, this will decrease the survival odds of people on the lifeboat. Should we take this risk to avoid moral qualms about judging people? Although there are some significant problems with adopting a utilitarian perspective on the lifeboat dilemma, it seems that it would be foolish to give no consideration whatsoever to maximizing the survival odds of those who will be on the lifeboat.

Property rights might also have some bearing on lifeboat ethics. Suppose that a rich man who is traveling with his wife happens to have brought along his own inflatable lifeboat precisely for situations like this one. The inflatable lifeboat can hold four people and he wants to use it to save himself and his wife, but no one else. Should that person be allowed to use his boat as he pleases or should his boat be confiscated and used as community property? According to libertarians, the boat is his property and he can do whatever he wants with it. He could donate the boat to the community or save two other people if he so desires, but his boat should not be taken from him. Kantians would also object to taking the boat from him on the grounds that this would be treating him as a mere means to achieve some goal and violates his dignity as a person. Utilitarians would favor taking the boat if this would save more lives. Egalitarians also might favor taking the boat and including it in a random drawing for lifeboat space.

The lifeboat dilemma is a fairly simple example, but many distributive justice issues are far more complex. The debate about health care reform in the United States affects hundreds of millions of people with trillions of dollars at stake. Many of the same theories and principles of justice we have mentioned here also have some bearing on this complex issue (Churchill 1987; Monheit 2008). Because most social justice issues are complex, it is not likely that a single theory will be able to address every problem or question related to justice that arises, and it may be desirable to consider multiple approaches (Barcalow 1994). As we shall see later in this book, questions of social justice also arise in environmental health.

ACTION GUIDANCE

Since Aristotle's time, philosophers have recognized that an important goal of any ethical theory is to guide human action (Barcalow 1994; Pojman 2005). To guide conduct, a theory should be able to 1) motivate people to act ethically; 2) apply to practical problems; and 3) solve difficult ethical dilemmas. The theories we have examined in this chapter differ in their ability to perform these tasks. Some perform some tasks well, but not others. No theory handles all of these tasks perfectly.

Consider motivating ethical conduct. To motivate conduct, a theory should latch onto people's emotions, desires, and other aspects of their psychology, which leads to action. One of the criticisms of Kantianism is that it has little connection with human psychology (Pojman 2005). Kantianism requires people to perform their duty for duty's sake, but most people are not so nobly motivated. Many people are motivated to behave morally so they can be happy or virtuous, have a meaningful life, or avoid guilt or punishment (Hauser 2006; Haidt 2007). Utilitarianism and social contract theories suffer from the same problem, because most people are not strongly motivated to promote the good of society or abide by some hypothetical social agreement. Virtue theories and religiously based ethical theories do a much better job of motivating conduct. Aristotle's ethics shows one how to achieve happiness by living a good (virtuous) life, which most people desire. Christian approaches hold that people can achieve salvation, enlightenment, spiritual growth, or connection with God by acting ethically. Christians may find ethical theories based on their doctrines or sacred texts to be more palatable than secular, philosophical theories (Pojman 2005). Natural rights views may also provide some motivation for ethical conduct because most people want to have their rights respected by others.

To be applicable, a theory should be fairly easy for ordinary people to understand and connect to real world problems. Virtue theories and Christian ethics have the advantage that they are easy to apply. Most people can readily understand and use phrases like, "be honest," "be brave," be kind," "love your neighbor," "forgive your enemies," and so on. Ross' ethical view, which states general rules concerning fidelity, beneficence, and so on, is not too difficult to apply, nor are natural rights approaches, which instruct people to avoid violating other people's rights. Likewise, some of the simple versions of utilitarianism, such as Mill's view, are not too difficult to apply because most people have a grasp of the possible benefits and risks of their actions. Kantianism may be difficult to apply, because the different versions of the CI are highly abstract and difficult for ordinary people to understand and use (Pojman 2005). It is not easy for most people to decide whether their actions could become a universal law that would be accepted by rational beings forming a society.

To solve difficult ethical dilemmas, a theory needs to have a decision-making procedure for describing these dilemmas, considering the different options, and settling conflicts among moral rules, values, or principles. One of the chief criticisms of virtue theories is that they do not provide people with much help when it comes to deciding what to do in ethical dilemmas (Pojman 2005). Consider the Trolley Problem again. Virtue theories would instruct us to be brave, kind, or just in the situation, but this advice would not tell us, specifically, what we should do. Virtue theories also would probably not help us to decide what to do in the lifeboat dilemma, because they do not provide us with a detailed account of how a just person acts. Some Christian ethical theories are also not very adept at solving ethical dilemmas

Table 3.1. *Action-Guiding Characteristics of Different Ethical Theories*

	Motivation	Applicability	Conflict Resolution
Virtue theories	√	√	X
Christian ethics	√	√	X
Natural rights	√	√	X
Kantianism	X	X	√
Mill's utilitarianism	X	√	√
Brandt's utilitarianism	X	X	√
WD Ross's view	X	√	X

because they do not give specific instructions about how to love someone in a particular situation, or how to settle conflicts between people. Though Ross' ethical theory is fairly easy to apply, it does not offer much help when it comes to dealing with ethical dilemmas because it advises us to appeal to our intuition when settling a conflict between *prima facie* rules, but different people may have different intuitions about what to do. Natural rights approaches may also not be very helpful at solving ethical dilemmas, because to solve conflicts among rights one needs a procedure for ranking different rights (Barcalow 1994).

One of the strengths of Kantianism is that it contains a decision-making procedure for solving ethical dilemmas. The different formulations of the CI can be used to generate specific rules that apply to particular actions (O'Neill 1990). These rules can be divided into perfect and imperfect duties. Perfect duties are duties we must always obey; imperfect duties are ones that may be disobeyed if the circumstances warrant (Kant 1964). For example, Kant held that we have a perfect duty not to break our promises but an imperfect duty to help others. If I am presented with a situation in which I must consider whether I should break a promise in order to help someone, my perfect duty to keep my promise trumps my duty to render aid. Utilitarianism also has a method for solving ethical dilemmas. According to Mill, one can always appeal to the principle of utility to decide what to do in a particular situation (Mill 2003). Table 3.1 provides an appraisal of some different ethical theories concerning action guidance.

To sum up this section, no ethical theory is perfect at guiding human actions. Some can motivate ethical conduct but not solve ethical dilemmas; some can solve ethical dilemmas but not motivate conduct; some are easy to apply; some are not easy to apply, and so on. What this suggests is that action guidance is another fundamental problem in normative ethics and that no single theory has the complete answer. This is another reason for considering multiple approaches when thinking about ethics.

VISIONARY VS. ORDINARY

The final fundamental problem in ethical theory is whether ethics should be visionary or ordinary. Should ethics criticize and reform our commonsense moral judgments and intuitions or codify and explain them? Different thinkers have approached this issue differently. Aristotelian ethics was, for the most part, ordinary not visionary. Aristotle was trying to carefully describe Greek notions of virtue and explain their philosophical underpinnings. He was attempting to show people how to live the good life, not to fundamentally alter human life. Jesus' teachings, however, were radical and visionary. Jesus introduced several ideas that were at odds with Jewish laws and teachings, such as forgiving one's enemies, and having compassion for all people, including Gentiles, criminals, tax collectors, and lepers (Lewis 1952).

Locke's ethical and political ideas were visionary as well. Though Locke focused on some issues that we would consider mundane, such as property rights, his ideas about property were visionary in his time. For many years in European countries all property was owned by the king or nobility: Common people were not lawful property owners. Kings asserted their absolute authority over people and property under a doctrine known as the Divine Right of Kings, which held that the king derives his moral and legal authority from God and can do no wrong. Locke provided a philosophical critique of the Divine Right of Kings that led people to abandon this doctrine. Locke also helped to establish lawful property ownership for ordinary people by writing about property as a natural right (Clapp 1967).

Kant's ethics was, for the most part, ordinary, not visionary. Kant was responding to Hume's attacks on commonly held metaphysical ideas, such as belief in God, the soul, freedom, and morality. Kant was concerned with showing how moral knowledge is possible, how we make moral judgments, and how we must conceive of ourselves if we are to act morally (Körner 1955). Mill, however, was a visionary philosopher. As noted earlier, he defended women's equality, a radical idea in the nineteenth century, and he also offered a strong defense of liberty. Philosophers since Mill have pointed out some of the radical implications of utilitarianism. Peter Singer has argued, on utilitarian grounds, that physicians should be allowed to kill patients to end their suffering and that people in developed countries should transfer most of their wealth to people who are dying from famine and poverty in developing countries (Singer 1979). Some philosophers have objected to utilitarianism that it has radical implications that we should not readily accept (Barcalow 1994).

Rawls' reflective equilibrium is essentially a method for codifying and explaining our moral judgments/intuitions, not for radically changing them. Though the method allows for the possibility that we may revise our judgments/intuitions as we eliminate biases and move toward reflective equilibrium, it is not designed to overhaul our current moral convictions. Empirical ethics research also tends to be ordinary insofar as it describes and explains the emotional and cognitive responses of ordinary (normal) human subjects to moral dilemmas.

Some of the recent critiques of traditional ethics, such as feminist theories and environmental approaches (discussed in more depth in Chapter 4), have offered radical alternatives to the status quo. Feminist scholars have argued that we need to reshape normative ethical theory to better reflect women's experiences, which would imply a significant change in ethical thinking and conduct.

The issue of whether ethics should be visionary or ordinary has no simple solution because there are valid reasons for adopting both approaches. On the one hand, one could argue that ethical theory should try to capture our commonsense moral intuitions because ethics should help us understand and justify our moral judgments and deal with practical dilemmas. If ethics is too radical, it may be rejected by ordinary people as irrelevant and out of touch with real, human experience. On the other hand, one could argue that ethics should do more than just make sense of our moral experience, because ethics should help us aspire to a higher law that transcends our social and cultural biases and commonsense assumptions. Ethics should not rationalize a corrupt status quo. Many times during human history, people have accepted social practices that were later regarded as immoral, such as slavery and racial and sexual discrimination. Without moral visionaries who were willing to challenge the status quo, these practices would have continued (Pojman 2005).

As we shall see in greater detail in the Chapter 4, the visionary vs. ordinary problem is a key issue in thinking about moral issues in environmental health, because traditional ethical theories pay scant attention to nonhuman species, ecosystems, or the environment. To find an appropriate balance between promoting human health and protecting other species and the environment, it may be necessary to revise and rethink traditional, ethical theories.

SUMMARY

Philosophers and theologians have proposed a variety of ethical theories in the last 2,500 years. There are several fundamental problems in ethical theory, such as the conflict between the individual and society, deciding what is just, providing effective guidance for human conduct, and determining whether ethics should be visionary or ordinary. Because no single theory has the perfect solution to all of these problems, it is useful to consider multiple approaches when attempting to answer ethical questions or solve ethical dilemmas. Chapter 4 will develop a method of ethical decision making that is based on giving fair and reasonable consideration to different approaches to morality. It will also consider the relationship between traditional ethical theories, the environment, and human health.

4

TOWARD AN ENVIRONMENTAL
HEALTH ETHICS

The previous chapter gave an overview of ethical theories, concepts, and principles. In this chapter, I will develop a method for ethical decision making that can be used to deal with questions concerning the relationship between human health and the environment. To do this, I need to first say a bit more about environmental ethics, because the theories and traditions discussed in the previous chapter have little to say about man's relationship to the environment, and it is important to incorporate environmental values into ethical decision making. I also will discuss health as a distinct value.

ETHICS AND THE ENVIRONMENT

Environmental ethics emerged as a distinct discipline in the 1970s as philosophers, theologians, attorneys, scientists, and political activists raised awareness about environmental issues such as pollution, species preservation, urban development, pesticide use, and hazardous waste disposal (Cochrane 2007; Brennan 2008). Many argued that traditional ethical theories did not have the conceptual tools to adequately deal with environmental problems because these theories are human centered (anthropocentric) and do not give adequate consideration to the value of other organisms, nonhuman species, ecosystems, and the biosphere (Attfield 2003). As we saw in the last chapter, traditional ethical theories emphasize the value of human happiness, virtue, dignity, rights, and justice, and address human moral obligations, duties, decisions, and rules. However, these theories do not explicitly mention the value of the environment or our obligations to the environment. Many argued that a radically new ethic was needed to deal with environmental issues (Johnson 1984).

The two central questions in environmental ethics are: 1) "do we have any moral obligations to other life forms and larger units of biological organization, such as populations, species, and ecosystems?" and 2) "if we have such obligations, what are they?" Our answers to these questions have implications for many different practices and policies concerning our relationship to the environment (Des Jardins 2005).

To address the first question, many philosophers, theologians, and ethicists have considered whether nonhuman biological systems, such as animals, plants, species, and ecosystems, have intrinsic value (Jamieson 2002; Attfield 2003; Brennan 2008). A value is something that one regards as worth having, pursuing, or protecting such as health, justice, virtue, or utility (Frankena 1988). If something has intrinsic value, then it is valuable for its own sake and merits special moral treatment (Attfield 2003; Brennan 2008). For example, laws against murder reflect the widespread conviction that human life is intrinsically valuable. Taking human life is not a trivial matter and requires extraordinary justification, such as self-defense. If something has only instrumental (or extrinsic) value, then it may be used as a means for promoting things that have intrinsic value without any special moral justification. For example, an ordinary rock has no intrinsic value. I do not need any special moral justification to toss or crush a rock. Many things have intrinsic and instrumental value. For example, one might consider a good marriage as inherently worthwhile and valuable as a means to promoting health and well-being. All of the moral theories examined in Chapter 3 posit some intrinsic values, such as moral agency (Kantians), happiness (utilitarians), and virtue (virtue theorists).

Anthropocentrism holds that only human beings or human traits (such as happiness, love, good will, or virtue) have intrinsic moral value and that other species and the environment are valuable only as a means to human needs, wants, and goals (Attfield 2003; Cochrane 2007). People require no special justification to exploit other species and the environment for food, water, clothing, and other resources (Passmore 1980). The creation story in the Bible's book of Genesis can be interpreted as endorsing anthropocentrism because it holds that man is created in the image of God and has been granted dominion over the fish, birds, and animals (White Jr. 2004; Holy Bible 2004). Until the modern environmental movement emerged in the 1960s, anthropocentrism was widely assumed to be the correct view of the relationship between man and nature.

Nonanthropocentrism emerged in response to critiques of anthropocentrism. Critics of anthropocentrism argue that it has been used to justify misuse of the environment with little concern for animals, species, ecosystems, or the biosphere as a whole and that human beings have a long and shameful history of environmental exploitation and mismanagement, including pollution, deforestation, destruction of wilderness, overfishing, and cruelty to animals (Naess 1973, 1986; Callicott 1989; Leopold 1989; Rolston III 1994). They argue that Western religious, philosophical, and cultural traditions have fostered these practices by placing man at the center of the universe, portraying animals as subject to human dominion, and viewing nature as a dangerous force to be conquered and used for economic gain. Because anthropocentrism encourages exploitation of the environment, it must be replaced by a nonanthropocentric ethics to ensure that the environment is adequately protected (White Jr. 1967).

Nonanthropocentrism holds that nonhuman biological systems have value in their own right and are not valuable merely as a tool for serving human ends (Naess 1973, 1986; Taylor 1986; Callicott 1989; Singer 1993; Varner 1998; Regan 2004). Many nonanthropocentrists hold that human activities, such as economic development, agriculture, and industry, need to be scaled back in order to protect nonhuman species, ecosystems, and other living things. Some have argued that the human population needs to be reduced and that meat-eating must stop (Naess 1986, Singer 1993). Nonanthropocentrism is a radical and visionary approach to environmental ethics, because it holds that many of our commonsense ideas about the relationship between human beings and the environment are mistaken.

There are different forms of nonanthropocentric ethics. Some, such as Singer (1993) and Regan (2004) argue that sentient, nonhuman animals have intrinsic value. Singer bases the intrinsic value of sentient animals on their capacity to feel pain and to suffer. Singer, a utilitarian, believes that animal welfare must be given equal consideration in any calculation of the overall utility of an action or policy. To decide whether to use animals in biomedical experiments, for example, one should consider not only the benefits to people but also the harm to animals. When the harm to animals of experimentation outweighs human (and animal) benefits, animal experimentation is immoral (Singer 1993).

Regan (2004) approaches animal ethics from a moral rights perspective. He argues that rights protect interests, such as the interest in life, health, freedom, pain avoidance, and property. Beings that are concerned about their lives have interests, and therefore, rights, according to Regan. Because sentient animals are concerned about their lives, they have rights, such as the right not to be harmed or exploited. According to Regan (2004) many of the ways we treat animals, such as using them in painful and deadly experiments or killing them for food, are immoral because they violate the rights of animals.

Others have argued that all life forms, not just sentient animals, have moral value. Hinduism teaches respect for all living things and recommends vegetarianism. Killing another living thing requires special justification (Perrett 1998). German-French physician and theologian Albert Schweitzer (1875–1965) held that all life is sacred and that we should avoid thoughtless injury to living things (Schweitzer 1959). Modern environmental ethicists, such as Taylor (1986), also endorse the idea that all living things have intrinsic moral value. Goodpaster (1978) argues that all living things have intrinsic moral value because they have needs and interests. If we grant moral value to sentient beings with interests, such as animals, then we should also assign moral value to nonsentient beings with interests, such as plants, bacteria, and so on.

Environmental philosophers have assigned value not only to individual organisms, but also to species, ecosystems, and the biosphere. A common way of defending the value of these larger units of biological organization is to argue that their moral worth derives from the individuals that compose them: The value of a species is based on the value of its members, the value of an ecosystem is based on the value of the different interacting species that compose it, and so on. Leopold (1949) argued that all members of the biological community, as well as the entire community, have moral value. Callicott (1980) expanded upon Leopold's idea but took a more radical approach by claiming that only whole ecosystems and not their parts (i.e., organisms, species) have intrinsic value. Organisms, including human beings, are valuable only insofar as they contribute to the functioning of an entire, unified ecosystem. Callicott (1989) later modified this view and recognized that parts of ecosystems also have intrinsic value.

Anthropocentrists have responded to nonanthropocentric views by arguing that an enlightened form of anthropocentrism provides sufficient recognition for the value of other species and the environment, and that there is no need to assign intrinsic value to non-human biological systems (Norton 1991; Brennan 2008). Enlightened anthropocentrists emphasize the importance of the environment for human well-being and they argue that traditional ethical theories, when understood properly, imply that we should have a great deal of care and concern for animals, other species, and ecosystems. Poor environmental stewardship can have a negative impact on human health, welfare, and moral development (Passmore 1980; Hill Jr. 1983; O'Neill 1997; Gewirth 2001) and can negatively impact human beings in many ways:

- Pesticides, pollution, and toxic chemicals cause human diseases;
- Excessive fishing and hunting reduces available food sources;
- Destruction of wilderness deprives people of areas for recreation and religious or philosophical inspiration;
- Damage to ecosystems deprives people of clean water and other ecological services;
- Loss of biodiversity deprives people of economically or medically valuable species and destabilizes ecosystems;
- Deforestation exacerbates global warming; and
- Mistreatment of animals and the environment can cause people to have less respect for human life.

Many different ethical theories, including utilitarianism, Kantianism, natural law theory, and virtue ethics, require us to refrain from engaging in activities that threaten human health and well-being. These theories recommend that we take care of animals, other species, ecosystems, and the biosphere in order to promote human interests. What's good for the environment is good for the human race. There is no need to develop a radically new ethic if we apply current ethical theories more diligently to environmental issues (Norton 1987; 1991).

Enlightened anthropocentrism represents an important advance. Broad recognition of the value of the environment for humanity has brought about important changes in attitudes, practices, and policies. But is enlightened anthropocentrism a satisfactory way of preventing environmental exploitation and degradation? Critics of anthropocentrism don't think so. As long as man is regarded as the moral center of the universe, the tendency toward exploitation of nature will be unavoidable. According to critics, enlightened anthropocentrism easily morphs into unenlightened, irresponsible anthropocentrism (Rolston III 1994). Furthermore, the critics argue that even enlightened anthropocentrists do not properly value other living things. Consider, for example, the enlightened slave owner who treats his slaves well. He feeds them, clothes them, educates them, and does not overwork them. Even if the enlightened slave owner is a kind master, he is still treating human beings as property. Enlightened anthropocentrism, like enlightened slavery, is a shallow theory, according to the critics, because it does not address the core assumptions at the center of our environmental problems (Naess 1973; 1986).

If we frame debates about environmental ethics in terms of questions of intrinsic value, it may be difficult to make significant headway in developing practical solutions to environmental problems because questions about intrinsic value can be intractable. For example, the two opposing sides of the abortion debate have very different views about the moral status of the fetus. Those who hold the "pro-life" view hold that abortion is immoral because the fetus has intrinsic moral value and should not be killed. Many of those who adhere to the "pro-choice" view hold that abortion is morally acceptable because the fetus does not have intrinsic moral worth (Pojman 2005). There has been little progress in the abortion debate in the United States since the 1970s, and the country is roughly evenly divided on this issue (PollingReport.com 2011).

One reason why debates about intrinsic value are difficult to settle is that intrinsic value usually plays a foundational role in ethical systems (Barcalow 1994). The best we can hope to do is to appeal to people's intuitions about value, and mention some considerations that should have an impact on those intuitions, but it is difficult to convince people about questions of intrinsic value by means of arguments. Aristotle (2003) explained what happiness is and how to obtain it by living a life of virtue, but he did not develop an argument to prove why we should want happiness. He assumed that everyone desires to be happy. Mill (2003) did not give direct proof for the principle of utility because he understood it to be a moral axiom that is beyond direct proof. He assumed that because everyone desires their own happiness they should also desire the general happiness. Rawls (1971) did not give a direct argument for why we should want primary goods and assumed that all people would recognize their worth (Rawls 1971).

If debates concerning intrinsic value must ultimately appeal to our moral intuitions, then it will be difficult to convince most people that they should regard nonhuman living things as having intrinsic moral worth, if they do not already share this intuition. If a person does not recognize the inherent value of a mouse, tree, mosquito, or wetland ecosystem, it will be difficult to convince him through words. We form intuitions about intrinsic value not by means of arguments but by experience (Audi 2004). We have no trouble appreciating the value of human beings because we have a full range of experiences concerning human relationships, and we have an evolved compassion for members of our own species. We also can appreciate the value of animals that we have relationships with, such as pets. Most people do not experience the value of nonsentient life forms, species, and ecosystems in that way that they experience the value of other human beings or pets. They may regard species, living things, and ecosystems as having some value, but not intrinsic value.

Because debates about intrinsic value can be very difficult to resolve, we should frame environmental ethics issues not in terms of dualistic choices, that is, intrinsic value versus no intrinsic value, but in terms of graduations in value (Norton 1991; Attfield 2003). We can recognize that foxes, ferns, forests, and even fleas have some value without claiming that they have a value equivalent to a human being. A scale of value approach is a useful way of dealing with conflicts among human beings, other life forms, species, and ecosystems

(Varner 1998; Attfield 2003). The scale of value approach recognizes that many different types of biological systems have value, but that there are differences in value. We can construct a scale (or ranking) of value to guide our decision making in complex problems involving value conflicts. The scale could be based on a number of different thought experiments designed to test conflicts of value. For example, suppose the trolley (discussed in Chapter 3) is heading down the tracks and is about to kill five dogs stuck on the tracks, but we can pull a lever that will divert the trolley so that it will save the five dogs but kill one human being. Most people would say that we should not pull the lever because one human being is more valuable than five dogs. Most people would probably also say that we should not pull the lever to save five chimpanzees if one human being will die. Other comparisons between organisms are also possible.

We could also develop thought experiments to ponder the value of larger units of organization, such as species and ecosystems. For example, suppose a mad geneticist has developed two types of viruses to release into the wild. One type of virus will eliminate a species that is harmful to human life, such as the parasite that causes malaria (*Plasmodium falciparum*), while another type will eliminate a beneficial species to human life, such as one of the forty-four species of honey bees, which pollinate fruiting plants. We only have the ability to stop him from releasing one of these types of virus. Most people would choose save the honey bee instead of the malaria parasite. Or imagine that an insane world leader has launched a missile armed with a 60-kiloton nuclear bomb (about five times the explosive power of the bomb dropped on Hiroshima) that is headed toward a large urban area with a population of 5 million people. We can allow the missile to run its course, or we can press a button that will jam its telemetry and cause it to explode in an ecologically important, but sparsely populated ecosystem, such as the Amazon jungle. It is likely that most people would save the 5 million people at the expense destroying a significant portion of the Amazon jungle.

We could, in theory, perform thought experiments like these to construct a *prima facie* scale of value, based on how we would rank different things when presented with conflicts. Most people would place intelligent beings at the top of the scale, followed by sentient beings (e.g., dogs and mice), nonsentient beings (e.g., plants and worms), and so on (Varner 1998). Placing ecosystems and other larger entities on the scale might require some complex maneuvering, but it could be done in principle. I use the phrase *prima facie* here to indicate that the scale would be based on value conflicts considered in the abstract, which would only provide us with some general guidance for decision making. To decide what to do in a real case involving value conflicts, such as the use of DDT to control malaria discussed in Chapter 1, we would need a considerable amount of information about the case, the various options, and the likely outcomes of different choices.

Later on in this chapter, I will describe three principles of ethical decision making that take into account insights from the scale of value approach. These principles help to ensure that adequate consideration is given to nonhuman interests, because they require us to consider how our choices may impact other life forms, species, and ecosystems.

THE VALUE OF HUMAN HEALTH

To make ethical decisions concerning environmental health, it is important to consider not only the environmental concerns, but also to sort through the different human interests and values, such as economic development, freedom, and health. Many discussions of environmental ethics tend to lump together all human-centered interests and values in framing environmental issues, but there are important differences between these interests that have implications for ethical decision making (Resnik 2009a). For example, people would probably think differently about damaging an ecosystem to build a hospital as opposed to a shopping mall. Thus, it is important to say a bit more about health as a distinct human value.

Traditional ethics theories said little about human health as a distinct moral value. For Aristotle, health was necessary for good functioning, but it was not a virtue. Some of the virtues, such as moderation, could help to promote health. Also, health was recognized as important for happiness, because poor health could cause pain and suffering (Aristotle 2003). Kant did not recognize health as a value, but he did acknowledge that people have duties of self-care, self-preservation, and self-improvement, which would imply a concern for one's own health (Kant 1964). Mill did not view health as valuable in its own right, though he recognized it as valuable as a means of promoting happiness, since illness can lead to unhappiness (Mill 2003). Health was not one of Rawls' (1971) primary goods, but one could argue that health is essential to obtaining some of these goods, such as wealth and income (Daniels 1984). An exception to this trend among moral philosophers can be found in the work of Frankena (1988), who listed health as an intrinsic moral value along with knowledge, happiness, freedom, virtue, life, and justice

Not surprisingly, medical ethicists have paid more attention to the value of health than traditional theorists. Most theories in medical ethics recognize health as a benefit (or good outcome) and hold that health care professionals have a duty to provide this benefit to their patients. The earliest medical ethics code, the Hippocratic Oath, which was developed by the followers of the Greek physician Hippocrates (460–370 BCE), held that physicians have a duty to benefit their patients and to not harm them, and to care for the sick (Hippocratic Oath 2002). Several influential, contemporary theories also hold that health care professionals should benefit their patients by promoting health and preventing disease (Gert et al. 2006; Jonsen et al. 2006; Beauchamp and Childress 2008).

Medical ethicists have offered some reasons to explain why health is a benefit. Caplan (1997) argues that health is beneficial because disease can cause suffering, pain, disability, and death, which most people wish to avoid. Health is also a social value because disease can cost society a great deal of money and undermine productivity and economic growth (Caplan 1997). Richman (2004) argues that health is beneficial because it helps people to achieve their life goals, such as happiness, career advancement, and fulfilling family relationships. Daniels (1984, 2008) incorporates concepts of health and disease into Rawls' theory of justice and argues that health is important for promoting equality of opportunity because diseases can limit the range of opportunities available to a person (Daniels 1984, 2008).

Even though health is widely recognized as an important value, it can conflict with other values. Sometimes, it is acceptable to place other values ahead of health (Callahan 2000). People choose to smoke, overeat, skydive, ride motorcycles, drink excessively, and engage in other risky behaviors for the sake of pleasure. People also place their health at risk in many occupations, such as coal mining, military service, firefighting, policing, factory work, and farming. People also disagree on how to balance health, pleasure, and work. Someone who skydives may think the enjoyment provided by the experience is worth the risk, while others may have a different view of the matter.

Many difficult choices involve conflicts between health and freedom or autonomy. Sometimes patients make decisions that are contrary to their own health, such as refusing potentially life-saving medical care. If a patient who has suffered acute trauma needs to receive a blood transfusion in order to live, and he refuses the transfusion on religious grounds, then medical professionals who are treating him must decide whether to honor his wishes. Transfusing the patient would promote his health but violate his autonomy, while not transfusing the patient would honor his autonomy at the expense of his health. Most theories of medical ethics hold that autonomy is generally more important than health: Patients with sound decision-making abilities should be allowed to make their own health care choices, even those decisions that are contrary to their health (Beauchamp and Childress 2008). However, matters are more complicated if the patient has compromised decision-making abilities due to immaturity, mental illness, and the influence of drugs or medications. Doctors might not honor the wishes of a delirious patient who refuses life-saving medical care.

Conflicts between freedom and health occur not only at a personal level, but also at a social level. Societies have implemented different policies that promote public health but also compromise human freedom, such as food and drug regulations, required vaccinations, workplace safety regulations, mandatory reporting of infectious diseases, and bans on public smoking. The argument for these policies is that they serve the public good by promoting human health and saving society money in medical expenses (Callahan 2000). However, these policies have been controversial. For example, in the United States, it is illegal to buy, sell, possess, or transport many different recreational drugs, such as marijuana, cocaine, heroin, and lysergic acid diethylamide (LSD). Citizens, scholars, and scientists have argued that some of these drugs, such as marijuana, should be legalized or decriminalized, because drug laws create a black market, efforts to enforce the laws are ineffective, and adults should be free to make decisions concerning the use of these substances (Grossman et al. 2002). This controversy illustrates the perennial tension between promoting public health and protecting human freedom, which mirrors the conflict between the good of society and the good of the individual discussed in Chapter 3. We will discuss the conflict between health and freedom again in Chapter 6.

How should we settle conflicts between health and other values? As noted earlier, many theorists have categorized values as having intrinsic or extrinsic worth. Thus, to think about the value of health we should ask whether it is valuable for its own sake or for the sake of something else, such as happiness, wealth, and freedom, or perhaps both (Frankena 1988). There is little doubt that health is extrinsically valuable because it plays a key role in obtaining employment and achieving happiness. The interesting question is whether it is only intrinsically valuable.

If health is only extrinsically valuable, then we may sacrifice health whenever we please without any special moral justification. However, one might argue that it would be unethical to intentionally damage our health without a good reason. To take an extreme case, suppose a healthy person decides to commit suicide, and he is not terminally ill or in great pain. Most people (and most moral theorists) would hold that it would be wrong to kill one's self in this manner. Deliberate harm to one's own health in other, less extreme cases, such as cutting off one's finger or drilling a hole in one's head, without good reason, is also morally problematic. Thus, one could argue that health is intrinsically valuable and that we should not sacrifice our own health (or the health of others) without good reason.

While an argument can be made that health has intrinsic and extrinsic moral value, I will not press that point further in this book because, as noted previously, I think the intrinsic versus extrinsic value distinction has limited applicability for handling complex practical problems, such as the conflict between human health and the environment. What matters is that health is a fundamental value that sometimes conflicts with other fundamental values. Conflicts between health and other values are not easily settled because they represent tensions inherent in our moral thinking. As mentioned in Chapter 3, different ethical theories take different perspectives on these conflicts, but all theories must come to terms with them in one way or another.

A PRINCIPLE-BASED METHOD FOR ETHICAL DECISION MAKING

As we have noted several times in this book, ethical dilemmas in environmental health involve conflicts among fundamental values, such as environmental preservation versus economic development, property rights versus the public good, promotion of human interests versus protection of animal welfare, and so on. The most important question in ethical decision making is how one should resolve such conflicts. Many moral philosophers believe that the key to ethical decision making is to develop a moral theory that provides a way of ranking conflicting values, rules, or obligations (Gert et al. 2006). When faced with an ethical dilemma, one could infer the correct choice from the dictates of the theory and the relevant facts. For example, in deciding whether to allow indoor DDT spraying to control malaria, utilitarians would estimate the potential benefits and risks to society. Conflicts between protecting the environment and promoting public health would be settled by appealing to utility. However, as argued in Chapter 3, there is currently no widely accepted ethical theory that can solve all conflicts among values, rules, or obligations. Philosophers and other scholars have developed many theories based on different insights into our moral experience, but so far no theory has emerged as clearly superior to the others. Additionally, moral theories tend to be highly abstract and are difficult to understand and apply to particular situations. People making real-world decisions do not have time to wait for theorists to reach some agreement: They need an approach to decision making that is practical and understandable.

In response to difficulties with using moral theories to resolve ethical dilemmas, some philosophers have argued that we should reach decisions by using a case-based approach (also known as casuistry). By carefully describing the facts and circumstances pertaining to a particular situation, and comparing the situation to similar ones, we will be able to reach a moral judgment (or intuition) about what to do (Jonsen and Toulmin 1988; Strong 2000). To decide whether to permit the indoor spraying of DDT, advocates of this method would hold that we should describe the situation in detail and compare it to similar situations involving pesticide use. If indoor DDT spraying is similar to another situation in which pesticide use was permitted, then it should be permitted; if it is similar to a situation in which DDT use was not permitted, then it should not be permitted. Decisions made in the past provide a precedent for future choices, under the casuistic approach.

Undoubtedly it is important to consider carefully the facts and circumstances of a case when making moral choices and to learn from the past, but the cased-based approach is not a satisfactory method for ethical decision making. First, casuistry has no procedure for determining what makes cases morally similar or different. For example, in comparing cases of pesticide use, we would need to determine whether the environmental and public health effects related to one type of use are similar to or different from the effects related to another type of use. But we cannot make this comparison unless we have rules or principles for deciding whether effects are similar or different. Second, casuistry does not offer a method of decision making that provides publicly defensible reasons for action. In explaining the rationale for a particular choice, the best the casuist can do is to appeal to judgments about particular cases. But most people would demand more than this: They want reasons for actions or policies grounded in moral rules, principles, or values. In response to these problems, some casuists have modified their view to include rules or principles for comparing cases (Strong 2000), but this reconfiguration of casuistry makes it less like a purely case-based approach and more like a principle-based approach.

I therefore view the best approach to ethical decision making to be a method that appeals to commonly accepted moral principles that can guide conduct and address conflicts between values, rules, and obligations (Beauchamp and Childress 2008). Moral principles are general rules for action that are supported by different ethical theories. Principles are easy to understand and apply to different scenarios. Moral principles imply specific rules for action that can be readily applied to particular situations (Richardson 2000). They are user-friendly. For example, the principle "respect human rights" is a highly general rule supported by Kantianism, utilitarianism, the social contract view, and other theories. The principle implies more specific rules, such as "do not kill human beings," "do not steal," "do not harm other people," "allow autonomous individuals to make their own decisions," and so on. Some of these specific rules may also imply other rules. For example, "do not steal," implies rules governing the acquisition and transfer of property. "Allow autonomous

Table 4.1. *A Principle-Based Method for Ethical Decision Making*

---

(1) State the question or problem.
(2) Gather relevant information.
(3) Explore different options.
(4) Apply ethical principles to the different options.
(5) Resolve any conflicts among ethical principles.
(6) Take action.

---

individuals to make their own decisions" implies rules for obtaining consent from research participants (discussed in Chapter 11).

The principle-based method (see Table 4.1) involves six steps: (1) state the question or problem; (2) gather relevant information; (3) explore different options; (4) apply ethical principles to the different options; (5) resolve any conflicts among ethical principles; and (6) take action (Fox and DeMarco 2000; Beauchamp and Childress 2008; Shamoo and Resnik 2009). The method is idealized because in real life people may not follow this precise order. For example, people may perform several steps simultaneously or go back and forth between steps. Sometimes there is barely enough time to perform any of these steps. Nevertheless, the method is a systematic, straightforward, and practical way of dealing with complex moral problems.

To illustrate the application of the method, consider the decision to burst open levees in Cairo, Illinois, mentioned in Chapter 3. The basic ethical problem could be stated as, "Should the Army Corps of Engineers break the levees in Cairo, Illinois to protect towns from flooding further downstream?" Some of the information relevant to this question includes the effects of bursting the levees on local human populations, wildlife, and ecosystems; the effects of not bursting the levees on human populations, wildlife, and ecosystems downstream; the economic costs of breaking the levees; the costs of not breaking the levees; and the basis for the Corps' legal authority to break the levees. Some of the options are: (1) break the levees; (2) don't break the levees; (3) wait and consider breaking the levees later. These options could also be refined. For example, once one has decided to break the levees, it would be necessary to decide where and how to break them. Some of the principles that apply to these different options include promoting utility (understood as maximizing good/bad outcomes for all people), protecting the property rights of people who would be affected by bursting the levees, and protecting species or ecosystems affected by flooding in Cairo or downstream.

Resolving conflicts among principles is often the most difficult step in the method, and involves a careful balancing of competing moral considerations in light of the facts and circumstances of the case (Fox and DeMarco 2000; Beauchamp and Childress 2008). Sometimes the balance will favor one principle over another, and sometimes the balance will shift the opposite way, depending on the facts and circumstances. For example, in deciding whether to break the levees in Cairo, Illinois, an important consideration would be the damage downstream caused by flooding. As the potential for downstream damage increases, the rationale for breaking the levees would increase. As the potential for local property damage increases, the argument against breaking the levees would become stronger. In deciding whether to permit indoor spraying of DDT, the balance of ethical principles depends on facts pertaining to the effects of DDT spraying on human health and the environment, and the effectiveness of other forms of malaria control. The case for DDT spraying will be stronger when the environmental and public health effects of DDT spraying are minimal and the other forms of malaria control are not effective, but this balance would shift the other way as the negative environmental and public health impacts of DDT spraying increase and other methods of malaria control become more effective.

The main reason why it can be difficult to resolve conflicts is that the principles are not ranked: They are fundamental moral imperatives that deserve to be considered in ethical decision making, and no principle always trumps the others. Although we tend to place a great deal of emphasis on respecting human rights, there are some situations in which concern for social utility would justify restricting human rights. For example, the right to free speech does not allow one to shout "fire!" in a crowded movie theater. In some situations, stewardship of biological resources and social utility might be given priority over property rights. For example, a society might decide that a land owner does not have the right to dump agricultural waste into a stream that runs through his property because of the adverse effects of contaminated water on human populations and wildlife.

Because the balance of ethical considerations largely depends on the facts and circumstances relating to a particular case, ethical decision making is partly "situational." The priority given to different principles can vary from one case to the next. However, viewing ethical decision making as partly situational does not imply that it is unprincipled or relativistic because principles and rules govern ethical decision making and help us think about the ethical significance of the facts and circumstances in particular cases (Beauchamp and Childress 2008).

Although there is no formula for determining the appropriate balance of competing principles in every situation, several factors should be considered when making decisions. First, the balancing should be consistent. If one principle is given priority over another in a particular case, then that prioritization should be the same in a similar case. The prioritization may be different in a different case. The consistency requirement is a direct application of the formal principle of justice discussed in Chapter 3, and is important for developing solutions that are rational and publicly defensible.

Second, the balancing should strike a fair and reasonable compromise, wherever possible, between conflicting principles. Compromises are often essential to effective moral and political decision making, because they allow disputing parties to work together toward mutually agreeable solutions (Gutmann and Thompson 1998; Rawls 2005). In a compromise, each side gives a little to the other to achieve a result that is acceptable to both, though not perfectly satisfactory to either. A compromise recognizes that different sides of the dispute have valid points that should be addressed. For example, economic growth and environmental protection are often portrayed as competing values, but it is often possible to achieve economic growth with minimal damage to the environment through technological innovations that increase the efficiency of production and make effective use of resources (Norton 2005; Czech 2008).

Third, the rationale for the balancing should be transparent, not mysterious. The public should be able to understand why this particular balancing of competing principles was adopted in this particular case. The balancing should also be able to withstand public scrutiny and criticism. Evidence presented in a defense of a particular position should be made available to the public and arguments should appeal to commonly accepted ideas and rationales (Gutmann and Thompson 1998). The facts and circumstances offered in support of a particular balancing of principles can assure the public that the chosen course of action is based on reasoning that is sound, not arbitrary or capricious.

While the procedure for balancing moral principles does not rely on moral theories, moral theories can still lend some insight into the reasons for giving priority to one principle over another because theories are useful in interpreting ethical concepts, principles, and values.

For example, in considering conflicts between property rights and the public good (discussed in Chapter 8), it will be useful to consider different theories of property rights in order to interpret this concept and to decide how to resolve conflicts. Theories of distributive justice can also play an important role in deciding how to interpret and apply the principle of justice (discussed later). In Chapter 10, I will consider how different theories of justice apply to environmental health issues. Thus, I will still refer to ethical theories from time to time in this book, even though I favor a principle-based approach to decision making.

I will apply the method described in this chapter to ethical and policy dilemmas discussed in this book. In some cases, I will work through each step of the method systematically and explicitly. In other cases, I will abbreviate the discussion of some steps (in the interests of time) and allow the reader to fill in some of the details and assumptions. It is important to stress, however, that the ethical and policy conclusions drawn in the book will be based on a careful consideration of the facts, options, and moral principles or rules that apply to the situation, and that the method described in this chapter will still operate in the background even when it does not appear in the foreground.

PRINCIPLES OF ENVIRONMENTAL HEALTH ETHICS

To apply the method described in the previous section to dilemmas in environmental health ethics and policy, it is necessary to articulate some principles for ethical decision making. As argued earlier in this chapter, ethical principles should extend beyond obligations to human beings one would find in traditional ethical theories and should also include obligation related to other life forms, species, ecosystems, and the environment. These principles are best understood as *prima facie* rules that guide conduct. When the principles conflict, one must decide which one should have priority.

HUMAN RIGHTS

This principle is similar to Kant's notion of respect for persons discussed in Chapter 3, except that it focuses on protecting the rights of people rather than on respecting human dignity. It builds on the commonly accepted idea that all people have a right to be treated with respect. The principle can be stated in the most general terms as "Respect human rights." Human rights include the right to life, liberty (freedom of thought, speech, religion, association, and action), property, bodily integrity, legal due process, and political participation. Scholars usually distinguish between negative and positive rights (Thomson 1992). Respecting negative rights only requires one to refrain from violating someone's rights, while respecting positive rights requires one to do something for someone else. For example, if the right to life is understood as only a negative right, it is simply a right not to be killed. The right to education, understood as positive right, implies that other people have a duty to provide education. Because positive rights require people to do things for others, usually often via government funding or regulation, they are more controversial than negative rights. Libertarians, for example, do not accept positive rights (Nozick 1974). While I will not argue for any positive rights in this book, I will hold that people deserve to have a decent level of education, health care, food, and other benefits. However, I do not believe that it is necessary to posit a right to these benefits in order to ensure that people have their fair share. Principles of justice require that citizens receive a fair share of the benefits of society (Rawls 1971; Daniels 1984). Respect for human rights implies numerous subsidiary principles, such as prohibitions against deception, theft, exploitation, murder, and rape.

UTILITY

This principle is similar to Mill's utilitarian principle, except that social utility is not defined in terms of a single value, such as happiness. The principle can be stated as follows: "Maximize social benefits and minimize social harms." Mill (2003) thought that all benefits and harms could be assimilated under the rubric of happiness: Things are good insofar as they are a part of happiness or contribute to happiness; things are bad insofar as they are a part of or contribute to unhappiness. However, Mill's theory of value was flawed. Philosophical thought experiments, such as the Trolley Problem, and real-life disputes, such as the abortion debate, demonstrate that we often find it difficult to resolve conflicts among basic values. Our moral indecisiveness in these tough cases strongly suggests that our values cannot be boiled down to a single one. There are a number of different things that we consider good, such as knowledge, virtue, pleasure, health, wealth, and economy, which cannot be defined or justified in terms of a single, overarching good, such as happiness. Because there are many different social values, there may be conflicts of values within the principle of utility itself. For example, economy may conflict with health and safety. The utilitarian principle implies a number of subsidiary principles, such as "Promote human health," "prevent harm to the public," "promote economic efficiency," and so on.

JUSTICE

This principle consists of procedural justice and distributive justice. Procedural justice can be stated as: "Use fair procedures to make social, political, and economic decisions." This principle has several subsidiary principles that spell out some of these fair procedures, such as "Treat similar cases similarly," "Allow citizens to participate in social, political, or economic decisions that affect them," "Make public decisions openly," "Protect due process rights," and "Provide people with equal protection under the law." The legal and political system should implement procedural justice (Rawls 1971, 2005). For example, open government laws make information about public decisions available to all, and laws governing criminal and civil procedures can protect peoples' rights to due process.

Distributive justice can be stated as: "Distribute the benefits and burdens of social cooperation fairly." Each person in society should have a fair share. Determining what counts as a fair share is a complex decision involving a careful consideration of different (and often conflicting) principles of distributive justice, such as "Distribute socioeconomic goods to promote equality of opportunity," and "Distribute socioeconomic goods to reward people for their ingenuity, labor, and contributions" (Beauchamp and Childress 2008). In Chapter 10, I will discuss how these principles apply to environmental policy debates.

Though justice has been treated traditionally as a national concern, since the 1980s, scholars have paid more attention to justice as an international issue. The Greeks viewed justice as a property of an individual or a nation/state. For Plato, a just state was well-ordered, with the ruling class in charge. For Hobbes, Locke, and other social contract theorists, justice was based on social cooperation within a civil society. In his *Theory of Justice* (1971), Rawls treated justice as a property of society. Rawls tackled the topic of international justice much later in his career (Rawls 1999). Because many environmental issues are global in scope, it is important to consider international justice in environmental health.

There are three positions concerning international justice: Skepticism, which denies that international justice exists; realism, which claims that international justice is a relationship among different nations; and cosmopolitanism, which holds that international justice is a relationship between people living in different nations (Beitz 1998). Skeptics claim that international justice is not possible because justice requires an agreement (or social contract) among people cooperating together in a common society, under the rule of law, backed by a stable government. There is no social contract binding all of the world's people and there is no international law backed by a global government. Hence, there is no international justice (Sandel 1981). Realists argue that there can be agreements among different nations to abide by international laws and treaties. Though there is no world government at present, a world government is not needed to enforce rules of international justice (Beitz 1998). Cosmopolitans reject realism on the grounds that many of the governments in power are illegitimate or corrupt, and that international laws and treaties are often impossible to enforce. Cosmopolitans also reject skepticism on the grounds that there can be a hypothetical social contract among the people of the world and hypothetical rules of justice, that is, what all people in the world would agree to. Cosmopolitans conceive of international justice as an ideal relationship among the people of the world, that is, what we owe each other as members of the human race, not as members of any particular nation or group of nations.

There is not sufficient space in this chapter to examine these different views of international justice in depth. However, I will briefly defend the realistic approach. My arguments for realism are twofold. First, if we are to make any significant progress in dealing with environmental (and other) issues that affect the entire planet, then we must reject skepticism as overly pessimistic. We should embrace a view that offers the hope of international solutions to global problems. Second, cosmopolitanism is a noble idea, but it may imply rules and obligations that are unenforceable. Suppose, for example, that some principles of distributive justice would promote equality of opportunity around the world. Because there are tremendous social and economic differences among people living in different nations, acceptance of this principle would require a massive transfer of wealth from developed nations to developing ones. Governments and citizens living in developed nations would not agree to this transfer of wealth in the absence of a powerful world government to enforce it. It is unlikely that we will have a world government with this kind of power for the foreseeable future (Rawls 1999). Individuals, foundations, companies, and even governments are free to donate their resources and wealth to developing nations to relieve human suffering and help build nations, but it is impossible to enforce these beneficent acts on a grand scale.

What would a realistic approach to international justice require? It would imply principles of procedural justice and distributive justice. The principle of procedural justice would be: "Use fair procedures to settle social, economic, and political conflicts among nations." This principle would imply subsidiary rules, such as "Respect national sovereignty," "Allow nations to participate in decisions that affect them," "Protect due process rights," "Make public decisions openly," and "Grant nations equal protection under international law." The principle of distributive justice would be: "Distribute the benefits and burdens of international cooperation fairly." Each nation should receive a fair share of relationships with other nations. This principle would not imply a massive transfer of wealth among nations, but it would require that nations receive a fair share of the benefits (and burdens) of international cooperation. For example, if two nations (or private companies based in particular nations) enter into an agreement concerning oil drilling, the nation drilling for the oil should provide a fair share of the benefits of this arrangement to the nation where the oil is located. The drilling nation should not exploit the nation where drilling occurs. As we shall see in Chapters 7 and 10, fairness concerning the distribution of benefits and burdens should also apply to international agreements, such as treaties designed to limit greenhouse gas emissions.

ANIMAL WELFARE

The first three principles – human rights, utility, and justice – have a solid basis in traditional ethical theories and traditions. The next three principles are important for giving fair consideration to nonhuman biological systems, including sentient animals, species, habitats, and ecosystems. The first of these is the animal welfare principle, which can be stated as: "Do not cause harm to sentient animals without good reason." Harm may include pain, suffering, disability, death, or psychological distress. The principle applies to many differ types of human activities, such as meat eating, hunting, fishing, pet ownership, animal experimentation, and zoo keeping. Two key questions arise in deciding how to apply this principle: "What is a sentient animal?" and "What is a good reason?"

Ethologists, neuroscientists, and other researchers who study animal behavior, cognition, and emotion can provide expertise useful for answering the first question. For several hundred years, scientists accepted French philosopher and mathematician Rene Descartes' (1596–1650) doctrine that animals did not have souls and were unthinking automatons. During this era, researchers performed vivisections on animals and interpreted their cries as reflex actions (Rollin 2006). The antivivisectionist movement of the nineteenth century led to a greater awareness of animal pain and suffering, and greater concern about the ethics of animal experimentation (Rollin 2006). During the first part of the twentieth century, a school of thought known as behaviorism dominated scientific thinking about animal sentience. Behaviorists held that scientific theories and hypotheses concerning human and animal psychology should be based on observable evidence, such as behavior. Because we cannot observe the mental states of animals, we should not regard them as having consciousness, emotions, or intelligence. All we can study scientifically is animal behavior (LaFollette and Shanks 1997). Toward the end of the twentieth century, scientists began to abandon their methodological commitments to behaviorism and began to undertake carefully controlled studies of animal cognition and emotion. Today, most animal researchers accept the idea that many different types of animals have consciousness, the capacity to feel pain, emotions, and that some, such as primates and dolphins, have more sophisticated traits, such as problem-solving abilities, intelligence, numerical concepts, and proto-linguistic communication (Griffith 2001; Beckoff 2002). These developments have important implications for how we should treat animals (Rollin 2006).

The second question, unlike the first, is not primarily a scientific issue, but a moral one. It is also a complex question, because what counts as a good reason for harming an animal depends on the nature of the animal, the nature of the harm, and the goal or purpose that justifies the harm. The nature of the animal is an important consideration because our moral attitudes toward animals should depend, in part, on the extent to which they possess humanlike traits, such as consciousness and intelligence. Animals that occupy a higher position on the scale of value should be treated differently than those that occupy a lower position. Chimpanzees deserve greater protection from harm than mice (LaFollette and Shanks 1997). The nature of the harm also needs to be considered because there is a moral difference between keeping an animal in captivity and inflecting severe pain, trauma, distress, or death. The purpose of the harm also matters because there is a moral difference between harming an animal for a goal that benefits many people in important ways and using an animal for a goal that only benefits a few. For example, there is a moral difference between using dogs in medical research and using dogs in brutal forms of entertainment, such as dog fighting (LaFollette and Shanks 1997). In Chapter 6, I will discuss how these considerations apply to environmental health debates.

STEWARDSHIP

Human beings should act as good stewards of natural resources, such as air, water, soil, species, ecosystems, biodiversity, and the biosphere as a whole. A steward is someone who is entrusted to care for someone else's property and has an obligation not only to prevent harm to what he (or she) is entrusted with but also to promote its overall good. For example, a property manager should ensure that the property is not damaged and should make improvements on the property. This principle can be stated as "Take good care of natural resources." Stewardship stands in sharp contrast to the exploitative approach to nature mentioned earlier in this chapter. Stewardship of natural resources is an important ethical principle because we depend on nature for our survival and well-being, and because biological resources have their own moral worth. As discussed in Chapter 2, various biological systems provide us with breathable air, potable water, a suitable climate, food, fuel, and medicine. Many different human activities, ranging from causing air and water pollution to pesticide use to land development can have adverse impacts not only on human health but also on the well-being of various biological systems. The stewardship principle implies a number of subsidiary ones, such as "Protect species and biodiversity," and "Avoid destruction of habitats and ecosystems." In Chapters 5 to 10, I will apply this principle to a number of different environmental issues. I will also examine conflicts between stewardship and other principles, such as promotion of human health.

SUSTAINABILITY

As mentioned in Chapter 2, ecological sustainability refers to the capacity of a biological system to endure over time (World Commission on Environment and Development 1987). Sustainability may also refer to the capacity of a society to develop economically and endure over time (Norton 2005). The sustainability principle can be stated as: "Practice sustainable uses of biological resources." A use of resources is sustainable if it causes no permanent change that disrupts ecological stability or decreases biodiversity. For example, fishing that does not involve overfishing is a sustainable use. Logging that involves replanting of trees and prudent timber management is sustainable. However, wanton destruction of valuable biological resources, such as a key predator or prey species, coral reefs and tropical forests, is not sustainable.

Sustainability is important for good stewardship of biological resources and for protecting the interests of future generations of the human race (Norton 2005). The idea that we have obligations to future generations has been disputed by some philosophers, who argue that we only have moral duties to existing people. The main argument against obligations to future generations is a philosophical paradox known as the nonidentity problem (Parfit 1986). The argument begins with the premise that the existence of any particular person is precarious, and depends on a number of different circumstances and events. For example, my son, Peter, would not have been born if I had not met his mother, Susan. Our actions today can affect who will be born tomorrow.

The next step in the argument against obligations to future generations is the premise, called the person-affecting principle, which holds that our actions are wrong only if they affect identifiable people. When I have done something wrong, I have wronged someone. The argument then concludes that we cannot act wrongly toward future people, because if we had acted differently, they might not have been born. People would have been born, but different people. If I decide that I should save gasoline to help future generations and decide not to drive forty-five miles to work and back today, different people may be born than if I had decided to drive to work. In my effort to make future people better off, I could cause them not to exist. To have a moral duty to a person, it must be possible me for me to act wrongfully toward that person. If I cannot act wrongfully toward future people, then I have no moral duties to them (Parfit 1986).

Philosophers have spent much time trying to unravel this paradox, and I will not review these debates here (see Roberts 2009). The most straightforward way to tackle this problem is to reject the person-affecting principle and accept the idea that we can have moral duties not only to specific people (or specific organisms) but also to nonspecific things (or aggregates), such as society as a whole, the human population, species, and ecosystems. We have a moral duty to promote the overall well-being of future generations, even if we do not have moral duties to any particular future person. One can argue that we have a moral obligation to ensure that future generations have environmental resources, such as clean air, drinkable water, food, and biodiversity, which they would need to promote their health and well-being (Baier 1984). The principle of utility provides support for duties to future generations, because it requires us to maximize good social consequences and minimize bad ones.

PRECAUTION

The principle of precaution is an overarching rule that may apply to almost any decision concerning risk taking and risk imposition. A great deal of ethical and policy decision making involves reasoning about benefits and risks. Risk/benefit reasoning includes three different steps: (1) identification of risks and benefits; (2) assignment of probabilities to risks and benefits, based on scientific evidence; and (3) management of risks and benefits, with an eye toward maximizing benefits and minimizing risks. Several ethical rules, such as the principles of utility and stewardship, involve a careful weighing of risks and benefits. Risk/benefit reasoning also plays an important role in decisions made by regulatory agencies. The FDA approves medical products only after careful assessment of their risks and benefits, based on scientific evidence from animal experiments, clinical trials, and other studies. The EPA uses risk/benefit assessment to make decisions concerning the sale and use of pesticides and the acceptable levels of air pollutants, such as ozone, based on industry data and other sources of evidence. Cost/benefit analysis, used by economists to understand the potential impact of business and government decisions, is also a type of risk/benefit reasoning (Resnik 2003a).

Though risk/benefit reasoning is a very useful tool for thinking about ethical and policy decisions, sometimes there is not always sufficient evidence to assess the risks associated with different options. We may not be able to assign an objective probability, that is, a probability based on scientific evidence, if a particular risk is indeterminate or unknown. For example, what is the probability that sending a radio signal to nearby stars will cause alien civilizations to attack us? What is the chance that drilling for oil off the eastern coast of the United States will lead to a major oil spill? These risks are real and significant, but we cannot use traditional risk/benefit analysis to deal with them, because we lack scientific evidence. Nevertheless, it is important to manage risks like these proactively, so that we may prevent, minimize, or mitigate disastrous outcomes.

In the 1970s, German legal and environmental scholars developed an approach to making decisions involving indeterminate risks known as the *Vorsorgeprinzip* or Precautionary Principle (PP) (Sandin 2004). The PP started to gain greater attention and influence when a version of it appeared as Principle 15 in the 1992 UN Rio Declaration on Environment and Development:

In order to protect the environment, the precautionary approach shall be widely applied by States according to their capabilities. Where there are threats of serious or irreversible damage, lack of full scientific certainty shall not be used as a reason for postponing cost-effective measures to prevent environmental degradation. (United Nations 1992)

This version of the PP emphasizes the need to take cost-effective measures to prevent threats that cause serious or irreversible damage to the environment, even when there is lack of scientific certainty about those threats. During the 1990s, environmentalists, policy analysts, concerned citizens, and others applied the PP to a variety of debates in which there was a scientific controversy concerning risks, such as climate change, Mad Cow Disease, and genetically modified crops, and urged society to take effective action to avert those threats (Goklany 2001). Other writers, scholars, and scientists were highly critical of the PP, and argued that it is a vague, risk-aversive doctrine that could be easily manipulated to suite various political ends. They also charged that the PP would stifle economic development and scientific and technological advancement (Sunstein 2005). Various authors and organizations responded to these critiques by refining the PP. They defined key terms and sought to dispel the claim that the PP is vague and unscientific (Resnik 2003a, 2004). Although the PP is still a controversial idea, it has gained some acceptance as many scholars and scientists have recognized that society needs a systematic way to make decisions about potential threats when traditional risk/benefit approaches are inadequate (Paterson 2007; Butti 2009; Diamanti-Kandarakis et al. 2009; Diffey 2009; O'Mathuna 2009; Ritter et al. 2009; Munthe 2011).

For the PP to serve as a useful guide to decision making, it must be clearly defined and carefully interpreted (Munthe 2011). First, there needs to be a clear understanding of what is meant by "lack of scientific certainty." As many philosophers and scientists have pointed out, science does not provide certainty. Scientific theories and hypotheses are based on empirical evidence. A scientific hypothesis is not proven to be certain, in the way that we way prove a theorem in mathematics, but it can be shown to be highly probable, given the evidence (Haack 2003). Probability depends on the degree of evidentiary support: The more evidentiary support for a hypothesis, the greater its probability. In risk/benefit reasoning, there is sufficient scientific evidence to assign probabilities to various outcomes. For example, when the FDA approves a new drug, it attempts to estimate the percentage of people in the population who are likely to benefit from the drug, the percentage of adverse reactions, and so on. If the probability of an outcome cannot be determined, we may still be able to decide whether the outcome is plausible (has some evidence in its favor) or is a mere possibility. If the PP addresses outcomes that are merely possible, instead of plausible, then it could lead to highly risk-aversive policies designed to avoid fanciful, nightmare scenarios (Resnik 2003a). So, the first condition for defining the PP is that the threats must be plausible.

Second, the PP needs to incorporate "reasonableness" in addressing threats. Some ways of managing risks may require us to forego important benefits or incur high costs. While it may be reasonable to forego important benefits and incur high costs to avoid severe threats, for other threats this degree of precaution may not be reasonable. The degree of precaution we employ must take such factors into account. A precautionary measure is reasonable, therefore, if it (1) is proportional to the severity of the threat, (2) carefully balances the competing values, and (3) is effective. For some threats, prevention (e.g., taking steps to avoid the threat) may be the most reasonable action. For other threats, mitigation may be reasonable (Munthe 2011).

To illustrate these points, consider some examples. Suppose that a friend offers to play a game of Russian roulette with you. You will use a pistol with six chambers but do not even know whether the gun is loaded, but it might be. The most reasonable course of action would be to prevent the threat by not playing the game at all. It is not worth possibly losing your life for this type of entertainment.

Suppose you are concerned about getting a flat tire on your way to work and your only means of transportation is by automobile, as there is no mass transit. You could prevent this threat by walking to work, but this would take too much time and you would be late for work. The most reasonable course of action would be to mitigate the threat by taking a spare tire and tire-changing equipment. You can also minimize the threat by making sure that your tires are well-inflated and have enough tread. Mitigation and minimization would seem to be the most reasonable course of action in this case.

To illustrate the importance of effectiveness, suppose that to address your concern about having a flat tire you do not take a spare tire but decide to avoid roads near construction sites, where there are likely to be nails or other items that can punch holes in tires. While this response might be helpful, it would not be very effective, because you could still run over nails

Table 4.2. *Principles of Environmental Health Ethics*

Human rights
Utility
Justice
Animal welfare
Stewardship
Sustainability
Precaution

on roads which you thought were safe, and other hazards and manufacturing defects might cause your tire to go flat. This would not be a reasonable method for dealing with the risk of a flat tire. See Table 4.2 for a summary of the principles of environmental health ethics.

The severity of a threat is a function of the quantity of harm and the quality (or type) of harm. For example, the threat posed by an occupational hazard that may kill 500 people per year is more severe than one that may kill up to fifty. An occupational hazard that may kill 500 people each year is more severe than one that may cause low back pain in 500 people each year. Severity should also take into account, as well as whether the harm will occur to people, sentient animals, ecosystems, or biodiversity. An explosion that could kill 500 people poses a more severe threat than one that could kill 500 horses. Though some versions of the PP hold that threats should be irreversible, I do not view this as a relevant condition because significant harms should be avoided, even if they are reversible. If a dam bursts and destroys dozens of houses but kills no people, we would still consider this a significant harm, even though the houses can be rebuilt.

Putting these points together, we can define the PP as: "Take reasonable measures to prevent, minimize, or mitigate severe, plausible threats." In Chapters 5, 6, 7, and 9, I will apply the PP to environmental health debates, such as controversies about genetic modified crops and nanotechnology.

OBJECTIONS AND REPLIES

Before concluding this chapter, I would like to address several objections. The first one claims that my view is a form of anthropocentrism because I place human beings at the top of the scale of value and include several ethical principles that focus on human concerns. Thus, my view is not much of an improvement over other anthropocentric views and doesn't give adequate protection to animals, other species, ecosystems, and so on.

The ethical position I have defended in this chapter is anthropocentric, but it is an enlightened form of anthropocentrism. Although I do place intelligent beings (such as humans) at the top of the scale of value, I hold that nonhuman biological systems, such as sentient animals, species, and ecosystems, have a value that is independent of human concerns or interests. I have also defended several ethical principles that focus on the environment, such as animal welfare, stewardship, and sustainability. These principles imply that human interests do not automatically take priority over the needs of other biological systems when a conflict arises. In dealing with ethical dilemmas pertaining to the human beings and the environment, one must carefully weigh and balance the different values at stake and reach a decision that is consistent, fair and reasonable, and able to withstand public criticism.

The other objections take issue with the principle-based method of ethical decision making I advocate. One might object that the principle-based approach may lead to inconsistency if different people who apply the method to the same set of facts and circumstances reach different conclusions because they weigh and balance principles differently. For example, one person could use the method to conclude that limited use of DDT is acceptable to control malaria, while another person could use the method to reach the opposite conclusion, even when presented with the same sets of facts and circumstances. A method for ethical decision making should not lead to inconsistency.

The principle-based method may indeed yield inconsistent results, but this possibility cannot be easily avoided, unless one adopts a single ethical theory that prioritizes all values, rules, obligations, and principles. As mentioned earlier, I have rejected this option because I am skeptical about the usefulness of moral theories for practical decision making, due to disagreements among theorists and the abstract nature of moral theories.

Even though the method may sometimes yield inconsistent outcomes when people rank principles and values differently, it can also produce a high degree of concurrence, because very often people with different rankings will agree that some options are not acceptable. For example, concerning the controversy over using DDT discussed in Chapter 1, both sides of this debate would agree that indiscriminate use of DDT (or any other pesticide) is not acceptable, and that failing to take effective action to combat malaria is unacceptable. As the parties in the dispute gather more information and seek mutual understanding and compromise, they may continue to narrow the range of acceptable options. Though this method may not always yield a single, best solution to an ethical dilemma or problem, it can produce a range of defensible solutions.

Another objection to the principle-based approach is that it is unsystematic: It is little more than a hodge-podge of conceptually diverse moral considerations. Ethical decision making should be based on a unified, philosophical system (Gert et al. 2006).

I agree that the principle-based approach is less systematic than an approach based on a unified moral theory, but this is fault I can live with. As mentioned before, I am skeptical about the usefulness of moral theories for practical decision making.

A third objection is that moral intuitions play a role in deciding how to balance ethical principles, which makes an important part of moral decision making a mysterious "black box." If people reach different conclusions, given the same principles, options, facts, and circumstances, all we can say is that they had different intuitions about which principle should have priority, which forestalls further rational debate.

While I recognize the significance of this problem, it is not unique to principle-based methods of decision making. As noted earlier, case-based methods of decision making rely heavily on intuitions concerning the morally relevant features of different cases. Even approaches that employ moral theories in decision making are ultimately founded on moral intuitions, because theories are justified insofar as they systematize and explain our intuitions concerning real cases and thought experiments, such as the Trolley Problem or the Lifeboat (Rawls 1971). Philosophers "test" moral theories by developing counterexamples that elicit our intuitions concerning right, wrong, and other moral concepts. If a theory cannot accommodate a counterexample, then it may be rejected or modified. Our moral theories can become better at systematizing and explaining our intuitions as we continue to test and modify them, but there is no complete escape from moral intuitions (Rawls 1971; Audi 2004).

SUMMARY

To deal with ethical issues in environmental health, it is important to understand the relationship between the value of human health and the value of the environment. Health is an important human value but it is not the only one. Others include autonomy, social utility, justice, and virtue. Besides human beings, a number of different biological systems also have value, including sentient beings, organisms, species, ecosystems, and the biosphere. A scale of value, with intelligent beings at the top, is a useful way of conceiving of the ethical relationship between human beings and other biological systems. A principle-based method for ethical decision making can help to resolve conflicts of moral values and principles. Some principles of environmental health ethics include respect for human rights, utility, justice, animal welfare, stewardship of biological resources, sustainability, and precaution. Ethical decisions should be consistent, fair and reasonable, and able to withstand public criticism. In Chapters 5 through 11, I will apply the method of ethical decision making described herein to different environmental health issues.

5

PEST CONTROL

Having explored the foundations of environmental health ethics in Chapters 2 through 4, I will examine some particular topics and controversies in Chapters 5 through 11, making use of the method for ethical decision making described in the previous chapter. This chapter will focus on the use of chemicals and other substances to control pests. I will give an overview of some of the salient facts before addressing ethical and policy issues. Other chapters will follow a similar pattern.

PESTICIDES

As noted in Chapter 2, a pesticide is a substance used to control, repel, or kill pest species. The term "pest" is anthropocentric: A species is considered to be a pest if it threatens human health and well-being (Robson et al. 2010). There are a variety of ways that pests harm human beings or human interests (Robson et al. 2010):

- Bacteria, fungi, and protozoa cause human, animal, and plant diseases.
- Mosquitoes, lice, flies, ticks, fleas, and pigeons serve as vectors for disease.
- Worms and flies infect humans and animals.
- Cockroaches can trigger allergies, exacerbate asthma, and contaminate food.
- Ants contaminate food, damage wood structures, and harm crops.
- Termites damage wood structures.
- Rats and mice serve as vectors for disease and contaminate food.
- Aphids, locusts, corn borers, Japanese beetles, Mediterranean fruits flies, corn earworms, and many other insects damage crops.
- Many different weeds interfere with the germination, growth and fruition of crops, and some, such as poison ivy, are harmful to humans.
- Coyotes, wolves, foxes, and snakes kill livestock and farm animals.
- Some species of spiders, insects, and venomous snakes have poisonous bites or stings that can cause pain, disability, or death.

It is worth noting that some species have both positive and negative impacts on human health and well-being. Bees, for example, can inflict painful stings. Though most people do not suffer any enduring ill effects from a bee sting, those who are allergic to bee stings can die from them. Bees are not considered pests, however, because they play an important role in agriculture by pollinating crops. Bats can carry diseases, such as rabies, but they also help to control mosquito populations and pollinate plants.

Human societies have tried to control pests for thousands of years but have only used pesticides since the 1800s. In the 1860s, farmers began using copper acetoarsenite to control the Colorado potato beetle (*Leptinotarsa decemlineata*) and fungi growing on plants. In the late 1800s, farmers used lead arsenite to control insect pests and fungi. The biggest event in the history of pesticide use was Paul Müller's discovery that DDT is an effective insecticide with low human toxicity, which was discussed in Chapter 1. From the 1940s until the 1960s, DDT was used to control a number of different insect pests, including mosquitoes and lice, which carry infectious diseases. Today, pesticides are used extensively to increase crops yields in industrial agriculture and to control pests in homes, schools, restaurants, and worksites. Pesticides are applied to crops, gardens, basements, foundations, baseboards, walls, alleys, streets, clothing, kitchens, closets, bedding, and even inside the passenger cabins in jets on some international flights. Over 5 billion pounds of pesticides are used worldwide each year, with over 1 billion pounds used in the United States (Robson et al. 2010). Thirty-five thousand commercial products are used as pesticides, with more than 900 active ingredients. Some of the common classes of pesticides and what they do are as follows (Robson et al. 2010):

- **Algicides** control the growth of algae in ponds, lakes, and water systems.
- **Antimicrobials** kill bacteria, protozoa, and other microorganisms.
- **Attractants** attract pests to traps.
- **Biopesticides** are pesticides derived from natural sources such as plants (**botanical pesticides**) and microorganisms (**microbial pesticides**). *Bacillus thuringiensis* (BT) toxins are chemicals derived from the *Bacillus thuringiensis* bacteria, which live in the soil, in the guts of some caterpillars, and on some plants.
- **Defoliants** cause leaves to drop from plants. Agent Orange is a code name for a defoliant used by the United States in the Vietnam War, which contained two different herbicides and dioxin (York and Mick 2008). According to the U.S. Department of Veterans Affairs (2010), Agent Orange exposure in American soldiers is associated with several types of cancer, Parkinson's Disease, diabetes, peripheral neuropathy, heart disease, and cloracne.
- **Disinfectants and sanitizers** kill or control pathogens on inanimate objects, such as surgical tools, hospital walls, and kitchen and bathroom areas. Some commonly used disinfectants and sanitizers include alcohols (ethanol or isopropanol), pine oils (contained in cleaning products), sodium hypochlorite (an ingredient in household bleach), calcium hypochlorite (used in swimming pools), chlorine (added to drinking water), hydrogen peroxide (used in medical treatment), chloroxylenol (an ingredient in some household cleaners), chlorhexidine (used in hand washes and mouthwashes) and o-phenylphenol (used in surgery) (McDonnell and Russell 1998).
- **Fumigants** are gases or vapors used to kill insects and other pests.

- **Fungicides** kill mold, mildew, blights, and other fungi.
- **Herbicides** kill weeds. Roundup, discussed in Chapter 2, is a widely used herbicide.
- **Insecticides** kill insects and other arthropods, such as spiders, ticks, mites, and centipedes. DDT is an insecticide that is no longer commonly used. Commonly used insecticides include organophosphates, carbamates, and pyrethroids. Organophosphates are neurotoxins that interfere with the function of acetylcholine, a neurotransmitter used by many species of insects and animals. Organophosphates are toxic to humans and have been used as nerve gases. Carbamates also interfere with acetylcholine, but they are less toxic than organophosphates (Robson et al. 2010).
- **Nematicides** kill nematodes, which are microscopic worms that feed on the roots of plants.
- **Pheromones** are chemicals that interfere with insect mating.
- **Plant growth regulators** change the flowering, growth, or reproduction of plants.
- **Repellants** repel pests. N,N-diethyl-3-methylbenzamide (DEET) is a chemical found in many commercial insect repellants. DEET is classified by the EPA as slightly toxic to humans because it can cause eye and skin irritation (Environmental Protection Agency 1998).
- **Rodenticides** kill rodents, such as mice, rats, and moles. Warfarin, an anticoagulant medication used to treat patients with clotting disorders, has been used for many years to kill rodents. Warfarin can be dangerous to humans and pets, and can cause internal bleeding if ingested in high doses.

PESTICIDES AND HUMAN HEALTH

People come into contact with pesticides in many ways. Inhalation of pesticides can occur when pesticides are sprayed on fields, parks, streets, or in home or work areas. Pesticides can enter the body through the skin when people apply liquid or dust pesticides to plants or areas in the home. Dermal exposure can also occur when people touch places that have been treated with pesticides. Pesticides can enter the body through the digestive system when people eat products that have pesticide residues, such as fruits or vegetables sprayed with pesticides. Oral exposure can also occur when people put their hands to their mouths after touching areas that have been treated with pesticides. Children tend to have higher pesticide exposures than adults living in the same environment, in part, because children come into contact with pesticides by playing on or near treated areas or by putting their hands into their mouths. Some of the highest pesticide exposures occur among farm workers, especially commercial pesticide applicators. Most states have passed laws designed to minimize dangerous exposures among commercial pesticide applicators, however these laws are often not well-enforced (Robson et al. 2010).

Because most pesticides have been developed to produce toxicity in target species, it is not surprising that these substances can produce acute and chronic toxicity in many other species, including human beings. There were over 22,433 accidental pesticide poisonings in the

United States in 1996: 32 percent of these cases occurred in children younger than six years old. More than 90 percent of these cases involved minor symptoms that could be treated at home, but some resulted in fatal injuries (Environmental Protection Agency 2008). The most common poisonings resulted from exposure to organophosphates, followed by pyrethrins and pyrethroids, pine oil disinfectants, and hypochlorite disinfectants. People also use pesticides to commit suicide. About 10 percent of pesticide toxicity cases in health care centers involve suicide attempts (Environmental Protection Agency 2008). Acute pesticide toxicity can result in permanent damage, including loss of cognitive and motor function (Kamel and Hoppin 2004). Pesticide poisonings are a significant problem in developing nations, due, in part, to lack of regulatory oversight and education on the safe use of pesticides (Pimental 1996).

Epidemiological studies have shown that long-term exposure to pesticides can increase the risk of several types of cancer, including non-Hodgkin's lymphoma, childhood leukemia, multiple myeloma, prostate cancer, pancreatic cancer, lung cancer, and ovarian cancer (Alavanja et al. 2004; Rudant et al. 2007; Wigle et al. 2009). Some of these studies have found associations between cancer risk and pesticide exposure, while others have linked cancer risk to exposures to specific substances, such as arsenic compounds, DDT, dioxin, organophosphates, and organochlorines. Long-term pesticide exposure also increases the risk of Parkinson's disease, amyotrophic lateral sclerosis (ALS), thyroid disease, and cognitive dysfunction (Kamel and Hoppin 2004; Kamel et al. 2007; Goldner et al. 2010). As mentioned in Chapter 1, DDT may disrupt human reproductive and endocrine functions (Longnecker et al. 1997). Some studies indicate that prenatal organophosphate exposure negatively affects cognitive development in children (Bouchard et al. 2011).

Insect repellants are products applied to human skin or clothing to prevent stings or bites from insects and other arthropods, such as mites or ticks. Insect repellants can play an important role in preventing insect-borne diseases, such as malaria, encephalitis, Lyme disease, Rocky Mountain spotted fever, and Yellow Fever. The environmental impact of repellants is generally low because they are not widely dispersed. Many different factors influence the effectiveness of repellants, such as temperature, humidity, wind speed, and the person's age and activity level (Robson 2010). Different repellants have different effects on insects and arthropods. Some repel some species but not others. Repellants made from naturally occurring chemicals include citronella, peppermint, and eucalyptus oils. Common synthetic chemical repellants include malathion, permethrin, and DEET, the most effective insect repellant. Though acute DEET toxicity is rare, exposure to high doses of DEET by itself, or in combination with chemical repellants, has been shown to cause neurological deficits in laboratory animals (Abdel-Rahman et al. 2004; Abou-Donia et al. 2004). Some commentators recommend moderate use of DEET to avoid health problems (Robson 2010).

PESTICIDES AND THE ENVIRONMENT

Pesticides can also have adverse impacts on nonhuman species and ecosystems. As noted in Chapter 1, DDT is harmful to a number of different species, especially those higher up the food chain, such as predatory birds. The decline of eagles, hawks, condors, and other birds in the United States in the 1950s and 1960s was due to widespread DDT use (Hamlin and Guillette 2010). DDT use can disrupt ecosystems by causing some species to decline or become extinct. For example, the decline or extinction of predatory birds could lead to overpopulation of prey species, such as field mice, rabbits, and squirrels. Because DDT is a persistent organic pollutant that can accumulate and concentrate in organisms and ecosystems, even moderate use of DDT can pose environmental problems.

Other pesticides also pose a risk to the environment. Pesticides have been identified as a potential cause of amphibian declines and deformities in the United States, have been detected in 80 percent of fish in major rivers and streams in the United States, and are a major factor in fish kills, that is, localized dying off of fish populations (U.S. Fish and Wildlife Service 2010a). Pesticides have also been implicated in bird kills (Pimental 1996). In Europe, over a hundred species of birds are threatened due to industrial farming practices, which involve habitat disruption, fertilizers, and pesticides (Krebs et al. 1999). Pesticides are a major factor in congenital defects and reproductive abnormalities in many different vertebrate species, including amphibians, reptiles, birds, fish, and mollusks (Hamlin and Guillette 2010). Aquatic animals are particularly vulnerable to the effects of pesticides, due to the runoff of pesticide contaminants into the water (Hamlin and Guillette 2010). One or more pesticides have been detected in 90 percent of major streams and rivers in the United States (U.S. Fish and Wildlife Service 2010a).

Pesticides also threaten beneficial insects and other invertebrate species (U.S. Fish and Wildlife Service 2010a). Evidence suggests that chronic pesticide exposure may contribute to low earthworm densities in some regions and declining butterfly populations in Europe (Longley and Sotherton 1997; Reinecke and Reinecke 2007). Pesticides can also lead to the decline of natural predators of insect pests, which can, paradoxically, increase pest populations (Pimental 1996). There has been a controversy concerning the hazardous effects of BT toxins in GM crops on the monarch butterfly (*Danaus plexippus*) and other nontarget insect species. A study published in 1999 showed that pollen produced from BT corn harms Monarch butterfly larvae under laboratory conditions (Losey et al. 1999). Because exposures to BT pollen in the field are much lower than the exposures produced in this study, the adverse impacts of BT pollen on monarchs are negligible (Sears 2001). However, additional research is needed (Romeis et al. 2006). Pesticides have been implicated in declining bumble bee populations (Goulson et al. 2008). Some researchers have presented evidence that pesticides may play a role in colony collapse disorder in honey bees along with several other factors, such as pathogens, parasites, and stress (Vanengelsdorp et al. 2009). However, others have presented evidence that colony collapse disorder is due to coinfection of two viruses affecting invertebrates (Bromenshenk et al. 2010). Additional research is needed to better understand colony collapse disorder (Environmental Protection Agency 2010j).

Many of the pesticides that pose the greatest threat to the environment are persistent organic pollutants (POPs), which do not break down easily in the environment. Some POPs, such as DDT, can accumulate and concentrate in the food chain. POPs can pose a threat to many different species, especially those higher up the food chain, such as predators (Hamlin and Guillette 2010). Organochlorines, such as DDT, are POPs. Because POPs pose a significant environmental hazard, 150 countries adopted the Stockholm Convention, mentioned in Chapter 1. POPs banned under the Stockholm Convention include DDT as well as aldrin, chlordane, dieldrin, endrin, heptachlor, hexochlorobenzene, and toxaphene (Robson et al. 2010).

PESTICIDE RESISTANCE

Pesticide resistance (mentioned in Chapter 2) has become a major concern for public health and agriculture. Hundreds of species of insects, mites, weeds, fungi, bacteria, nematodes, and rodents have become resistant to different pesticides. Scientists have known about the potential for pesticide resistance since the early 1900s, but the problem became much more common during the 1950s, due to the intense use of synthetic chemicals in industrial agriculture. Pesticide resistance has stabilized since then as a result of the development of improved chemical and biological methods of controlling pest species. Some arthropods, such as insects and mites, have become resistant to DDT and organophosphates. Resistant species include mosquitoes, flies, beetles, true bugs, and moths (Georgehiou 1986). Resistance often tends to be a local and dynamic phenomenon.

Insecticide resistance may soon become a significant problem for controlling mosquito-borne diseases, such as malaria (Ranson et al. 2009; van de Berg 2009). DDT-resistance has been observed in *Anopheles* mosquito populations in Ethiopia, Uganda, Cameroon, Sudan, Zimbabwe, South Africa, India, Vietnam, and China (van den Berg 2009). DDT is still effective even if the insects have developed resistance because it may be used as a repellent. Some *Anopheles* populations in Vietnam and Africa have developed resistance to pyrethroids (Van Bortel et al. 2008; Ranson et al. 2009).

There is also a growing concern that insect species will become resistant to BT toxins, which are applied to crops. These toxins are also secreted by genetically modified (GM) plants, such as BT corn and BT cotton, which have been genetically engineered to produce BT toxins as a form of protection against many species of insect pests. Agricultural researchers have been exploring different ways of avoiding BT resistance, such as selective use of BT (Soberón 2007). (GM crops will be discussed in more depth in Chapter 6.)

Herbicide resistance is becoming a major problem in industrial agriculture. Many weed species have become resistant to glyphosate, as a result of intense selection pressures created by widespread use of this herbicide (Owen and Zelaya 2005; Owen 2008). Glyphosate-resistant weeds are found in the United States, Australia, China, and Brazil. Glyphosate resistance has been described as the biggest threat that industrial agriculture has ever seen (Neuman and Pollack 2010). Weeds have developed resistance to other herbicides, such as atrazine, simazine, paraquat, propanil, and triallate (Gressel 2009).

When antibiotics were first discovered in the 1930s, they were hailed as miracle drugs that could cure many infectious diseases. In the last few decades, however, antibiotic resistance has become a major public health concern (Levy 1992). Antibiotic resistance occurs because bacteria that survive exposure to antibiotics transmit this trait to next generation. Over time, resistance genes can become prevalent in the population as a result of natural selection. Bacteria can also transfer resistance genes to each other through nonhereditary processes, such as conjugation and the exchange of plasmids. Antibiotic resistance is a problem for the treatment of a number of different bacterial infections, including *Tubercles bacillus* or tuberculosis (TB), *Staphylococcus aureus*, and *Streptococcus pneumoniae*. Drug resistance is also a problem for the treatment of malaria, which is caused by a plasmodium, a single-celled parasite (Centers for Disease Control and P revention 2009a).

TB is one of the most significant global health problems. It is estimated that one third of the world's population is infected with TB, and that 2 million people die from this disease annually (Centers for Disease Control and Prevention 2010). Various TB strains have become resistant to antibiotics, including isoniazid, rifampicin, floroquinolone, amikacin, kanamycin, and capreomycin. Multidrug-resistant TB is resistant to isoniazid and rifampicin, and extensively resistant TB is resistant to these two drugs as well as floroquinolone and one other drug used to treat TB (Centers for Disease Control and Prevention 2009a).

Methicillin-resistant *Staphylococcus aureus* (MRSA) has been a major concern in hospitals and nursing homes since the 1960s, but it is now also prevalent in the greater community. The elderly and people with weakened immune systems are especially susceptible to MRSA (Klevens et al. 2007). MRSA causes skin infections, can lead to pneumonia, and is often fatal. In 2005, 18,650 people in the United States died from MRSA infections (Centers for Disease Control and Prevention 2009a). In 2007, the U.S. mortality rate for MRSA was 6.3 deaths per 100,000 people (Klevens et al. 2007). MRSA is resistant to methicillin, oxacillin, penicillin, and amoxicillin (Centers for Disease Control and Prevention 2009a, Klevens et al. 2007).

Several factors contribute to the problem of antibiotic resistance. First, antibiotics have been overused and inappropriately used. For example, physicians often prescribe antibiotics to treat viral infections, such as the common cold, which do not respond to antibiotics. Although most physicians know that it is inappropriate to use an antibiotic to treat a viral infection, they sometimes prescribe antibiotics to satisfy their patients' demands (Selgelid 2007). The average person in a developed country receives ten to twenty courses of antibiotics during childhood (Blaser 2011). Overuse of antibiotics may also harm beneficial bacteria that live in our gastrointestinal system. Bacteria in our intestines help with digestion and absorption of food, vitamin synthesis, and proper immune system functioning. Antibiotic overuse may increase the risk of obesity, type II diabetes, asthma, and inflammatory bowel disease (Blaser 2011).

Second, patients who are prescribed an antibiotic for a bacterial infection often do not complete the entire course of treatment, because their condition improves after a few days and they think they do not need to keep taking the medication (Selgelid 2007). Failing to complete the entire course of antibiotics can leave the infection weakened but not eradicated, which allows resistant strains to proliferate.

Third, many farmers add subtherapeutic doses of antibiotics to animal feed to promote growth. According to some studies, this practice can lead to the evolution of resistant bacteria that can infect farm animals and humans (Selgelid 2007). (This issue is discussed in more depth later.)

Fourth, research on new antibiotics has dwindled since the 1970s. Only two new classes of drugs have been developed in the last three decades (Aiello et al. 2006). Some U.S. lawmakers have introduced legislation to provide incentives for drug companies to develop new antibiotics (Pollack 2010).

INTEGRATED PEST MANAGEMENT

Public health officials, scientists, and government organizations have developed strategies for minimizing resistance to pesticides. Integrated pest management (IPM) is a strategy for minimizing the environmental impact of pesticides used in agriculture, which can also counteract pesticide resistance (Stern et al. 1959; Bentley 2009; Naranjoa and Ellsworth 2009). The IPM approach employs a number of different strategies for controlling pest populations, including (Committee on the Future Role of Pesticides in U.S. Agriculture 2000; Robson 2010):

- Active monitoring of pesticide use patterns and emerging resistance;
- Judicious use of synthetic and natural pesticides;
- Manipulation of the environment, such as removal of standing water, careful storage of food, pruning, selective fertilization and watering, to make it unattractive for pests;
- Sanitation and solid waste management;
- Structural maintenance, such as fixing leaks and repairing openings;
- Physical controls, such as keeping refuse containers off the ground, using bug zappers or traps to kill insects, and regular plowing of fields to disrupt weed life cycles;
- Biological controls, such as using natural predators to kill pest species;
- Consumer education to increase awareness of IPM techniques.

To combat antibiotic resistance, the CDC and other public health organizations have taken measures to educate clinicians and the public about the problem of antimicrobial resistance and how to counteract it. The CDC's Campaign to Prevent Antimicrobial Resistance emphasizes prevention of infection, early diagnosis and effective treatment, wise use of antimicrobials, and prevention of disease transmission. The campaign includes recommendations to minimize microbial resistance in hospitals, dialysis centers, and long-term care facilities. The campaign also emphasizes partnerships among clinicians, patients, and health organization; distributes educational materials; and outlines evidence-based strategies to prevent antimicrobial resistance in specific patient populations (Centers for Disease Control and Prevention 2005).

PESTICIDE REGULATION

Pesticides have been regulated in the United States since 1910, when a law was passed to protect consumers from ineffective products and inaccurate labeling. Congress passed the Federal Insecticide, Fungicide, and Rodenticide Act (FIFRA) in 1947. FIFRA required registration of pesticides with the U.S. Department of Agriculture and accurate product labeling. The law did not regulate pesticide use, however. FIFRA was rewritten in 1972 to regulate pesticide use and has been amended numerous times since then. FIFRA authorizes the EPA to regulate pesticides but also allows state and local governments to adopt their own pesticide rules, as long as they are not weaker than the federal law (Environmental Protection Agency 2010d). Pesticide companies must register their products with the EPA prior to manufacture, sale, or transport. Companies must submit data to the EPA pertaining to their product's chemistry as well as its impacts on human health, the environment, and nonhuman species (Environmental Protection Agency 2010d).

The EPA weighs the benefits of the pesticide against the risks to human health and the environment when deciding whether to approve a product registration. The EPA approves products for specific uses, which are stated on the product label, along with other safety information. The EPA also regulates composition, packaging, distribution, and disposal of products. The EPA has the authority to require companies to submit additional data, and it can suspend or cancel the registration of a product to protect human health or the environment. The EPA has an appeals process for its decisions (Robson et al. 2010).

When a pesticide is registered, the EPA decides whether it may be sold for general or restricted use. If a pesticide is sold for general use, then anyone may purchase and use the product. If a pesticide is sold for restricted use, however, only registered pesticide applicators may purchase and use the product. Registered pesticide applicators must receive training in the proper use of pesticides and demonstrate their knowledge of these products. They must pass an examination, receive continuing education, and apply for recertification. Restricted use pesticides tend to be more toxic than general use pesticides and require additional safety measures. Some pesticides are sold for general use at low concentrations and restricted use at higher concentrations (Robson et al. 2010).

Another important law affecting pesticide regulation is the Federal Food, Drug, and Cosmetic Act (FFDCA). Although the FFDCA applies primarily to the FDA, which regulates foods, drugs, and cosmetics, this legislation authorizes the EPA to establish maximum levels (or tolerances) of pesticide residues on foods and animal feed (Robson et al. 2010). Pesticide tolerances are based on two safety factors of ten applied to NOAEL studies in animals (discussed in Chapter 2). The FDA and the U.S. Department of Agriculture help to enforce tolerances by monitoring pesticide levels in fruits, vegetables, seafood, meat, milk, poultry, and eggs (Robson et al. 2010).

The Food Quality Protection Act (FQPA) amended FIFRA and FFDCA, and set more stringent safety standards for pesticides. The FQPA requires the EPA to consider aggregate exposures when establishing tolerances, not just particular dietary exposures. The EPA must also take into account the cumulative effects of pesticides that affect similar biochemical pathways, and consider the endocrine-disrupting effects. The FQPA established an additional ten-fold safety factor to protect children and infants, which means that the allowable human exposure on food residue is 1/1000 the NOAEL in animals, unless there is reliable evidence that this ten-fold safety factor can be reduced. The FQPA also requires the EPA to rereview pesticide registrations every fifteen years and reassess tolerances on a regular basis (Robson et al. 2010).

ETHICAL AND POLICY ISSUES

The use of pesticides raises a number of ethical and policy issues. Because pesticides can harm sentient animals, threaten species, reduce biodiversity, and disrupt ecosystems, the use of pesticides poses the dilemma of human interests versus the environment. Because pesticides can also have adverse impacts on human health, the use of pesticides also creates conflicts among different human interests, such as public health, agricultural productivity, and economic development. There are three basic ethical/policy viewpoints regarding pesticides:

(1) Unrestricted use of pesticides.
(2) No use of pesticides.
(3) Judicious use of pesticides with regulatory oversight.

The unrestricted use view prevailed in the United States prior to the revision of FIFRA in 1972, and still operates in countries that have not adopted pesticide laws. Someone who is opposed generally to government regulation of commerce and industry, such as a libertarian, might support the unrestricted use of pesticides. However, few environmental scientists or scholars consider this viewpoint to be a defensible position, given the well-documented environmental and public health threats posed by pesticides. The ethical debate is mostly between those who favor some form of restricted use and those who oppose any use of pesticides. Beyond Pesticides' mission is to eliminate the use of toxic pesticides around the world (Beyond Pesticides 2010), and Pesticide Action Network seeks to eliminate the use of dangerous pesticides (Pesticide Action Network International 2010). Health and Environment Alliance (2010) and the Sierra Club (2010) want to reduce radically the use of pesticides.

In this chapter, I will defend the judicious use of pesticides: Pesticides may be used for an important purpose, provided that potential threats to public health and the environment are understood and minimized. Pesticides should be regulated and carefully controlled, and some pesticides may need to be banned. The strongest argument for using pesticides judiciously is to promote a goal that is universally recognized as important, such as human health. One might argue that public health uses of pesticides, such as employing pesticide to prevent infectious diseases, repel parasites, sterilize surgical instruments, or sanitize hospitals and homes, are more justifiable than other uses, because public health uses save human lives.

PESTICIDES AND MALARIA VECTOR CONTROL

One of the most compelling reasons for using pesticides is to prevent the spread of a devastating infectious disease, such as malaria. As noted in Chapter 1, the WHO has endorsed limited use of DDT, such as indoor spraying. However, this use of DDT, even to fight malaria, remains controversial, and many people do not support the WHO's recommendations (Berenbaum 2005; Pesticide Action Network of North America 2007; Sierra Club 2010). The principles and methods for decision making, described in Chapter 4, can yield some insights into this dispute. The first step of the analysis would be to frame the ethical question. It could be stated as, "Should the limited use of pesticides be allowed to control malaria?"

The next step would be to gather the relevant information, such as:

- The impact of limited use of pesticides on human health;
- The impact of limited use of pesticides on sentient animals, other species and the ecosystem;
- The impact of limited uses of pesticides on pest resistance;
- The history of pesticide use and resistance in the region;
- The prevalence of malaria in the region, and its social, economic, and health impacts on the population;
- The mortality and morbidity due to malaria
- The social and economic burden of malaria;
- The financial costs and effectiveness of limited use pesticides in preventing malaria;
- Other forms of malaria prevention, such as protective netting and clothing, and insect repellants;
- The financial costs and effectiveness of other forms of malaria prevention;
- The costs and availability of malaria treatment.

Though I will not address all of these factual issues here, a few points are worth mentioning. First, as noted in Chapter 1, malaria is a devastating disease in tropical regions, especially sub-Saharan Africa, with significant social and economic impacts (Kapp 2004).

Second, forms of malaria prevention that do not involve pesticides, such as protective netting and clothing, are not completely effective. As long as *Anopheles* mosquitoes are in an area where malaria is endemic, people are likely to get bitten and contract malaria. Controlling *Anopheles* mosquito populations would seem to be an essential part of any malaria prevention strategy (Kapp 2004). If this is the case, then a key question is, "What is the most effective way of controlling *Anopheles* mosquito populations?" DDT has proven to be one of the most effective pesticides at controlling *Anopheles* populations. It has low resistance and minimal human impact. It is also inexpensive, which is an important consideration in developing nations (Kapp 2004). However, the costs of DDT are increasing. DDT is not the only pesticide that could be used, and other chemicals may offer some advantages over DDT, such as less environmental impact or less resistance.

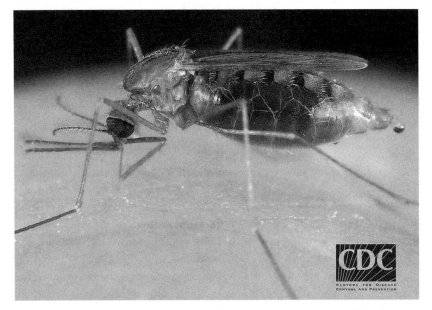

Figure 5.1. *Anopheles freeborni* Mosquito Taking a Blood Meal (photo courtesy of the U.S. Centers for Diseases Control and Prevention).

Third, prevention is preferable to treatment when it comes to malaria, due to the mortality and morbidity associated with the disease, and the limited availability of treatment, due to costs and lack of health care infrastructure, in areas where malaria is a problem (Kapp 2004). See Figure 5.1 for a photo of an Anopheles mosquito.

Fourth, as discussed earlier in this chapter, pesticides can have acute and chronic adverse effects on human health. However, unless a person receives a toxic dose from improper pesticide use, the adverse health effects of pesticides are generally much less harmful than the adverse effects of malaria.

After gathering the relevant information, the next step is to consider the different options. The two most basic options would be: A) limited use of pesticides and B) no use of pesticides. Option A may include different suboptions differentiated according to how pesticides are used. For example, pesticides could be applied to different areas of the home, applied to areas where mosquitoes breed, used in some parts of the country but not in others, or applied during specific times or dates, or for a limited period.

Applying ethical principles to the different options, in light of the relevant information, is the next step in the decision-making process. The principles of utility and justice would favor pesticide use that has a minimal impact on human health because malaria prevention can save human life and promote the good of society. An important consideration concerning justice would be that the burden of malaria tends to fall most heavily on socioeconomically disadvantaged people, who may lack the resources to take effective measures to prevent mosquito bites or to receive treatment for malaria. Principles of international justice would support national sovereignty concerning pesticide use, which would imply that each nation should be allowed to use pesticides to protect its own population from malaria, provided that the use of these chemicals does not adversely impact other nations.

Animal welfare, stewardship, and sustainability would not favor pesticide use, however. The animal welfare principle would recommend against pesticide use, if it adversely impacts the welfare of sentient animals, such as predatory birds. The stewardship principle would strongly condemn using pesticides to control malaria, if introducing these chemicals into the environment contributes to the decline or extinction of species or disrupts ecosystems. If pesticide use resulted in the elimination of several species of predatory birds, for example, this would lead to overpopulation of prey species, which would disrupt the ecosystem. Extinction of these predator species would also be a significant loss of biodiversity. Pesticide use might also lead to the extinction of some mosquito species, which could also disrupt the ecosystem because various species of insects, fish, amphibians, bats, and birds feed on larval and adult forms of this organism. However, loss of these species might not adversely impact the ecosystem if there are other mosquito species that fill a similar ecological niche. The sustainability principle would caution against any use of pesticides that is not sustainable over time. Even if limited pesticide use promotes human health with minimal environmental damage in the short run, repeated use of pesticides over a longer period of time could cause significant environmental damage, because some of these chemicals, such as DDT, persist in the environment and can accumulate and concentrate in species and ecosystems. Repeated use of pesticides could also lead to pesticide resistance, which would reduce the effectiveness of these chemicals, and could lead to increased uses of pesticides.

The precautionary principle would urge us to take reasonable measures to prevent, minimize, or mitigate harms from pesticide uses that are plausible and severe. Some of these harms would include loss of species and biodiversity, disruption of ecosystems, and adverse human health impacts. The PP, rather than other risk management principles, would be an appropriate way of thinking about the hazards of pesticide use, because we cannot, at present, assign an objective probability to the harms resulting from pesticide use. The PP could yield different recommendations, depending on how we decide to interpret and apply it. On the one hand, one could argue that the PP would recommend that we avoid all pesticide use, because this is the only way to avoid harms to the environment and human health. On the other hand, one could argue that the PP would not recommend that we avoid all pesticide use because reasonable precautions should take into account the various values at stake, such as human health, protection of species and ecosystems, economic growth, and so on. One could argue that the PP might favor limited uses of pesticides to avoid the devastating impacts of malaria on human health, society, and the economy. Refusing to use any pesticides to control malaria would be an overreaction to threats posed by these chemicals.

Once we have considered how these different principles apply to options concerning the use of pesticides to control malaria vectors, the next step is to resolve conflicts among them.

Several of these principles conflict with each other. For example, utility and justice conflict with animal welfare and stewardship. In Chapter 4, it was noted that one should settle conflicts among principles by reaching decisions that are consistent, fair and reasonable, and transparent. Integrated pest management, discussed earlier in this chapter, offers an approach to malaria vector control that may be able to satisfy these conditions (Robinson et al. 2009). The use of pesticides, within an IPM framework for malaria vector control, would involve a number of different methods, such as:

- Active monitoring of the use pesticides, such as organophosphates, pyrethroids, and DDT, with special attention to any emerging resistance;
- The use of protective clothing, bed nets, and mosquito repellants;
- Careful and controlled use of synthetic or natural pesticides;
- Development of new pesticides;
- Indoor or outdoor spraying of pesticides;
- Manipulation of the environment to control *Anopheles* populations, such as removal of standing water;
- Structural maintenance (where appropriate), such as repairing homes to prevent mosquitoes from entering and installing mosquito netting;
- Physical controls, such as bug zappers placed near homes (if electricity is available);
- Biological controls, such as deploying mosquito predators; or genetic modification of mosquitoes, which will be discussed in Chapter 6;
- Sterilization of mosquitoes;
- Consumer education to increase awareness of these techniques.

The IPM approach would be consistent, fair and reasonable, and transparent, because it is a cohesive set of strategies that can be used to manage many different pest populations. The principles that apply to control of malaria vectors also apply to control of corn borers, aphids, mice, and so on. IPM also strikes a fair and reasonable compromise among conflicting ethical principles by controlling pest populations with minimal environmental damage. Finally, IPM is transparent because the public can understand the methods used in IPM and their rationale. IPM is a publicly defensible approach to pest control.

One of the advantages of the IPM approach is that it would not rely entirely on pesticides to control the *Anopheles* populations. Limited use of pesticides would be one strategy among many. The IPM approach could also lead to a reduction in pesticide use if other pest management strategies prove to be effective. Although there are many advantages to IPM, it does involve a substantial commitment of time, money, and resources, which developing nations may lack (Robinson et al. 2009). Widespread DDT spraying is a relatively inexpensive way of controlling malaria vectors (Walker 2000). The Roll Back Malaria partnership, consisting of over 500 academic institutions, governments, private foundations, nongovernmental organizations, and private companies, can help developing nations obtain the resources needed for effective malaria vector control. Founded by the WHO, the World Bank, the United Nations Children's Fund (UNICEF), and the United Nations

Development Program (UNDP) in 1998, the Roll Back Malaria partnership aims to eradicate malaria throughout the world (Roll Back Malaria 2010). The Bill and Melinda Gates Foundation is also an important contributor to the effort to eliminate malaria (Bill and Melinda Gates Foundation 2010).

Any pesticide policies that are implemented should be revised in light of new scientific findings. If it turns out, for example, that even limited DDT use has significant adverse impacts on human health or the environment, or leads to resistance, then it may be advisable to stop using DDT to control malaria vectors. Because we may not fully understand the impacts of limited DDT use for many years, precaution is advisable. New scientific findings concerning the harmful effects of other pesticides could also lead to policy revisions. It is imperative that environmental health researchers continue to study the effects of pesticides on human health and the environment and the feasibility of pest control measures that do not involve the use of these chemicals.

Government agencies should make regulatory decisions based on the best available scientific evidence concerning the effects of pesticides on human health and the environment and take precautionary measures, when appropriate. Government officials need to be aware of new scientific findings and be prepared to make necessary changes in policies or regulations.

PESTICIDES AND AGRICULTURE

If limited uses of pesticides can be justified to promote public health goals, such as malaria vector control, can other uses also be justified, such as the use of pesticides in agriculture? Some of the relevant information might include:

- The current patterns and practices of pesticide use in industrial agriculture, including the types and quantities of pesticides used, methods of application, target crops, and target organisms;
- The impacts of agricultural uses of pesticides on human health;
- The impacts of agricultural uses of pesticides on species, biodiversity, and ecosystem;
- The contribution of pesticides to productivity, efficiency, and low cost in agriculture, and the role of pesticides in helping alleviate the world hunger problem;
- The relationship between pesticide use and food exportation, importation, and food security;
- The extent of the world hunger problem and its principal causes;
- Alternative forms of agriculture that do not use pesticides, including estimates of their productivity, efficiency, and cost;
- The feasibility of dealing with the world hunger problem without pesticides.

Some of these facts have already been discussed in a general way, but more information about the effects of different chemicals would be useful.

First, agriculture produces food, which is essential to human life and health. Over one billion people in the world do not have enough food to sustain a healthy life. Each year, nearly six million children die from starvation, malnourishment, or diseases related to inadequate food or nutrition. Hunger and malnutrition can also exacerbate other diseases, such as HIV/AIDS, TB, and malaria. People who do not have enough to eat get sick more often than people who have enough to eat, and they also have a more difficult time getting well (Bread for the World 2010).

Second, although hunger is a major global concern, the world currently produces enough food to feed the human population adequately (World Food Programme 2010; World Hunger Education Service 2010). The principal causes of world hunger are poverty, lack of local arable land, natural disasters (such as droughts and floods), inefficient food distribution, and military conflicts (World Food Programme 2010; World Hunger Education Service 2010). According to the World Bank (2010a), 1.4 billion people live on $1.25 or less per day, an amount of money that is not enough to purchase an adequate amount of food. Prolonged droughts in Kenya, Somalia, Ethiopia, and other parts of Africa have led to crop failures and livestock losses (World Food Programme 2010). Each year, military conflicts displace millions of people. Refugees often lack access to the basic necessities, such as food, water, and shelter. Some developing countries are ruled by military elites, who seize food shipments from foreign countries and use food as a means of suppressing the population (World Food Programme 2010).

Third, the world's food output currently depends on modern, industrial farming practices implemented during the Green Revolution (circa 1940s-1980s), such as irrigating land; planting selectively bred, disease-resistant crops; and applying chemical fertilizers and pesticides. These practices increased agricultural productivity dramatically (Food First 2000; Borlaug 2002,). The Green Revolution spread from the United States to Mexico, Europe, India, Pakistan, Brazil, Australia, and China, and the world's grain output nearly tripled, using roughly the same amount of arable land (Borlaug 2002). The father of the Green Revolution, Norman Borlaug, received the Nobel Peace Prize in 1970 for his efforts to feed the hungry people of the world. From 1961–2005, cropland grew by only 27 percent, but yield increased by 135 percent (Burney et al. 2010). Production of the equivalent grain output without implementing Green Revolution techniques would lead to massive deforestation because cropland would have need to increase by 171 percent (Borlaug 2002). Deforestation has adverse environmental consequences, such as exacerbation of global warming, habit and species loss, and ecosystem disruption. Even though modern farming practices produce significant amounts of greenhouse gases, such as methane, ammonia, and carbon dioxide, they more than compensate for this environmental impact by making efficient use of the land and preventing deforestation (Burney et al. 2010).

Fourth, organic farmers, who reject the use of pesticides, chemical fertilizers, antibiotics, and genetically modified crops, have developed pest control methods that do not involve pesticides, such as the use of natural predators and parasites, insect traps, plowing, manual removal of weeds, mulching, and crop rotation and diversification (Zehnder et al. 2007; Bale et al. 2008; Small-Farm-Permaculture-And-Sustainable-Living.com 2010). Although only a small percentage of the world's food is produced by organic farming, it has become increasingly popular over the last decade, due to growing concerns about the effects of industrial farming practices on human health and the environment (U.S. Department of Agriculture [USDA] 2009, 2010). It is not known whether alternatives to industrial agriculture, such as organic farming, will be able to provide the world's population with an adequate supply of low-cost food. It may be the case that organic farming can supplement but not replace industrial farming (Food and Agriculture Organization of the United Nations 2007). Because it is so labor-intensive, organic food is usually 20 percent to 100 percent more expensive than nonorganic food (Martin and Severson 2008; U.S. Department of Agriculture 2009).

Fifth, the price of food is a major factor in world hunger because the poor can ill afford significant increases in food prices. A recent increase in corn prices, caused by high demand for this grain as a substrate in ethanol production, alarmed many international economists, who warned that using corn to produce fuel could starve the poor (Brown 2006). Increases in food prices exacerbated world hunger from 2007 to 2009 and led to riots. If the elimination of pesticides leads to dramatic increases in food prices, this could significantly increase world hunger (von Braum 2010).

Sixth, expected population growth is a factor that must be considered in any policy related to food production (United Nations 2009). Farming methods will need to keep up with the world's increasing demands for food. (Ethical and policy issues related to population growth and control will be discussed in more depth in Chapter 9.)

Seventh, the world is divided into net exporter and net importer nations when it comes to food. Some of the top exporters include the United States, China, Brazil, and India, Argentina, and France (Food and Agriculture Organization of the United Nations 2005). Many countries are unable to produce enough food to feed their populations. Some of these countries export oil or other desired commodities, which they can use to purchase food, while others, such as developing nations in sub-Saharan Africa, do not. The division between food importer and exporter nations creates potential problems for national security (food security), international trade, economic development, and world hunger (World Health Organization 2010d; von Braum 2010). The farming methods adopted by various nations need to address these issues.

After reviewing the facts related to this controversy, the next step is to consider the different options, of which there are many, such as: limited use of pesticides in agriculture; use of only certain types of pesticides on certain types of crops; use of pesticides in agriculture in some countries but not others; or no pesticide use at all in agriculture. Organic farming is one possible option, but so is IPM, which minimizes the environmental impact of pesticides.

Turning to the application of ethical principles to the issue of pesticide use in agriculture, it would appear that utility and justice would favor limited use, assuming that health benefits of pesticides outweigh the health risks and farming methods that do not employ pesticides are unable to provide an adequate supply of food at a low cost. The main utilitarian argument for pesticide use is that it helps combat world hunger. A key concern related to justice is that the burden of hunger tends to fall most heavily on socioeconomically disadvantaged people, such as people in developing nations, who may lack the resources to grow or obtain their own food. Pesticide use could help to relieve this burden by helping to secure an adequate supply of low-cost food. Principles of international justice would support national sovereignty concerning pesticide use, which would imply that each nation should be allowed to use pesticides to produce food for its own population, provided that the use of pesticides does not adversely impact other nations.

Other principles probably would not support pesticide use in agriculture, however. The animal welfare principle would recommend against pesticide use, if it adversely impacts the welfare of sentient animals, such as predatory birds. The stewardship principle would oppose pesticide use that contributes to the decline or extinction of species or disrupts ecosystems. Loss or decline of target and nontarget species could disrupt ecosystems and lead to loss of biodiversity. The sustainability principle would caution against any use of pesticides in agriculture that is not sustainable over time. Even if limited pesticide use promotes human health with minimal environmental damage in the short run, repeated use of pesticides over a longer period of time could cause significant environmental damage, because some of these chemicals may persist in the environment and accumulate and concentrate in species and ecosystems, and pesticide use might need to increase to overcome pest resistance.

Turning to the PP, this principle would urge us to take reasonable measures to prevent, minimize, or mitigate harms from uses of pesticides that are plausible and severe. Some of these harms would include loss of species, loss of biodiversity, disruption of ecosystems, and adverse human health impacts. It is safe to say that we cannot, at present, assign an objective to the occurrence of all of these undesirable outcomes as a result of limited pesticide use in agriculture, so the PP would be a useful way of thinking about these potential hazards to the environment and human populations. The PP could yield different recommendations, depending on how we interpret and apply it. On the one hand, one could argue that the PP would recommend that we avoid all pesticide use, because this is the only way to avoid harms to the environment and human health. On the other hand, one could argue that the PP would not recommend that we avoid all pesticide use because reasonable precautions should take into account the various values at stake, such as human health, agricultural productivity, economic growth, and protection of species and ecosystems. One could argue that the PP might favor limited uses of pesticides in agriculture to avoid the devastating impacts of food shortages on human health, society, and the economy. A reasonable policy would be one that makes careful and controlled use of pesticides, such as IPM.

Once we have considered how these different principles apply to options concerning pesticide use in agriculture, the next step is to resolve any conflicts among them. Several of these principles conflict with each other: If utility and justice support a policy of judicious pesticide use, but animal welfare, stewardship, and sustainability do not. The PP could yield different outcomes, depending on how we interpret and apply it in a particular situation. The IPM approach, which was recommended for malaria vector control, could also play a key role in agriculture. IPM could provide a way of settling conflicts between human-centered and nonhuman centered principles that is consistent, reasonable, and transparent. The use of pesticides in agriculture, within an IPM framework would involve a number of different methods, such as:

- Active monitoring of the use pesticides, with special attention to any emerging resistance;
- Careful and controlled use of synthetic or natural pesticides;
- Development of new pesticides;
- Manipulation of the environment to control pests populations, such as plowing, manual weeding, mulching, crop rotation, and crop diversity;
- Physical controls, such as insect traps positioned near crops;
- Biological controls, such as deploying predators or parasites that attack agricultural pests;
- Sterilization of pest species;
- Consumer education to increase awareness of these techniques.

As noted earlier, one of the advantages of IPM is that it would not rely entirely on pesticides to control agricultural pests. Limited use of pesticides would be one strategy among many. IPM could also lead to a reduction in pesticide use if other pest management strategies prove to be effective. Some pesticides that are deemed to be too dangerous could be banned, and others could be significantly restricted. As mentioned earlier, pesticide policies should be revised in light of new scientific findings. If it turns out, for example, that even limited use of a particular pesticide in agriculture has significant adverse impacts on human health or the environment, or leads to resistance, then it may be advisable to stop using this pesticide. Acceptable levels of pesticides could also be lowered in response to new scientific evidence. Environmental health researchers should continue to study the effects of pesticide use in agriculture on human health and the environment, as well as the feasibility of pest control measures that do not involve the use of these chemicals. Government regulation (discussed earlier) should also play a fundamental role in pesticide management and policies in agriculture. The public should provide sufficient funding for pesticide research and oversight.

OTHER USES OF PESTICIDES

There are many other uses of pesticides, which I will discuss only briefly in this chapter. For example, people use pesticides to control rats, cockroaches, bed bugs, ants, lice, mold, bacteria, flies, termites, and other species that invade the home; to repel chiggers, ticks, fleas, and mosquitoes; to control insects and weeds in gardens and lawns; and to sanitize bathrooms, kitchens, restaurants, health care facilities, and schools. Some of the key questions that need to be addressed for these other types of pesticide use are similar to those we addressed with regard to using pesticides in malaria vector control and agriculture:

- What is the purpose of the use of pesticides? How important is this purpose?
- What are the effects of these pesticides on human health?
- What are the effects of these pesticides on other species and the environment?
- What are the alternatives to pesticide use?
- Are the alternatives efficacious and cost effective?
- Can the use of pesticides be minimized or reduced effectively?

I will not address the ethical issues concerning all of the different uses of pesticides in this chapter, but I will suggest that IPM may provide a useful, consistent, and responsible way of addressing these questions.

ANTIBIOTIC RESISTANCE ISSUES

Before concluding this chapter, I will discuss some ethical and policy issues related to antibiotic resistance. As mentioned previously, antibiotic resistance has become a significant public health problem, which threatens our ability to treat bacterial infections in human beings. As we saw earlier, antibiotic resistance is a major problem related to the treatment of MRSA, TB, and other diseases. Unless we take some effective measures to address this problem, we could face a dire predicament related to the prevention and treatment of infectious diseases.

One of the main reasons why antibiotic resistance has developed is that individuals do not have sufficient incentives to curtail their use of antibiotics (Aiello et al. 2006). When a mother asks a pediatrician for an antibiotic to treat her child's ear infection, she is mainly concerned with her child's health, not with the impact of antibiotic treatment on public health. The pediatrician may have some concern for the public health impact of antibiotic misuse or overuse, but his focus is also primarily on the health of the patient. He may also want to maintain a good relationship with the child and parent. When a farmer puts antibiotics in cattle feed, his main concern lies with the welfare of his animals, not with the impact of this practice on public health. When a pharmaceutical company decides to spend money on developing a new medication, its primary concern is to achieve a reasonable return on this investment, not necessarily to improve the public health (Resnik 2007a). At its core, the problem of antibiotic resistance represents a conflict between individual rights/welfare and the public good (Aiello et al. 2006). Without appropriate incentives, social controls, or laws, individuals seeking their own good may take actions that lead to antibiotic resistance and undermine public health.

To address the problem of antibiotic resistance, individuals and organizations must be motivated to take actions that they do not necessarily view as in their interests. The CDC's Campaign to Prevent Antimicrobial Resistance (mentioned earlier) uses education to change the behavior of health care professionals, patients, and health care institutions. But is education enough? Should society adopt policies or laws designed to control the behavior of individuals? Some of these social controls/incentives might include:

- A ban on the use of antibiotics in farm animal feed;
- Punishments for physicians who prescribe antibiotics inappropriately;
- Additional government spending on the development of new antibiotics;
- Additional financial incentives for companies to develop antibiotics, such as increased patent protection or limitations on legal liability;
- Taxes on some antibiotics;
- Rationing of some antibiotics.

I will not examine all of these policy options in this book. Instead, I will use the method of ethical decision making described in Chapter 4 to consider the merits of a ban on antibiotics in animal feed. In 2006, the European Union (EU) banned adding antibiotics to farm animal feed to promote growth. Sweden has banned this practice since 1986 (Dibner and Richards 2005). The United States and many other countries do not have a ban (Union of Concerned Scientists 2006).

The general ethical question related to this issue would be, "Should there be a ban on adding antibiotics to animal feed?" Some of the factual issues that need to be addressed include:

- The nature and scope of adding antibiotics to animal feed. How common is this practice? Which antibiotics are used? What are the dose levels? Which species of farm animals are fed antibiotics?
- The benefits of adding antibiotics to feed for the health of animals and agricultural productivity. How effective are antibiotics in feed at preventing disease and promoting growth?
- The role of antibiotic feeding in antibiotic resistance in animal and human diseases. Can resistant bacteria that infect animals transfer genes to bacteria that infect humans? Does eating antibiotic-fed meat pose any health risks?

I will briefly touch on some of these relevant facts.

In the United States and many other countries, most industrial farmers have been adding antibiotics to animal feed ever since the growth-promoting effects of these drugs were discovered in the 1940s. Twenty-three different antibiotics are used, including many with human applications, such as: penicillins, sulphonamides, tetracyclines, macrolides, lincosamides, streptogramins, and quinolones. The dose levels are generally low (i.e., subtherapeutic). Antibiotic-fed animals include poultry, cattle, and swine (Phillips et al. 2004). Antibiotics promote growth in farm animals by controlling gut microbiota and improving the absorption and metabolism of food, and by preventing bacterial infections when immunization is not effective. Antibiotics can improve growth rates by an average of 16.9 percent in pigs (Dibner and Richards 2005). There is also evidence that antibiotics in feed help protect farm animals against some diseases, and that bans on antibiotics in feed have led to increases in colitis and necrotic enteritis (Bywater 2005). However, some studies suggest that the impacts of antibiotics on animal growth and health are minimal (Wegener 2003).

There is currently a scientific dispute about whether antibiotic feeding contributes to antibiotic resistance in humans. Most scientists agree that antibiotic feeding can lead to the evolution of resistant strains of pathogens in animals, such as *Escherichia coli (E. coli),* *E. faecium, Salmonella,* and *Campylobacter,* and that human beings can contract these antibiotic-resistant diseases from contact with animals or eating uncooked meat (Phillips et al. 2004; Bywater 2005). However, there is disagreement about whether antibiotic resistance in animals poses a significant risk of antibiotic resistance in human diseases, because there is no conclusive evidence that resistant strains in animals have become prevalent in human populations or have transferred genes to bacteria that infect people (Bywater 2005; Matthew et al. 2007). Additionally, most of the antibiotic resistance in human diseases can be explained by the inappropriate use of antibiotics by physicians and patients (Phillips et al. 2004). However, many scientists assert that the risks of antibiotic resistance in human diseases are real and worrisome, even if they cannot be quantified at this point (Engberg et al. 2001; World Health Organization 2002; Jensen et al. 2004; Union of Concerned Scientists 2006).

After examining the relevant facts, the next step is to consider the different options. Some of these include: no ban on feeding antibiotics to farm animals (current U.S. policy); a total ban on feeding antibiotics to farm animals (the EU approach); and a partial ban (e.g., a ban on feeding antibiotics with human applications to farm animals).

Turning to the application of ethical principles to the issue, the human rights principle would support allowing farmers to feed antibiotics to their animals. According to this argument, animals are the farmers' property, and farmers have a right to take care of their property. Another argument against a ban would be that antibiotics in feed promote the welfare of sentient farm animals by preventing disease and promoting growth. The principle of utility might support or oppose a ban, depending on the risks and benefits of antibiotic feeding for society. If the benefits of antibiotic feeding outweigh the risks, it would oppose a ban; if the opposite is the case, it would favor a ban.

The PP may lend some insights into this issue. Few people would dispute the claim that the potential harms of antibiotic feeding are plausible and significant. The PP would recommend that we take reasonable precautions to address these risks, even though the scientific evidence concerning them is not conclusive. A reasonable precaution would be one that takes appropriate measures to prevent harm while giving ample consideration to the values at stake (e.g., public health, animal welfare, agricultural productivity, and farmers' rights). The EU has decided that a reasonable precaution in this case is a total ban on feeding antibiotics to farm animals. However, one might argue that a total ban is an overreaction to the threat of antibiotic resistance, and that a more appropriate response would be to only ban the use of antibiotics with human applications. Allowing antibiotics to be used in animal feed that have no human applications would help to promote the health of animals and agricultural productivity without significantly jeopardizing human health. A total ban could be implemented if additional research demonstrates that such a policy is necessary to avoid antibiotic resistance in human diseases.

The Preservation of Antibiotics for Medical Treatment Act (H.R. 1549) would be an important step toward a partial ban on the use of antibiotics in animal feed in the United States. This legislation would prohibit applications for new animal drugs unless the applicant can show there is a reasonable certainty that no harm to human health will occur as a result of antibiotic resistance. The legislation would also allow critical, human antimicrobial drugs to be withdrawn from use in animal feed unless specific safety requirements are met (Preservation of Antibiotics for Medical Treatment Act 2009). (The Preservation of Antibiotics for Medical Treatment Act had not become law as of the writing of this book.)

SUMMARY

Pesticides have a variety of effects, positive and negative, on human beings and the environment. High-dose, short-term exposures to pesticides can cause acute toxicity in human beings. Long-term, low-dose exposures can increase the risk of a number of different diseases. Pesticides can harm sentient animals, threaten some species, and disrupt ecosystems. Persistent organic pollutants, such as DDT, pose significant risks to the environment because they accumulate in ecosystems and concentrate in organisms, especially those higher up the food chain. Extensive pesticide use leads to pesticide resistance. Antimicrobial resistance is now a significant public health problem. A ban on all pesticides would be an overreaction to the risks posed by these chemicals, and would threaten human health and well-being. A better approach is to use pesticides judiciously, within an integrated pest management framework and with rigorous government oversight. The next chapter continues the discussion of agricultural practices and policies.

6

GENETIC ENGINEERING, FOOD, AND NUTRITION

This chapter expands on some themes from the previous chapter and examines several different issues related to the production and consumption of food. Food ethics is much broader than issues related to the use of pesticides and fertilizers, and encompasses such topics as genetic engineering, meat eating, hunting and fishing, and growing food locally. As in the previous chapter, the discussion will include a description of some facts relevant to the ethical and policy issues.

GENETIC ENGINEERING

Heredity is controlled by an organism's genes, made up of deoxyribonucleic acid (DNA) and located in the chromosomes of every cell. DNA is a long, double-stranded molecule that carries genetic information in the form of linear sequences of four chemical compounds termed *nucleotides* linked together into long stretches. The four nucleotides (also called *bases*) are: adenine (A), which pairs with thymine (T), and cytosine (C), which pairs with guanine (G). Because of this unique base-pairing rule, DNA is capable of self-replication because either strand can serve as a template for synthesis of the other strand.

At intervals along the DNA, long stretches are arranged in a specific sequence, and the cell can use each sequence to direct the construction of proteins. Thus, a region of DNA that carries all the encoding information for a protein is called a "gene." Genes range in size from a few hundred to a few thousand DNA base pairs in length. Most of the cell's DNA does not consist of genes; the function of these "spacer" regions is varied, and need not concern us for the purposes of this introduction. Each human cell contains billions of bases, arranged to form roughly 23,000 distinct genes. The entire set of an organism's nuclear DNA is known as its genome (Nichol 2008; Dolan DNA Learning Center 2010).

In higher organisms, such as animals and plants, chromosomes reside in a membrane-bound cellular structure known as the nucleus. Organisms with a cell nucleus are termed *eucaryotes*. In eucaryotes, DNA is packaged into long structures called *chromosomes*. DNA is coiled around proteins called *histones*, which give the chromosomes their structure. The number of chromosomes is one type of distinguishing characteristic of each species. Human beings have forty-six chromosomes: twenty-two pairs (known as autosomes) plus two additional chromosomes, "X" or "Y" (known as sex chromosomes). Cells of females contain two X chromosomes; male cells contain one X and one Y chromosome. Other organisms have different numbers of chromosome pairs, up to over 100 in the case of some plants.

Most of the DNA in eukaryotic organisms is contained in the nucleus, but some DNA (less than 1 percent) resides in the mitochondria, which are organelles responsible for metabolic processes in the cell (Nichol 2008; Dolan DNA Learning Center 2010). Some organisms, such as bacteria, have a single chromosome to house their DNA. Many lower organisms, such as bacteria, lack a nucleus to house chromosomes. These organisms are termed *prokaryotes*.

Cells use the information contained in DNA to form proteins, which regulate many important cellular functions including cell division, shape, differentiation (turning from one cell type into another), migration, movement, and death. Proteins are formed through processes called transcription and translation. DNA is transcribed into a single-stranded messenger ribonucleic acid (mRNA), using the base-pairing system mentioned earlier, so that each RNA transcript carries the same base-sequence information as the gene's DNA did. RNA is comprised of the same bases as DNA, except uracil (U) is substituted for thymine.

Messenger RNA is translated into proteins by organelles called ribosomes. Ribosomes translate mRNA by reading the RNA sequence three bases at a time. Each three-base portion is termed a *codon*. Different codons represent the instruction to incorporate a single protein building unit – one of twenty chemicals called *amino acids*. Certain three-base sequences also tell the ribosome how to start and how to stop translation.

For example, G-G-G codes for incorporation of the amino acid glycine; whereas A-C-T codes for the incorporation of threonine. After the ribosome forms the basic structure of a protein (the amino acid sequence) the protein undergoes additional processing in the cell.

Knowledge of – and the ability to experimentally manipulate – this DNA-RNA-protein system led scientists to look for ways to alter DNA sequences on purpose. Whereas spontaneous mutations of the DNA involve errors that alter one DNA base into a different base, experimental alterations can be made to purposefully alter a DNA sequence in numerous positions. Some purposeful DNA mutations can thereby result in encoding for proteins with different amino acid sequences. The process of carrying out this kind of purposeful alteration of cellular DNA is termed *genetic engineering*.

Genetic engineering began in the early 1970s when scientists discovered how to insert DNA into bacteria. Scientists took advantage of the natural ways that bacteria acquire DNA, such as direct exchange of DNA during physical contact with other bacteria, or by infection by viruses that specifically infect bacteria (called *bacteriophages*). Alternatively, short custom-designed DNA molecules could be assembled easily into circular DNA termed *plasmids*. Plasmids can be introduced into cells by many different means, and thus became the standard vectors to transfer DNA into different types of bacteria or other types of cells.

Scientists have developed techniques to isolate DNA and use enzymes to cut DNA and insert it into bacterial or viral plasmids. Plasmids can be placed into different cells through a variety of techniques called *DNA transformation* (for bacteria) and *DNA transfection* (for

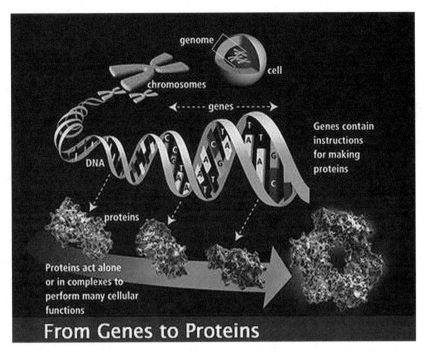

Figure 6.1. From Genes to Proteins (image courtesy of the U.S. Department of Energy).

eukaryotic cells). In some cases, the plasmid can recombine into the host cell's nuclear genome or it can exist as a separate piece of DNA. Viruses that infect bacteria can also transfer their DNA into the host's genome (Nicholl 2008). See Figure 6.1 for a depiction of how genes code for proteins.

When scientists insert DNA into an organism, they may also include other sequences that code for specific proteins as well as sequences that control where the DNA will be inserted into the chromosome and/or when the DNA will be expressed as a protein. Scientists may also insert pieces of DNA that function as markers for the purposes of verifying gene transfer. Organisms that have been genetically engineered are called *genetically modified organisms* (GMOs) (Nicholl 2008). Recently, scientists have also developed a method for constructing a whole bacterial genome from DNA sequence data. Although this technique is still in its infancy, researchers hope that it will greatly increase their ability to genetically engineer organisms. Instead of inserting one gene at a time into a cell, whole genomes could be designed in the laboratory (Gibson et al. 2010).

Cloning plays an important role in animal genetic engineering. Since the 1970s, scientists have used bacteria to copy (or clone) DNA, ribonucleic acid (RNA), and proteins (Nicholl 2008). Other forms of cloning make copies of a whole organism. Twinning occurs naturally during mammalian reproduction, when an embryo splits in half, and two embryos with the same genome implant in the uterus. Scientists have discovered how to artificially split embryos. Embryo splitting is frequently used in cattle reproduction, because it allows breeders to produce copies of animals with desirable traits, such as increased milk production (Hasler 1992). To clone a plant, all one needs is a cutting, which can be cultured and grown into a new plant genetically identical to the cutting.

The most controversial form of cloning involves making a copy of a large adult animal. In the 1990s, scientists developed a process, known as nuclear transfer, in which a nucleus is removed from a cell of an adult animal and transferred into an egg that has had its nucleus removed. The zygote is then implanted in a womb. If all goes well, the offspring will be virtually identical, genetically, to the adult. The two animals will not be fully genetically identical because they will have different copies of mitochondrial DNA (Human Genome Project 2009). The most famous clone was Dolly, a sheep born in 1996. Dolly had six offspring, but had to be euthanized at six years of age, due to debilitating arthritis and lung disease. It has been theorized that Dolly became ill because she was born as old as the cell she was cloned from, which was six years old. As cells age, their telomeres (structures at the end of chromosomes that prevent DNA from unraveling) become shorter. When telomeres become too short, cells die, which leads to age-related functional decline. Since Dolly, scientists have cloned many other mammals, including mice, dogs, cats, horses, goats, and cows, but not human beings (Human Genome Project 2009).

Cloning can play an important role in genetic engineering because it is useful in reproducing genetically modified (GM) animals. If researchers create a GM mammal with desired traits, they may want to clone the mammal to ensure that those traits are passed on to the next generation because normal breeding could produce an animal that lacks those traits. Dolly's creator, Ian Wilmut, wanted to develop cloning techniques to reproduce genetically engineered sheep that produce medicines in their milk (Resnik et al. 1999).

When genetic engineering methods were first developed, scientists, journalists, citizens, and political leaders were concerned about the possible risks of accidental contamination from GMOs. Many people feared that scientists would create a "superbug" that would escape the laboratory and wreak havoc on the world (Barinaga 2000). In February, 1975, the top scientists in the emerging field of molecular biotechnology held a conference in Asilomar, California to discuss the safety hazards of recombinant DNA research and develop recommendations to protect laboratory workers, the public, and the environment from biohazards. The scientists recommended that recombinant DNA experiments only use organisms that are unable to survive outside of the laboratory, and vectors that are only able to grow in specific hosts. They also recommended a number of different safety procedures, such as physical containment techniques, adherence to good laboratory practices, and education and training for personnel. They thought that recombinant DNA research should move forward cautiously, and that certain experiments should not be undertaken (at that time) because they were deemed too risky (Berg et al. 1975).

Government agencies also took steps to minimize the risks of genetic engineering research. The NIH established the Recombinant DNA Advisory Committee (RAC) in 1974 to provide oversight and guidance for NIH-funded recombinant DNA research.

Guidelines, first published in 1976, and revised since then, apply to institutions that receive NIH funding for recombinant DNA research. The guidelines include a number of different measures for minimizing the risks of recombinant DNA research, including the requirement that organizations receiving NIH funds establish institutional biosafety committees (IBCs), which provide local oversight for recombinant DNA research. Although the RAC's guidelines do not apply to industry-funded research, most private companies that sponsor recombinant DNA research have opted to follow the guidelines. In addition to issuing guidelines, the RAC has also reviewed proposed recombinant DNA experiments and held educational forums to discuss scientific and ethical issues related to recombinant DNA research (National Institutes of Health 2009).

The biotechnology industry has blossomed in the United States and other developed countries since the 1980s as a result of the development of genetic engineering. According to industry estimates, biotechnology companies supported 3.2 million jobs in the United States in 2006. U.S. biotechnology jobs increased at a rate of 7.3 percent per year from 1996 to 2006. Job growth is expected to continue with the development of new products, such as biofuels and biopharmaceuticals (Biotechnology Industry Organization 2011). Many nations and states are trying to attract biotechnology companies to spur economic growth and job creation.

Today, there are many different scientific and practical applications of genetic engineering, such as (Nicholl 2008):

- GM bacteria that clean up oil spills, manufacture hydrocarbon fuel, sequester carbon, and produce medicines;
- GM cell lines, tissues, or laboratory animals that can serve as models for human diseases, such as diabetes, heart disease, stroke, obesity, dementia, Parkinson's disease, and various forms of cancer;
- GM plants that produce crops, fuels, medicines, and help with pollution control (discussed further below);
- GM animals that produce food and medicine (discussed further below);
- Genetic modification of human somatic cells to treat inherited diseases and cancer.

Because genetic engineering of human beings raises issues that go beyond the scope of this book, this chapter will focus on ethical issues concerning the genetic engineering of plants and animals. For further discussion, see Resnik et al. 1999; Fukuyama 2003; and Rasko et al. 2006.

OBJECTIONS TO ALL FORMS OF GENETIC ENGINEERING

Some people argue, based on philosophical or theological considerations, that genetic engineering is inherently wrong, regardless of its consequences for society or the environment. They reject genetic engineering as a matter of principle (Rifkin 1984, 1985). Opponents have developed two in-principle arguments against genetic engineering, the argument from nature and the "playing God" argument. According to the argument from nature, genetic engineering is wrong because it changes species. Why is it wrong to change species? According to the theological version of the argument, species were made by God, who has endowed them with intrinsic goodness (Ramsey 1980). Changing a species goes against God's will and demonstrates an ungrateful attitude toward his gifts (Ramsey 1980). According to the secular version of this argument, species are natural patterns of biological organization, and what is natural is good. Changing or destroying species is a rejection of nature (Bovenkerk 2002; Kass 2008).

Theological versions of the argument from nature are problematic because they appeal to particular religious worldviews, which may not be widely accepted. Someone who is an atheist or does not embrace the specific religious doctrine employed in the theological argument will not view it as very convincing. Though some of the world's religions reject all forms of genetic engineering as against God's will, many do not (Cole-Turner 1997). The Catholic Church is not opposed to genetic engineering as a matter of principle, but opposes applications of genetic engineering that harm the environment or human health, or violate human dignity (such as human cloning) (Allen 2008). Judaism also does not oppose genetic engineering as a matter of principle. Though Judaism holds that God created the world, man has a role as cocreator and steward of nature. Judaism opposes genetic engineering that is harmful to human life, animals, or the environment (Wolff 2001). Islam does not oppose genetic engineering as a matter of principle, and supports medical applications of genetics. Islam also condemns applications of genetic engineering that are harmful to human life (Al Aqee 2007). Finally, Buddhism does oppose genetic engineering as a matter of principle, but takes a precautionary approach. Buddhism opposes applications of genetic engineering that have harmful effects on human or animal life (Epstein 2001).

Secular versions of the argument from nature also have significant shortcomings. First, they make the controversial assumption that species should not be changed. One obvious flaw with this viewpoint is that it contradicts the widely established scientific fact that species are in a constant state of flux due to natural selection, random genetic drift, and other evolutionary mechanisms (Reiss and Staughan 1996). Because the human population is part of the biological world, it is impossible for us not to impact other species. How we eat, work, play, and live inevitably affects other life forms. Species that are able to adapt to human activities will thrive, while those that cannot adapt may become extinct (Rollin 1995).

Second, secular versions of the argument from nature assume that all species have intrinsic value, but this is a dubious claim. Consider the thousands of species of bacteria, viruses, and other pathogens that have caused tremendous human suffering. Do these species have intrinsic value? Would it be wrong to eradicate smallpox, polio, or malaria? An argument can be made that nonhuman species have value insofar as they contribute to human well-being or ecosystem functioning (Norton 1987). For example, causing a mosquito species to become extinct is not wrong as a matter of principle, but it may be wrong if loss of this species has adverse effects on other species that prey on the mosquito.

Third, secular (and religious) versions of the argument from nature imply that the widely accepted practice of selective breeding is immoral (Rollin 1995). For thousands of years, farmers and agricultural scientists have used selective breeding to improve crop yields, to domesticate animals, and to enhance the flavor, texture, and nutritional value of fruits and vegetables. Most people have no ethical qualms about selective breeding, even though it changes species. How can one consistently maintain that selective breeding is acceptable but that genetic engineering is wrong as a matter of principle?

Opponents of genetic engineering might argue that genetic engineering is inherently wrong because it is significantly different from selective breeding (Thompson 2010). First, genetic engineering is capable of transferring genes across unrelated species, whereas selective breeding operates on genes that are within the same species or closely related species. For example, genes from fish have been spliced into tomato plants to promote longer shelf-life of harvested fruits. Second, because genetic engineering can transfer genes between very different species, it can bring about radical transformations that would not be possible by means of selective breeding, such as pet fish that glow in the dark. Third, opponents could also argue that genetic engineering is more difficult to control – and therefore more risky – than selective breeding because genes might not insert into the genome properly, and might not be appropriately regulated or expressed in the recipient organism (Thompson 2010).

While these differences are important, none of them justify treating genetic engineering as unethical as a matter of principle. Genetic engineering may be more innovative, radical, and risky than selective breeding, but that does not make it inherently wrong. One could argue that the unique features of genetic engineering justify precautions, but not outright prohibition (Nuffield Council 1999). What matters from a moral perspective is not how the genome is manipulated, but the results of that manipulation. Genetic manipulation that causes harm to human beings, animals, or the environment is ethically problematic, regardless of whether the manipulation occurs through selective breeding or genetic engineering.

The second in-principle argument is that human beings should not "play God" with life (Ramsey 1980; Rifkin 1985). "Playing God" is probably one of the most overused expressions in bioethics (Boone 1980). It has been employed to condemn euthanasia, abortion, and many other activities that people find morally objectionable. Though the phrase has some visceral appeal, it is vague. On one interpretation, the phrase means that human beings should not do things that properly belong only within God's dominion. If "playing God" is understood in this fashion, then it is just another way of stating the theological version of argument from nature, which was discussed earlier (Boone 1988; Peters 2002).

On another interpretation, the phrase means that humanity lacks the knowledge and wisdom to make profound decisions concerning life and death. Because we do not have God-like knowledge and wisdom, we should practice humility and refrain from making these decisions. To "play God" is to engage in the vice (or sin) of hubris (Ramsey 1980; Rifkin 1985; Kass 2008). The second interpretation of "playing God" is more like a stern warning than an in-principle critique of genetic engineering because it is possible that one day we will acquire enough knowledge and wisdom to make some types of genetic manipulations. The argument makes unreasonably pessimistic assumptions that contravene the modern worldview. One could argue that advances in science, technology, ethics, and policy can provide us with the knowledge and wisdom to manage the benefits and risks of genetic engineering.

To summarize this section, both in-principle arguments against genetic engineering have serious weaknesses. Though they may appeal to people who oppose genetic engineering for religious or philosophical reasons, they are not likely to have widespread acceptance. The ethical analysis of genetic engineering should focus on how this technology will impact the environment, public health, society, and the economy.

GENETIC ENGINEERING OF PLANTS

As mentioned earlier, recombinant DNA techniques have been used to develop different GM plant crops, including corn, wheat, potatoes, soybeans, rice, cotton, sugar beet, cantaloupe, and tomatoes (Whitman 2000). Different types of GM crops have been designed to offer distinct advantages over traditional crops, such as increased yield; disease and pest resistance; drought, heat, cold, and salt tolerance; support of nitrogen-fixing bacteria, which produce fertilizers; and enhanced nutritional content and shelf-life (Whitman 2000; Falk et al. 2002).

There are many potential benefits of GM plants. GM crops can help reduce world hunger and can play an important role in the development of sustainable agriculture (Borlaug 2000; Nature 2010). GM crops may also benefit the environment by reducing the use of pesticides and fertilizers and improving the efficiency of agricultural land use, which helps to minimize deforestation (Wolfenbarger and Phifer 2000; Brookes and Barfoot 2006). GM crops may also have significant economic impacts by contributing to agricultural income and productivity (Brookes and Barfoot 2006).

GM crops have steadily increased in market share since the mid-1990s. Global GM crop plantings have grown from 1.67 million hectares (16,700 square kilometers) in 1996 to 87.16 million hectares (or 871,600 square kilometers) in 2005 (Brookes and Barfoot 2006). The United States has been the leading nation in GM crop planting. 57.7 percent of the global GM crop acreage is in the United States, followed by Argentina (19.1 percent), Brazil (15 percent), Canada (7 percent), India (6.2 percent), and China (3.8 percent) (World Resources Institute 2008). In the United States, 93 percent of soybean, 79 percent of cotton, and 52 percent of corn crops are genetically modified (World Resources Institute 2008; U.S. Department of Agriculture 2011b). The most popular GM crops are soybeans (58 percent of GM plantings), corn (25 percent), cotton (12 percent), and canola (5 percent) (Brookes and Barfoot 2006). Most of the GM crops have been developed and patented by multinational biotechnology companies, such as Monsanto and Syngenta (World Resources Institute 2008).

Scientists have also engineered plants for nonagricultural purposes. For example, trees have been engineered to extract heavy metal pollutants from the soil, sequester carbon efficiently, and produce wood and fuel (Mann and Plummer 2002; Rosner 2004).

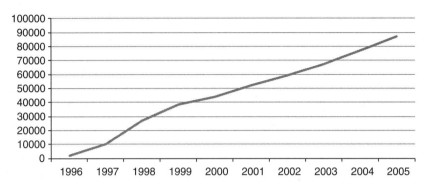

Figure 6.2. Global GM Crop Plantings, 1996–2005 (thousands of hectares, based on data from Brookes and Barfoot 2006).

Tobacco plants are being engineered to detect explosives and toxic chemicals (Potera 2011). Medicinal and aromatic plants have been genetically manipulated to increase their production of medically useful compounds, and other plants have been modified to produce anticancer drugs (Gibbs 1997; Gómez-Galera 2007). Grasses have been genetically modified to tolerate drought and herbicides, and to require little mowing (Barboza 2000). Researchers are also studying ways to genetically modify algae to make it an efficient biofuel producer (Radakovits et al. 2010). (Biofuels will be discussed in more depth in Chapter 9.) See Figure 6.2 for a summary of global GM crop plantings.

Two of the most common types of GM crops are BT and Roundup Ready crops. As mentioned in the previous chapter, BT crops are plants that secrete BT toxin, a chemical which is toxic to many different insect pests, including moths and beetles. BT degrades quickly in the environment and poses no significant risks to human beings. BT crops also pose minimal risks to nontarget insect species, birds, fish, and mammals, and are safer for the environment than chemical alternatives (Mendelsohn et al. 2003). One of the advantages of BT crops is that they produce their own insect poison, which reduces the need to treat the crop with insecticides. To prevent BT resistance from becoming common in insect populations, farmers can plant a non-BT crop near the BT crop, which provides a refuge for insects. Planting a refuge crop allows insects that are not resistant to BT to survive and keeps the population from being overtaken by BT-resistant insects (Pinstrup-Andersen and Schiøler 2000). BT crops can benefit non-BT crops planted in the same area by helping to suppress pest populations (Huchison et al. 2010).

Roundup Ready crops are genetically modified plants that are resistant to the herbicide glyphosate, a chemical contained in Monsanto's herbicide Roundup (discussed in Chapter 2). Monsanto developed these plants so that farmers could make effective use of Roundup. As noted in Chapter 5, many species of weeds have begun to develop resistance to glyphosate. If farmers plant Roundup Ready crops, they can increase the amount of this herbicide that they use, which kills a larger percentage of resistant weeds while sparing the crop. Many scientists and environmentalists are concerned that the use of Roundup

Ready crops will unnecessarily increase the amount of this herbicide that is used, which will cause adverse effects on other plants species and the environment (Union of Concerned Scientists 2010a).

In the 1990s, researchers developed gene use restriction technologies (GURTs), also known as "Terminator Technologies" or "Terminator Genes," which could have had many uses in GM agriculture. Ever since GM crops were first developed, there have been concerns that these crops would contaminate other species through fertilization or other natural forms of gene transfer. For example, glyphosate resistance could spread from GM crops to other plants through interbreeding. GURTs were developed to help contain GM crops by preventing the formation of fertile seeds. GURTs can render hybrids of GM and non-GM plants infertile, assuming that the hybrids contain the terminator genes. Many scientists, consumer advocates, and environmental groups objected to the introduction of terminator genes into commercial agriculture, because this would prevent farmers in the developing world from growing crops from seeds they have saved. Farmers in the developing world, unlike those in the developed world, do not have enough money to buy new seeds each year, so they save seeds (Ban Terminator 2007). In 2000, the UN Convention on Biological Diversity recommended that countries not approve terminator GM crops. In 1999, Monsanto pledged not to develop terminator GM crops, but then it appeared to revoke this pledge when it purchased a company that owns patents on GURTs in 2005. In 2009, Monsanto reaffirmed its commitment not to develop terminator GM crops, while reserving the right to revisit this issue in the future (Monsanto 2009).

Another important innovation that could occur in the next twenty years is the development of perennial grain crops. Perennial grains would have many advantages over current crops, which need to be replanted each year. Perennial grains use less water, pesticides, fertilizer, labor, and fuel than annual crops. They also have a longer growing season and help prevent soil erosion. Genetic engineering holds the key to developing perennial grains, because it would allow researchers to transfer genes into grain crops that cannot be introduced using conventional breeding techniques (Glover et al. 2010).

Although GM plants and crops offer many potential benefits, they have some risks. GM crops have been controversial in Europe since they first went on the market in the 1996 (Butler and Reichhardt 1999). Numerous citizens, farmers, and environmental groups staged protests against "Frankenfoods" and petitioned their governments to ban GM crops, which the EU did from 1998 to 2007. In March 2010, the EU approved the first type of GM crop for cultivation in Europe, a species of potato (Phillips 2010). The EU allows member states to decide whether to permit GM crops within their borders, requires mandatory labeling of GM foods, and has stringent regulations designed to prevent contamination of non-GM crops by GM crops (Chipman 2010; Ramessar et al. 2010). The EU also allows member nations to ban GM crops, which Austria and Hungary have done. In 2006, the World Trade Organization ruled that bans on GM maize in six European countries were illegal because they were not based on scientific evidence (Cendrowicz 2010). Other countries have also banned the commercialization or importation of all GM crops or foods, including Algeria, Benin, Croatia, Ghana, Malawi, Saudi Arabia, Thailand, Zambia, and some countries have banned particular types of GM crops or foods (Center for Food Safety 2006a). Regions and counties in various countries throughout the world have banned GM crops or foods (Center for Food Safety 2006b).

The United States did not adopt any laws dealing specifically with GM crops when products were first introduced. The rationale for this policy, according to government scientists, is that GM crops do not raise any unique risks that require new laws or regulations. Three different agencies – the EPA, the FDA, and the USDA – are responsible for regulating GM crops, foods, and products (such as medicines). The EPA regulates GM crops that produce their own pesticides, such as BT corn or cotton; the FDA handles GM food, food additives, animal feed, and medicines; and the USDA oversees GM meat, dairy products, poultry, and eggs (Whitman 2000). A bill was introduced in Congress to require the FDA to treat genetic modifications to food products as food additives, which would have required extensive safety testing on GM foods before they could be marketed. A food additive, unlike a food, is presumed to be unsafe, and the FDA requires manufacturers to submit extensive safety data. The bill did not pass, however. Another bill, which also failed, would have required mandatory labeling of GM foods (Goldman 2000). The FDA does not require GM foods to be labeled as such, unless the food contains a known allergen (such as peanut or shellfish proteins) or the composition of the food differs substantially from a non-GM equivalent (Food and Drug Administration 1999). Even though the U.S. government does not require labeling of GM foods, many food producers have labeled their foods, "organic," "natural," and "not genetically modified," to appeal to the consumer demand for non-GM foods (Haslberger 2000).

When GM crops were first developed, critics speculated that GM foods would be unsafe because inserting DNA into the genome would result in mutations or changes in gene regulation that would produce toxic, allergenic, or carcinogenic compounds. Others worried that the ingestion of DNA, or virus vectors used to insert DNA, could have adverse health impacts. Some were concerned that GM foods would have less nutritional value than regular foods, or would be more difficult to digest. Critics also speculated that GM crops resistant to certain types of bacteria could contribute to antibiotic resistance by transferring antibiotic resistance genes to microbes living in the human mouth, nose, or gut (Butler and Reichhardt 1999; Teitel 2001; Batista and Oliviera 2009).

While it is impossible to prove that all GM foods are perfectly safe, the evidence indicates that the GM foods developed thus far are no more dangerous to human health than non-GM foods (Lemaux 2008; Batista and Oliviera 2009; World Health Organization 2010e). Industry and nonindustry scientists have been studying GM foods for over two decades. GM foods have undergone extensive safety testing before being introduced to the market. Foods are chemically analyzed to determine whether they are substantially equivalent to comparable non-GM foods already on the market. Foods are deemed to be substantially equivalent if they have the same content of proteins, fats, carbohydrates, vitamins, minerals, or other nutritive compounds (Lemaux 2008). GM foods are fed to a variety of animals to study their potential toxicity and allergenicity, and to better understand their digestibility and nutritional value (Lemaux 2008). Animal testing involves the testing of whole foods as well as the testing of individual genes or gene products introduced into the foods (Lemaux 2008).

One product that failed safety testing was a type of soybean with genes from Brazil nuts that code for the amino acid methionine, which is not found in soybeans. The GM soybean produced allergic reactions in people with allergies to Brazil nuts, so the manufacturer decided not develop the product (Nordlee 1996). While it is reassuring that the safety system worked in this instance and the product was not introduced to the market, this example demonstrates the potential that some types of GM foods can induce allergic reactions in some people. GM food researchers and manufacturers need to take appropriate steps to minimize this risk, such as avoiding the introduction of known allergens into foods (Lemaux 2008).

Many consumer and environmental groups who dispute the scientific evidence concerning the safety of GM foods warn that products should be thoroughly tested before they are deemed safe for human consumption. They are also concerned that GM foods have not been on the market long enough for long-term health risks to materialize (Whitman 2000, Teitel 2001).

The environmental hazards of GM crops pose a more serious concern than the health risks, at this point in time. Perhaps the most significant environmental risk is that GM crops (and other GM plants) could become invasive species that disrupt the ecosystem, destabilize agriculture, and threaten biodiversity. Biodiversity could be impacted if GM crops out-compete native plants and cause them to become extinct or in decline. For example, perennial grains grown for human or animal consumption could out-compete native grasses. GM grass grown on golf courses and lawns could become an invasive species with widespread environmental impacts (Dale et al 2002; Conner et al. 2003; de Melo-Martín and Meghani 2008). For thousands of years, human activities have resulted in the transport of nonnative species to areas in which they have become invasive. In the United States some common invasive (non-GM) plants species are Kudzu (*Pueraria montana var. lobata*), Russian Olive (*Elaeagnus angustifolia*), and Scotch Broom (*Cytisus scoparius*) (U.S. Department of Agriculture 2011a). Human activities will continue to produce invasive species irrespective of whether GM plants are developed.

There are several ways to minimize the risks to native species from GM crops. First, crops could be self-contained in an artificial environment. GM bacteria that produce biopharmaceuticals and other compounds are grown in bioreactors and are not released into the wild (Keasling 2010). Other types of GM crops could be grown indoors. Second, plants can be sequestered from native species and non-GM crops. While containment is not likely to be 100 percent effective, it can reduce the impact of GM crops on native and domesticated species (Conner et al. 2003). Third, GM crops can be rendered infertile so they will be unable to reproduce in the wild. As mentioned previously, "terminator technologies" prevent plants from developing fertile seeds. Though these technologies may not be appropriate for use in developing countries, they may have applications in the developed world, which would help control GM crops (Dale et al. 2002). Fourth, GM crops could be designed to be susceptible to chemical agents that are not dangerous to other plants. These chemical agents could be used to kill stray GM crops without harming other plants.

GM plants could also impact native and domesticated species through interbreeding and horizontal gene transfer, a process whereby pathogens acquire genes from one host and transfer them to a different host (Dale et al 2002; Conner et al. 2003; Keese 2008). Some studies have shown that GM crops can hybridize with other crops (Wolfenbarger and Phifer 2000). Interbreeding and horizontal gene could form hybrids with unpredictable environmental effects. For example, transfer of glyphosate-resistance genes from GM crops to native plants could increase glyphosate resistance, which is already becoming a problem for commercial agriculture in some areas. Glyphosate-resistant "superweeds" could cause significant problems for farming (Powles 2008). However, glyphosate resistance is not likely to confer a significant adaptive advantage to species outside of agriculture. Other traits transferred to native plants, such as drought tolerance or increased growth, may have a more widespread impact on ecosystems. It is important to note that interbreeding and gene transfer also occur when non-GM crops are grown (Dale et al. 2002; Conner et al. 2003).

There are some methods that can help prevent gene transfer from GM crops to other species (Conner et al. 2003). First, GM crops could be sequestered from other plants by use of physical or geographic barriers or containment systems. However, sequestration is not likely to be perfect if plants are grown outdoors, as pollen and pathogens can travel from GM plants to other species (Stokstad 2011). Second, the development of procedures to render GM crops infertile, such as GURTs, discussed earlier, can help to prevent interbreeding, although these methods are not likely to be 100 percent effective (Stokstad 2011). There are no effective methods of preventing horizontal gene transfer, which will occur regardless of whether GM crops are planted (Keese 2008). Also, current methods for detecting horizontal gene transfer are not sensitive enough to monitor the potential ecological effects of GM crops on native plant populations (Heinemann and Traavik 2004).

Another environmental risk is that GM crops designed to produce insecticides could harm nontarget species. Nontarget species could be exposed to insecticides by feeding on GM crops or pollen. Exposures could also occur if insecticides from GM crops enter the soil or water. As noted in Chapter 5, there has been a dispute about whether BT corn poses a threat to the Monarch butterfly. Though current evidence suggests the impact of BT corn is negligible, more research is needed (Romeis et al. 2006). Impacts of pesticides produced by GM plants on nontarget species can be minimized by carefully tailoring desired traits in GM plants to affect only target species. To do this, it is necessary to understand how different species are affected by toxic chemicals, and how these chemicals are dispersed in the environment. Though the evidence suggests that the risks of BT toxins to nontarget species are minimal, this issue merits further study (Romeis et al. 2006). It is also important to note that pesticides sprayed on non-GM crops also threaten non-target species, and that exposures from pesticide spraying are likely to be greater than exposures from GM crops, because spraying introduces a larger quantity of a chemical into the ecosystem (Romeis et al. 2006).

Another environmental risk is that planting GM crops that secrete BT toxins could increase resistance to BT toxins among various insect species, which would require farmers to use other pesticides, which might be less environmentally friendly. However, BT toxins sprayed on crops can also lead to resistance among insects, so the effects of GM crops may make little difference. Indeed, one of the reasons why crops that secrete BT toxins were developed was to minimize the spraying of BT toxins and other pesticides. The risk of BT toxin resistance can be minimized through crop management. For example, farmers can plant crops that do not secrete BT toxins alongside those that do, which reduces the adaptive advantage of BT toxin-resistance and maintains nonresistant insects in the population (Dale et al. 2002).

Disagreements about policies relating to GM crops and plants can have a significant impact on world trade and international relations. As noted earlier, the EU banned GM foods and crops for a period of time and some European countries still have bans. The EU now requires mandatory labeling of GM foods. Zambia, Namibia, and Mozambique banned the importation of GM foods or crops to safeguard their ability to sell their own agricultural exports to European nations. Some African nations even refused food donations provided by the United States because they were concerned about importing GM foods or crops (McDowell 2002). The United States protested the EU's ban on GM foods as a restriction on free trade.

Having reviewed some of the important background information related to GM plants, we can apply the method of ethical decision making described in Chapter 4 to the issues. The first step is to specify the ethical question. The most general ethical question is: "Should the genetic engineering of plants be allowed?" However, there are also many other specific questions one could ask, such as:

- Should genetic engineering of plants for human consumption be allowed?
- Should genetic engineering of plants to produce fuel be allowed?
- Should genetic engineering of plants to produce medicines be allowed?
- Should genetic engineering of specific species of plants (such as corn or soybeans) with specific genetic alterations (such as herbicide resistance genes or terminator genes) be allowed?

There are important differences between these questions because some types of genetic engineering of plants, such as designing plants to produce fuel, may have a minimal impact on human health and the environment, while other types of genetic engineering, such as developing food crops, may have a greater impact. Some types of genetic engineering, such as rendering crops infertile, may have significant negative consequences for farmers in developing nations, while other types, such as making crops drought resistant, may not. In this book, I will address only the general ethical question concerning GM plants.

Once we have specified the ethical question concerning the genetic engineering of plants, the next step is to review the relevant information, including:

- Impacts of plant genetic engineering on agriculture, the food supply, and world hunger;
- Impacts on human health;
- Effectiveness of methods, such as safety testing, which can be implemented to protect human health;
- Environmental impacts, including not only risks but also potential benefits;
- Effectiveness of methods that can be implemented to reduce environmental risks;
- Social and economic impacts;
- Implications for world trade and international relations.

Much of this information has already been reviewed here. Although scientists have learned a great deal about the impacts of GM plants on human health, the environment, the economy, and society, more research is needed. Because GM crops have been grown for only about fifteen years, it is difficult to assess their impacts on human health and the environment. While there is little evidence at this point that GM crops produce acute human toxicity, except for possible allergic reactions in rare cases, they could still produce chronic toxicity, which might not be detectable for years or decades. Animal studies may help scientists to understand the potential for chronic human toxicity related to GM food ingestion, but they have significant limitations due to differences between humans and animals. Computer simulations can help scientists to understand how a GM crop might affect the environment, but it still may take years or decades to observe adverse environmental impacts, such as species decline or ecosystem disruption.

There are three basic policy options concerning GM plants: 1) allow genetic engineering of plants with no regulation, 2) allow it only with regulation, and 3) don't allow it. There are a variety of regulations that might be adopted under option 2, such as: mandatory human health and environmental impact assessment prior to introduction of GM plants, mandatory labeling of GM foods, monitoring of GM plants, and containment of GM plants.

Turning the application of ethical principles to the different options, the principle of utility would favor the development of GM plants, provided that the benefits to society outweigh the risks. As noted earlier, the benefits of GM plants include production of food, fuel, and medicines. GM plants may also contribute to economic development. The risks include potential adverse health impacts. Currently, the benefits of GM plants would seem to outweigh the risks, but our knowledge of the risks of GM crops is incomplete, and more research is needed. The principle of justice would also favor the development of GM crops, if this enhances agricultural productivity and helps to address world hunger, which has its most significant impact on poor people in developing nations. The principle of justice would also require that communities and nations affected by the introduction of GM plants participate in policy decisions. The principle of stewardship, however, would caution against the development of GM plants, on the grounds that they may have adverse impacts on species, ecosystems, and biodiversity. The principle of sustainability would also caution against the use of GM plants, if the environmental impacts of GM plants are not ecologically sustainable.

Because our ignorance of the potential human health and environmental risks of GM plants is significant, the precautionary principle provides the best way of addressing these potential hazards and balancing the different values at stake. The PP would recommend that we take reasonable measures to prevent, minimize, or mitigate the risks of GM plants. Forbidding the genetic engineering of plants would protect the environment at the expense of other values, such economic and agricultural development, and promotion of human health (assuming the GM plants help address world hunger and they pose minimal health risks). Allowing genetic engineering of plants to take place without regulation would promote agricultural productivity and economic development, but would fail to protect human health or the environment. The most reasonable choice would be to allow genetic engineering of plants, but with some form of regulation (Nuffield Council 1999; Weale 2010).

The key questions are, therefore, what form should regulation take and how restrictive should it be? The EU now requires mandatory labeling of GM foods. While manufacturers have complained that this is inconvenient, expensive, and potentially confusing to consumers, this type of regulation is not unduly restrictive, because it does not prevent GM crops or foods from entering the market. The FDA has taken the position that labeling should not be required, unless a GM food contains allergens or has nutritional properties that are different from a non-GM equivalent food. One could argue that health and safety are not the only reasons for labeling foods as GM. Consumers have a right to be informed about information that is relevant to their purchasing decisions. Since many consumers would like to know whether foods being sold are GM, one might argue that GM foods should be labeled as such. Product labeling can enhance consumer knowledge and autonomy without keeping GM foods off the market. However, it may be more difficult to provide accurate labeling to inform consumers whether foods contain GM ingredients, due to the mixing of GM and non-GM products in food manufacturing. For example, a breakfast cereal may be composed of GM and non-GM corn, sugar, or rice. Percentages of GM and non-GM ingredients may also vary from one formulation to another or from package to package. For this reason, it may not be very useful to apply GM labeling to manufactured foods, such as cereals, crackers, soups, or breads. Labeling may be more helpful with regard to whole foods, such as apples, tomatoes, corn on the cob, and so on.

Requiring GM foods to undergo the same type of safety testing as is required for new medical products would be an unduly restrictive form of regulation. Consider the FDA's testing requirements for approval of a new drug, biologic, or medical device. The FDA requires manufacturers to present data on medical products from in vitro chemical analyses, animal studies, and three phases of clinical trials involving human subjects. The FDA also requires manufacturers to monitor their products once they enter the market, and may recall or relabel products for safety reasons. It typically takes over eight years and more than $500 million to bring a new drug to market (Resnik 2007). Applying these stringent safety requirements to GM foods/crops would significantly impede and deter their development.

Countries apply stringent safety standards to new drugs, biologics, and medical devices because these products are regarded as inherently risky. Medical products cannot be marketed until they are proven to be safe and effective. If GM foods were as dangerous as new medical products, then stringent safety testing prior to approval would be appropriate. However, the best evidence is that GM foods are much safer than medical products. A new drug, even when used correctly, often produces many known side-effects. If the drug is used incorrectly, it can produce adverse reactions or even death. The FDA approves a new medical product not because it is completely safe, but because the benefits outweigh the risks. According to Potrykus (2010), drugs or biologics produced by genetically engineered plants should undergo similar safety testing that the FDA applies to other drugs and biologics, however this level of testing is not appropriate for GM foods or other products.

According to Potrykus (2010), the most appropriate way to regulate GM foods would be to subject them to some degree of safety testing less stringent than the FDA's requirements for new medical products. Companies could perform in vitro chemical analyses of GM foods as well as some animal and human studies, without conducting three phases of clinical trials. If a company can prove that a GM food is substantially equivalent to another safe food that is already on the market, then the company should be able to market the food. For example, to market GM corn, a company would need to generate data showing that its corn is substantially equivalent to non-GM corn. For GM foods that are not equivalent to foods already on the market, additional data concerning safety and nutritional content would be required.

Another important issue related to GM plants is what steps should be taken to prevent environmental harm. As noted above, there are a variety of strategies for minimizing the environmental impact of GM plants, such as sequestering and containing crops or rendering them infertile. The most appropriate way of minimizing environmental harm would depend on the type of plant grown, how it is cultivated, and its potential interactions with other plants. Extensive control measures will be needed for crops that are grown outdoors, whereas minimal control measures may be needed for plants that are grown in self-contained areas, such as algae cultivated for biofuels. Careful monitoring should be an integral part of any risk management plan, so that scientists can obtain information about how GM plants are affecting the environment. This information can be used to improve risk management procedures. Companies seeking approval of GM plants or crops should address potential environmental impacts when providing data to oversight agencies. Oversight agencies should not approve GM plants or crops if there are significant environmental impacts that cannot be satisfactorily controlled.

Additionally, regulations may need to be expanded or clarified to cover GM plants not currently covered. In July 2011, the USDA determined that it does not have the authority to regulate a type of herbicide-resistant GM grass developed by Scotts. In the past, the USDA has been able to regulate GM plants because they were developed using plant pests, such as bacteria or viruses, to deliver genes. Scotts developed its grass using a gene-gun, which inserts DNA directly into a plant. Scotts decided to evade the USDA regulations because USDA approval was being held up by a lawsuit (Waltz 2011). The USDA might still be able to regulate the grass if it determines that it is a noxious weed. However, USDA regulations may need to be expanded to cover all GM plants, regardless of the mode of gene transfer (Waltz 2011).

GENETIC ENGINEERING OF ANIMALS

Scientists have applied genetic engineering techniques to animals since the 1980s, when researchers from Harvard University and DuPont developed a transgenic mouse model for human cancers. The animal, known as an "Oncomouse," has been used to test the efficacy of different drugs in cancer treatment and prevention (Margawati 2003). Since then, scientists have developed transgenic mice, rats, rabbits, and monkeys to serve as models for a variety of human diseases. Today, transgenic animals play an important role in helping scientists understand physiological mechanisms, disease pathology, gene-environment interactions, and behavior. Transgenic animals are also used in toxicology and pharmaceutical testing (Chan and Yang 2009).

Scientists have also developed animals that produce drugs or biologics, including human hormones, such as insulin; other human proteins, such as clotting factors; and other medicinal compounds. The animals produce these substances in their blood, milk, or eggs (Stokstad 2002; Margawati 2003; Lillico et al. 2005). One of the main reasons why scientists have developed transgenic animals for these purposes is that these compounds can be difficult or expensive to synthesize in the laboratory.

Scientists have developed transgenic animals for agricultural purposes, including GM pigs, sheep, cows, goats, fish, and chickens. Animals have been engineered for enhanced growth, nutritional value, and disease-resistance (Magawati 2003). Researchers have also cloned animals to produce meat low in fat (Weiss 2008).

Pigs have been genetically engineered to serve as potential organ donors for human beings, which could reduce the shortage of vital human organs for transplantation. To make these animals immunologically compatible with human beings, researchers have inserted genes into pigs that code for human histocomptability proteins. To date, no pig-human whole organ xenotransplants (transplants between species) have been attempted, though there have been successful xenotransplants between pigs and primates (Ekser et al. 2009).

GM animal food products (such as meat, eggs, or milk) have important implications for human health. So far, no GM animal food products have been introduced into the market, though this may change soon. GM fish, designed to contain increased amounts of tri-omega fatty acids (which protect against heart disease), may be the first products on the market. Cow's milk with enhanced nutritional value or less lactose may also be marketed soon (Food and Agricultural Organization of the United Nations 2010). Chickens with resistance to the avian flu could have uses in agriculture and help prevent the transmission of pandemic influenza to humans (Enserink 2011).

Some of the safety issues related to GM animal food products are the same as those that occur in GM crops and foods, such as risks related to the unintended expression of novel proteins or other toxic compounds, and allergens in food (Committee on Defining Science-Based Concerns Associated with Products of Animal Biotechnology 2002). Some organizations have recommended that animal food products undergo thorough safety testing before entering the market. Because some products may be inherently riskier than others, safety assessment should be performed on a case-by-case basis (Food and Agriculture Organization of the United Nations 2010).

The environmental risks of GM animals are potentially of greater concern than the human health risks (Committee on Defining Science-Based Concerns Associated with Products of Animal Biotechnology 2002). GM animals released into the environment, intentionally or accidentally, can threaten existing species through predation, parasitism, consumption, or direct competition. They can also disrupt habitats, food webs, and ecosystems. Some recent examples of invasive animal species that have caused environmental havoc in the United States include African honeybees, the Southern fire ant, Japanese beetles, and Mediterranean fruit flies. Some of the factors that increase the environmental risks of a GM animal include: 1) how easily it can become feral; 2) its mobility; and 3) whether it has caused damage in the past. Some of the most environmentally hazardous GM animals would include rats, mice, fish, shellfish, and insects. Dogs, horses, and rabbits pose some concerns, while chickens, cattle, and sheep pose minimal concerns (Committee on Defining Science-Based Concerns Associated with Products of Animal Biotechnology 2002).

AquaBounty Technologies has developed transgenic salmon, which can grow twice as big as normal salmon in the same amount of time. AquaBounty has submitted environmental, nutritional, and safety data to the FDA concerning its GM salmon. The FDA held public hearings on AquaBounty's application in September 2010. An FDA panel that reviewed that scientific data determined that AquaBounty's GM salmon are just as safe to eat as Atlantic salmon (Pollack 2010a). Transgenic salmon have raised significant environmental concerns, however, due to their size, mobility, and aggressiveness. They are also higher in PCBs than wild salmon. In an experimental stream study, the number of native salmon decreased by a third when transgenic salmon were added. In the past, imported salmon that have escaped from fish farms have outcompeted native species (Stokstad 2002). AquaBounty would address this problem by selling sterile female eggs to be raised only on salmon farms. However, it is uncertain whether this method for ensuring sterility would be 100 percent effective. If only 1 percent of the salmon released into the wild are fertile, they could cause environmental disruption. As of the writing of this book, the FDA was still deciding whether to approve transgenic salmon (Pollack 2010a; Taylor 2010). Some commentators have argued that the FDA should consider the full scope of environmental and public health impacts of transgenic salmon when deciding whether to approve this product (Smith et al. 2010).

Genetic engineering may one day be an effective tool in the prevention of mosquito-borne diseases. Since the 1990s, researchers, private companies, and nongovernmental organizations, such as the Bill and Melinda Gates Foundation, have been working together to develop GM mosquitos. In the fall of 2009 and summer of 2010, Oxitec, a private company, released GM mosquitos into the wild on an island near Grand Cayman, in the Caribbean. The mosquitos were all male members of the species *Aedes aegypti*, which carries dengue, a disease that infects over 100 million people each year, mostly in tropical regions (Centers for Disease Control and Prevention 2011). The male mosquitos have a gene that causes offspring to die in the larva or pupa stage. The GM males mate with the native females, which adversely impacts reproduction. The trial reduced the local mosquito population by 80 percent. These techniques could be applied to reduce populations of mosquitos that carry other disease, including malaria. Oxitec announced its successful trial at a meeting of the American Society of Tropical Medicine and Hygiene in November 2010. The announcement of the release of GM mosquitos upset some scientists because they felt that the research had been kept secret and they believed that the release was premature. Some scientists argue that more research on the environmental impacts and public dialogue is needed before releasing GM mosquitoes into the wild (Enserink 2010). Other genetic modifications being explored include designing mosquitoes that resist malaria, dengue, and other diseases, so they cannot serve as vectors (World Health Organization 2010i).

The environmental concerns related to GM mosquitos are different from those raised by GM salmon. There are no plans to release GM salmon into the wild. The main environmental risk would be the effects of accidental release on native salmon populations and other species. GM mosquitos would be released into the wild, however. Environmental risks include the impact on mosquito populations and species that feed on mosquitos. Driving a mosquito species to extinction could have adverse impacts on insects, amphibians, fish, birds, and other predator species. Another environmental risk is the possibility of accidental transmission of genes to other species. Because local human populations will be directly impacted by the release of mosquitos in the wild, community engagement and discussion should be a key part of any GM mosquito program (World Health Organization 2010).

Genetic engineering also poses risks to the animals themselves. Laboratory animals have been genetically modified to develop many different diseases that cause pain and suffering, such as cancer, Parkinson's disease, hypertension, diabetes, arthritis, inflammatory bowel disease, cystic fibrosis and morbid obesity. Additionally, researchers often delete particular genes in animals to study their effects. These experiments may or may not cause significant suffering, and it is often difficult to predict how they will affect animal welfare. Additionally, laboratory animals may also suffer from various problems related to accidental mutations caused by genetic engineering. Researchers must address these concerns when developing GM animals (Rollin 1995; Buehr and Hjorth 2003).

Large offspring syndrome is a significant risk for calves produced by *in vitro* fertilization. Calves that are too large at birth often have congenital abnormalities, double muscling, joint problems, heart failure, and enlarged organs (Fiester 2005). Large calf size can also lead to difficult births and necessitate C-sections. Large offspring syndrome is thought to be caused by chromosomal abnormalities or disturbances in early gene expression (Committee on Defining Science-Based Concerns Associated with Products of Animal Biotechnology 2002). Another concern is the number of animals needed to produce a successful transgenic animal. Less than 1 percent of livestock embryos that are genetically manipulated survive to birth, and of those, less than 50 percent express the gene. Thus, it takes hundreds of embryos and dozens of embryo recipients (mothers) to produce a successful GM animal. Mutation is another significant concern. Five to ten percent of transgenic mice have mutations that prevent the expression of functional genes. About 75 percent of these mutants die prenatally, but those that survive can have abnormalities, such as muscle weakness, missing kidneys, behavioral problems, seizures, sterility, limb deformities, and inner ear problems. Mutations often do not produce adverse effects until the next generation (Committee on Defining Science-Based Concerns Associated with Products of Animal Biotechnology 2002). Problems with gene expression can also be a concern. For example, improper growth hormone expression can produce a variety of physiological abnormalities. Finally, some potentially useful genetic modifications, even if successful, could cause harm to animals. For example, chickens could be designed to have massive breasts or lack feathers, which would enhance productivity but adversely impact their quality of life (Bovernkerk et al. 2002). To minimize harms to animals, it is important for scientists to take appropriate steps to promote the quality and reliability of gene transfer methods and to understand the potential impact of genetic modifications. Animal welfare should be of paramount concern when designing animals for use in laboratory testing or agriculture (Committee on Defining Science-Based Concerns Associated with Products of Animal Biotechnology 2002, Rollin 1995).

In the United States, the FDA regulates GM foods fed to animals, GM animals that produce drugs or biologics for human use, GM animals used as research tools, and GM animals that provide food products for human consumption, such as milk or eggs. On January 15, 2009, the FDA issued industry guidance on transgenic animals. The FDA stated that it will not allow food produced from GM animals to enter the market unless it has determined that the food is safe. The FDA will make decisions about GM animals on a case-by-case basis, based on their potential human health risks. The FDA does not require pre-market approval for animals deemed to be low risk, such as transgenic mice used in biomedical research (Food and Drug Administration 2009). Other agencies with some jurisdiction over GM animals include the USDA, which regulates GM livestock, meat, and poultry; and the Office of Laboratory Animal Welfare at the NIH, which oversees transgenic animals produced for NIH-funded research projects. Also, academic institutions have animal care and use committees, which oversee research involving animals, such as genetic engineering research (Committee on Defining Science-Based Concerns Associated with Products of Animal Biotechnology 2002).

We can also use the method for ethical decision making described in Chapter 4 to examine the controversies concerning GM animals. The most general ethical question would be, "Should genetic engineering of animals be allowed?" There are also specific questions, such as:

- Should genetic engineering of animals for research be allowed?
- Should genetic engineering of animals for agriculture be allowed?
- Should genetic engineering of animals for drug production be allowed?
- Should genetic engineering of animals for xenotransplantation be allowed?
- Should specific types of genetic modifications of animals, such as featherless chickens, or mosquitoes that do not transmit malaria, be allowed?

There are important differences between the ethical concerns related to these questions. For example, genetic engineering of animals for research poses virtually no risks to human health, but genetic engineering of animals for xenotransplantation poses significant health risks, such as organ rejection and zoonoses (animal infectious diseases transferred to humans) (George 2006). Genetic engineering of animals for research poses minimal risks to the environment, while genetic engineering of animals for food does not.

Some of the information relevant to addressing the general ethical question concerning GM animals would include:

- The benefits of GM animals used in biomedical research;
- The benefits of GM animals used in agriculture;
- The benefits of GM animals used to manufacture drugs or biologics;
- Other social or economic benefits of GM animals;
- The human health risks of GM animals, such as the risks of consuming GM food or the risks of zoonoses;
- The risks to sentient animals of genetic manipulation, such as diseases caused by mutations, or intentionally produce traits that cause harm to animals;
- The environmental risks of GM animals, such as decline or loss of native species, reduction of biodiversity, and ecosystem disruption.

Though we have discussed some of this information in this chapter, there is much we do not know at this point in time, and researchers continue to study the effects of genetically modifying animals.

The principle of utility would favor the development of GM animals if the benefits to human beings outweigh the risks. So far, some of the most important benefits of genetically modifying animals have come from advances in biomedical research made possible by developing animal models of human disease. Because these animals are kept in laboratories, it is unlikely that they will harm the environment. As these animals are not intended for human consumption, it is also unlikely that people would develop diseases from eating them. The benefits of animals used to manufacture drugs or biologics would also seem to outweigh the risks because these animals will also be sequestered from the environment, and they are not intended for human consumption. Drugs or biologics produced by GM animals will also undergo rigorous safety testing before they enter the market. The benefits of GM animals used in agriculture may or may not outweigh the risks because these animals could pose significant risks for human health and the environment. Because they will be raised on farms, there is a significant chance that they could escape and cause environmental damage. Opposition to GM animals would come from other ethical principles.

The principle of respect for animal welfare would strongly caution against genetic engineering of animals (Thompson and Hannah 2008). As noted earlier, GM laboratory animals may experience considerable pain or suffering as a result of genetic modifications. Animals used in agriculture may also be adversely affected by genetic engineering. Genetic engineers must be mindful of animal welfare issues. The stewardship principle would caution against the genetic engineering of animals that are likely to have a significant impact on other species, ecosystems and the environment. As noted earlier, deliberate or accidental release of animals into the wild could have significant environmental impacts.

Because our ignorance concerning the potential human health and environmental risks of GM animals is significant, the precautionary principle provides the best way of addressing these potential hazards and balancing the different values at stake, that is, biomedical research, agricultural productivity, economic development, human health promotion, justice, animal welfare, and environmental protection. The PP would recommend that we move forward with genetic engineering by taking reasonable measures to prevent, minimize, or mitigate the risks of GM animals, such as:

- Diligent regulation of the genetic engineering of animals by government agencies with oversight authority;
- Rigorous testing (i.e. testing requirements equivalent to those applied to drug development) of GM animal products used in medical treatment prior to introduction to the market;
- Safety evaluation of GM animal food products, such as meat, milk, and eggs, prior to introduction to the market; GM food products should be at least as safe as equivalent non-GM products;
- Monitoring of the health impacts of GM animal products;
- Monitoring of the welfare of GM animals;
- Careful attention to welfare concerns for GM animals used in research, agriculture, medicine, and other applications;
- Control over GM animals to prevent environmental contamination;
- No intentional release of GM animals into the wild without a thorough environmental impact assessment and plans in place to control the animals;
- Monitoring of any GM animals released into the wild.

ETHICS OF EATING MEAT

We will now switch gears a bit and examine some other ethical issues related to agriculture, the environment, and human health. The first of these is the ethics of eating meat. Human beings are omnivores, capable of surviving on a diet with or without meat. Meat eating raises some obvious animal welfare concerns. Not only are animals killed for their meat, but they are raised in conditions that are often inhumane. In industrial farms, thousands of chickens, turkeys, cows, and pigs are kept together in close quarters, with little room to move. They may live in crates, sheds, or feed lots, often surrounded by feces and filth. They are usually given hormones to induce growth and meat production. Some become so large that they break bones or collapse under their own weight. They often suffer from diseases and distress related to crowded living conditions. When animals are slaughtered, they may experience severe pain before dying. Many people have decided to become vegetarians out of concern for the welfare of animals (Singer and Mason 2007; GoVeg.com 2010). Two and one-half percent of the people in the United States are vegetarians (American Dietetic Association and Dieticians of Canada 2003).

There are other reasons for adopting a vegetarian lifestyle. Many people abstain from eating meat to derive health benefits such as reduced risk of obesity, heart disease, hypertension, type II diabetes, prostate cancer, gallstones, rheumatoid arthritis, diverticular disease, and colon cancer. Vegetarians tend to have lower levels of blood cholesterol and saturated fat, as compared to meat eaters, and higher levels of carbohydrates, dietary fiber, and antioxidants, which can lower the risk of cancer. Because some essential nutrients are difficult to obtain on a vegetarian diet, people who do not eat meat must plan their diet carefully to make sure that they meet the nutritional requirements. The use of fortified foods or supplements can help vegetarians obtain enough protein, iron, zinc, calcium, vitamin D, vitamin B-12, iodine, and fatty acids (American Dietetic Association and Dieticians of Canada 2003).

Meat eating also has more adverse environmental impacts than vegetarianism. The production of food for a typical meat eater's diet uses 2.9 times more water, 2.5 times more primary energy (e.g., fossil fuels), 13 times more fertilizer, and 1.3 times more pesticides than the production of food for a vegetarian diet (Marlow et al. 2009). Meat production also yields animal waste products, such as feces, carbon dioxide, methane, and nitrous oxide. Hog farms, for example, produce waste products that can adversely impact human health and water quality. People who live near hog farms have a higher incidence of headaches, respiratory illnesses, and diarrhea as compared to people who do not live near hog farms (Wing and Wolf 2000). According to a study sponsored by the World Watch Institute, 51 percent of the human-caused greenhouse gas emissions are due to the industrial production of meat. The study included greenhouse gases produced by livestock and the machinery used in meat production, processing, and transportation. The report also examined the loss of carbon sequestration capacity due the conversion of forestland into areas for grazing (Goodland and Anhang 2009). An earlier report by the Food and Agriculture Organization of the U.N. (2006) had placed the greenhouse gas emissions due to industrial meat production at 18 percent. According to some authors, the percentage of meat in the human diet needs to be reduced to 2005 levels to help combat global climate change (McMichael et al. 2007). Meat eating has increased dramatically in the last decade as citizens in developing countries, such as China and India, have increased the percentage of meat in their diets. (Climate change will be discussed in greater depth in Chapter 9.)

Given the environmental and health impacts of meat eating, and animal welfare considerations, a strong case can be made for vegetarianism. Are there any plausible arguments for meat eating? There would seem to be at least two. First, not all meat that people consume is produced by the food industry. For millions of years, hunting and fishing were the main sources of meat in the human diet. In some hunter-gatherer societies they still are. Even people in advanced nations sometimes hunt or fish for their meat. Although hunting and fishing can cause pain and suffering to animals, they do not produce the environmental damage created by industrial meat production, as long as people avoid over-hunting and over-fishing. Indeed, in some instances hunting can have beneficial environmental effects by controlling populations of prey species, such as deer (Varner 1995). Meat raised on small farms, using organic methods, also produces less environmental damage than industrial meat. Second, in some areas of the world it may be extremely difficult to receive adequate nutrition without eating some meat. In the arctic it may not be possible to grow enough food to subsist on vegetables. For thousands of years, the Eskimo diet has consisted mostly of meat and fish (Gadsby 2004). It is impossible for Eskimos to adopt a vegetarian lifestyle without destroying their way of life and culture.

While there are sound ethical reasons for vegetarianism, it may be difficult to change peoples' dietary habits, because cultural, economic, and psychological factors reinforce a preference for meat. First, in many societies, meat eating is associated with status and wealth. As per capita incomes increase in poor nations, people are able to afford meat. Red meat and dairy consumption have risen 33 percent in the last ten years in developing countries like China, India, and Brazil (Rosenthal 2008). Second, meat eating plays an essential role in many ethnic traditions, family events, and religious rituals. Who can imagine Thanksgiving without turkey, the 4th of July without hot dogs or hamburgers, or southern cooking without barbequed meat? Third, many people enjoy eating, preparing, and sharing meat dishes. For many people, meat eating is an important part of their quality of life that they do not want to relinquish. The principles of respect for human rights and utility would support meat eating insofar as it is tied to cultural traditions because people have a right to practice their culture and culture plays an important role in well-being.

Although vegetarianism is a morally commendable choice for an individual to make, it would be unwise and arrogant to enforce vegetarianism as a matter of social policy, because many people would oppose such as policy for many different reasons. Trying to use the coercive power of the state to make people convert to vegetarianism would be similar to the prohibition of the sale, transport, consumption, and manufacture of alcohol in the United States from 1920 to 1933, which was, by most accounts, a disastrous social experiment. The prohibition of alcohol created a large black market for alcohol, which supported organized crime. Because there was no legal oversight of the underground alcohol industry, the alcohol that was sold often contained impurities, such as lead, which posed a threat to human health. Prohibition also made people into criminals who would ordinarily obey the law, and did not even succeed in reducing alcohol use (Thornton 1991).

One lesson to learn from alcohol prohibition is that it is unwise to mandate behaviors that are not widely accepted. However, this is not the only lesson from this failed social policy. Though banning alcohol was unwise, other forms of government action concerning alcohol can be appropriate and effective. The government should enforce laws concerning alcohol use because alcohol abuse is an important public health concern. Abuse of alcohol leads to adverse health outcomes, such as liver cirrhosis, diabetes, and depression (Medline Plus 2009b). Drunk driving is one of the leading causes of automobile wrecks, and alcohol use is involved in a large percentage of violent crimes. The United States and many other countries have adopted regulations designed to promote the responsible use of alcohol (Thornton 1991). Many governments have also developed educational programs to inform people about the medical and psychological risks of excess alcohol consumption.

Strict enforcement of regulations designed to promote the welfare of animals used in agriculture would be an appropriate way of addressing some of the vegetarians' concerns without prohibiting meat consumption. Educational programs can encourage people to reduce their consumption of meat for health reasons. Additionally, society can promote alternatives to meat, such as artificial meat produced from animal cell lines cultured in the laboratory. Though researchers have made some progress in developing artificial meat, there are still a number of technical problems that need to be solved before these products are ready to bring to the market, and the process needs to become more cost-effective. Also, it is not known whether consumers would find the taste and texture of the meat to be palatable. Some may also object to artificial meat on the grounds that it is an unnatural meat product. However, because consumers willingly eat bologna, fish sticks, hot dogs, chicken nuggets, and other highly processed meats, most people will probably have few qualms about eating unnatural meat. In 2008, the People for the Ethical Treatment of Animals announced it would award a $1 million prize to the first group to bring artificial chicken to the market in six U.S. states (Jones 2010). Artificial meat would still need to undergo appropriate safety testing in order to receiver market approval by relevant regulatory agencies.

FOOD AND NUTRITION POLICY

The relationship between diet and health is well documented. Though many people in developing nations struggle to find enough food to survive, people in developed nations have the opposite problem. Excessive caloric intake is one of the chief causes of obesity. In the United States, 34 percent of adults and 17 percent of children are obese (Belluck 2010). Although obesity rates are highest among developed nations, obesity is now increasing in developing nations, such as China, India, and Brazil, and is becoming a global health problem (World Health Organization 2010f). Obesity increases the risks of many diseases, including type II diabetes, heart disease, hypertension, stroke, arthritis, sleep apnea, gall bladder disease, and cancer. The United States spends $92.6 billion to treat diseases directly related to obesity each year, or about 9 percent of total health care costs (Nguyen and El-Serag 2010). Obesity may soon overtake tobacco use as the most significant lifestyle related public health problem (Marshall 2004; World Health Organization 2010f).

Specific types of food are associated with adverse health outcomes. For example, artificially produced trans fatty acids increase the risk of heart disease (Woodside et al. 2008), sugared beverages increase the risk of obesity and type II diabetes (Hu and Malik 2010), processed meats increase the risk of heart disease and type II diabetes (Micha et al. 2010), red and processed meats increase the risk of colon cancer (Ferguson 2010), and sodium intake increases the risk of hypertension (Mohan and Campbell 2009). Also, eating improperly prepared or stored food can lead to microbial infections that cause food poisoning, such as salmonella, botulism, *E. coli*, campylobacter, and Hepatitis A (FoodSafety.gov 2010). In the United States, there are more than 70 million cases of foodborne illness each year, resulting in 5,000 deaths (McSwane 2010).

The ethical principles of utility and justice imply that society should adopt policies to ensure that food is safe, nutritious, and distributed fairly. Food policies can enhance social utility by promoting health and preventing disease, and also by saving money in health care costs. Socioeconomically disadvantaged people often have difficulty obtaining food that is safe and nutritious due to lack of income or access to high quality food. Food policies can help ensure that people have a fair share of food that is necessary for survival. Some food policies supported by utility and justice include (Fortin 2009):

- Monitoring of food for safety and quality;
- Development of food safety and quality standards;
- Inspections of restaurants, grocery stores, slaughterhouses, meat processing plants, and other commercial organizations involved in food production and distribution;
- Labeling of food for nutritional content;
- Issuing nutritional guidelines;
- Regulation of chemical food additives;
- Sponsorship of research on the relationship between diet, health, and disease;
- Government food assistance programs, such as food stamps, school lunches for low-income children, and so on.

Although the above policies have been fairly noncontroversial, other policies that have been proposed or implemented in recent years have generated considerable debate, such as:

- Bans on artificial trans fats in restaurant food and commercial food products (Resnik 2010a);
- Taxes on sugared drinks and snack foods (Jacobson and Brownell 2000; Chaufan et al. 2009);
- Imposing higher insurance or tax rates on obese people (Johnson 2009; Leonhardt 2009);

- Public health surveillance of diabetes patients (Gostin 2007a);
- Tort liability for fast food restaurants (Gostin 2007a);
- Restrictions on marketing of food to children and adolescents (Gostin 2007a);
- Regulation of the sodium content in commercial food products (Moss 2010);
- Banning of the selling of snacks high in sugar at public schools, including items sold at bake sales (Gostin 2007a; Brown 2008);
- Zoning laws that limit the percentage of fast food restaurants in areas with higher rates of obesity (Gostin 2007a; Hennessy-Fiske and Zahniser 2008).

The reason why these policies have been controversial is that they create conflicts between the promotion of public health and other important values, such as human rights and justice (Gotsin 2007a; Resnik 2010a). Food and nutrition policies can interfere with the freedom of consumers to choose what they want to eat, and the freedom of manufacturers to produce and market their products. As we saw earlier, food plays an important role in cultural, religious, and ethnic traditions and has an important bearing on quality of life. Although people want to enjoy food that meets safety and quality standards, most do not want their dietary choices significantly controlled by the government (Resnik 2010). Many people would view a ban on cookies at school bake sales as an example of health promotion that has gone too far (Brown 2008). Food manufacturers have argued that, while it is possible to remove some sodium from processed foods without affecting quality, significant reductions in sodium levels are likely to radically alter the texture, taste, and freshness of their products, which would lead to consumer dissatisfaction and loss of business (Moss 2010).

Food policies can have implications for social justice, because some types of taxes or restrictions can make it more difficult for economically disadvantaged people to obtain food. Food taxes tend to be regressive, because poor people spend a larger percentage of their income on food than rich people (Resnik 2010a). Zoning laws that limit the percentage of fast food restaurants in a particular area might decrease the availability of food, if other types of restaurants or grocery stores do not take the place of fast food establishments. Food zoning laws may also constitute a form of racial discrimination because they have been implemented in minority neighborhoods but not in white ones (Saletan 2008). Higher insurance or tax rates for obese people may seem unfair to many because genetic factors beyond the control of the individual influence weight. Also, some people with a high body mass index, a common measurement of obesity, are actually in very good health, because their excess weight is due to muscle development, not fat (Leonhardt 2009).

The key to developing ethical food policies is to forge a reasonable balance between health promotion, human freedom, and justice. Because health promotion is a social goal that could be used to justify many different food policies, the potential for excessive government regulation of the human diet is a serious concern. Few people would want to live in a society in which unhealthy foods they like to eat are banned or heavily taxed. The freedom to make lifestyle choices – even unhealthy ones – is an important liberty that should be respected. Though some policies are necessary to protect people from unsafe foods that produce acute toxicity or death, the government should refrain from banning or taxing foods that merely increase the risk of disease if eaten for many years (i.e., foods that may lead to chronic toxicity), unless these foods pose serious public health concerns and less coercive strategies for controlling consumption of these foods, such as mandatory labeling or educational campaigns, have proven to be ineffective (Resnik 2010). Additionally, any tax on food must be carefully assessed for its potential regressive effects.

Recall the discussion of paternalism in Chapter 3. Paternalism involves protecting people from self-inflicted harm and promoting their welfare. Mill held that people should be allowed to make their own choices, even foolish ones, provided that they do not cause harm to others (Mill 2003). Some of the food and nutrition policies in the United States are paternalistic. For example, the FDA regulates chemicals added to foods to enhance taste, color, texture, appearance, or freshness. The FDA requires manufacturers to submit data concerning their products to the agency prior to approval. The FDA will allow a food additive to be marketed only if there is a reasonable certainty of minimal harm to consumers. The FDA can take a product off the market if new evidence emerges concerning its risks (Food and Drug Administration 2010a). According to some scholars, the regulation of food additives, like the regulation of drugs, biologics, or medical devices, is an acceptable form of paternalism, because these products are potentially hazardous and most consumers do not have sufficient knowledge concerning benefits and risks to make autonomous choices concerning these products (Childress et al. 2002; Gostin 2007b).

What about other food products? If government paternalism is acceptable for food additives, shouldn't it also be extended to other potentially dangerous foods, such as artificial trans fats, processed meats, and sugared drinks? There is an important difference between food additives and other food products, however. Though many food additives are perfectly safe to eat, others are not. Some food additives, such as ethylene glycol and yellow dye 3, can cause acute toxicity, and others, such as cyclamate and green dye 1, are carcinogenic (Center for Science and the Public Interest 2009). While some foods can also produce toxicity if eaten in sufficient quantities or prepared improperly, and some can increase the risk of cancer if eaten for many years, they are generally much safer than food additives. Paternalism is justified only to protect competent adults from eating dangerous foods when they do not understand the benefits and risks of those foods. It is not justified as a general strategy for making people eat only healthy foods.

SUMMARY

In this chapter, I have examined a variety of issues related to agriculture, the environment, public health, food, and nutrition. I have argued that genetic engineering of plants and animals is acceptable provided that reasonable precautions are taken to prevent harm to human health and the environment, such as regulation, safety testing, labeling, containment methods, and environmental and health monitoring. Regulations may need to be expanded or clarified to cover all GM plants and animals, regardless of the mode of gene transfer. Additionally, scientists must attend to animal welfare concerns when developing GM animals. I have examined the ethics of meat eating and argued that vegetarianism is a commendable choice for an individual to make, but that it should not be enforced as a matter of social policy. I have also argued that societies should adopt policies to ensure that food is safe, nutritious, and distributed fairly. Bans on particular types of food should not be implemented, unless the food poses a serious public health threat and consumers are not likely to understand the benefits and risks associated with eating the food. Food taxes should be avoided because they are regressive. In the next chapter, I will examine ethical issues related to pollution and hazardous wastes.

7

POLLUTION AND WASTE

This chapter will discuss issues related to the dispersal of pollutants and wastes into the environment. It will describe common types of pollution and waste, and how they impact human health and the environment. It will also discuss pollution issues related to nanotechnology.

AIR POLLUTION

Air pollution has caused health problems for urban populations for hundreds of years. In the 1200s, a commission established in London to deal with pollution emitted from kilns, furnaces, and fireplaces recommended restrictions on coal burning, which were largely ignored. As noted in Chapter 2, pollution from coal-burning factories and steam engines during the Industrial Revolution in nineteenth-century England did not trigger any air quality legislation. Several events in the twentieth century led many countries to adopt air pollution regulations. A severe air pollution episode killed sixty people in Meuse Valley, Belgium in 1930, and, in 1948, an industrial air pollution event killed twenty people in Sonora, Pennsylvania. In December 1952, a dense cloud of air pollution from the burning of coal to heat homes settled over London. The cloud, known as the London Fog, contained sulfur dioxide and particulate matter. During a two-week period in which sulfur dioxide levels tripled, the mortality rate tripled. It is estimated that as many as 12,000 people died as a direct result of the London Fog (Bell and Davis 2001; Bell and Samet 2010).

Air pollution can occur both outdoors (e.g., automobile exhaust) and indoors (e.g., tobacco smoke). Sources of air pollution may be stationary (e.g., factories) or mobile (e.g., automobiles). While exposure to high levels of air pollution can produce acute health problems, such as respiratory infections, decreased lung function, and death, exposures to lower levels of air pollution over the long term can cause or exacerbate many different respiratory diseases, including asthma, bronchitis, emphysema, lung cancer, and chronic obstructive pulmonary disease. Chronic exposure to air pollution has been also linked to kidney, liver, and nervous system damage; cardiovascular disease; birth defects; and reproductive problems. Air pollution can also cause unwanted symptoms, such as eye and throat irritation, nausea, and sinus congestion (Environmental Protection Agency 2007; Bell and Samet 2010).

Types of air pollution that pose significant problems for human health and the environment include:

- **Particulate matter (PM)**, is solid or liquid particles suspended in the air. PM includes particles produced from the combustion of fossil fuels, organic material, or industrial activity. It also includes pollen, dust, and mold. PM is classified according to the size of the particles. While larger particles are stopped by the nose and mucous membranes, fine particles (diameter of 2.5 microns or less) and ultrafine particles (0.1 microns or less) can penetrate deep into the lung alveoli (Bell and Samet 2010). Exposure to larger, fine, and ultrafine PM matter can cause respiratory inflammation and irritation and decreased lung function; increased risk for cardiovascular disease and mortality; and can exacerbate lung diseases, such as asthma (Laumbach 2010). Exposure to the PM in tobacco smoke is a major health concern. It has been established that smoking greatly increases the risk of lung cancer, cardiovascular disease, and emphysema. Recent evidence suggests that exposure to second-hand smoke also increases the risk of cardiovascular and pulmonary disease (Pope et al. 2010).
- **Sulfur dioxide (SO_2).** Sulfur dioxide is produced from the combustion of coal or metal ores. In the United States, electric power plants are the main sources of SO_2. Other sources include the burning of coal in cooking and heating, metal processing, factories, and volcanic activity. SO_2 is converted into sulfuric acid in the atmosphere, which dissolves in water droplets and forms acid rain. Acid rain has widespread adverse impacts on vegetation and animal life, and can lead to species decline and loss of biodiversity (Lovett et al. 2009). Inhaled SO_2 can contribute to various respiratory problems, such as reduced lung function and airway constriction. SO_2 was a major component of the London Fog of 1952 (Bell and Samet 2010).
- **Nitrogen oxides** (e.g., NO_2, NO also known as **NOx**). Nitrogen oxides are formed during combustion, when atmospheric nitrogen is oxidized. Anthropogenic sources of nitrogen oxides include automobile engines, industrial processes, electric utilities, tobacco smoke, and kerosene and gas stoves and heaters. Nitrogen oxides are toxic gases, which are soluble in water. They can cause irritation of the eyes, nose, and throat; increased susceptibility to respiratory infections; and decreased lung function. Nitrogen oxides play a key role in the formation of tropospheric ozone (Bell and Samet 2010).
- **Carbon oxides (CO_2, CO).** CO_2 is a gas produced by combustion of fossil fuels and organic matter, industrial processes, cement manufacturing, production of metals (such as steel and iron), and animal respiration. Most of the anthropogenic CO_2 is produced by production of electricity and transportation. CO_2 is a major contributor to global warming, which can have major impacts on human health and the environment (Environmental Protection Agency 2010e). (Climate change issues will be discussed in more depth in Chapter 9.) CO is gas formed by the incomplete combustion of fossil

fuels and organic materials. Most of the atmospheric CO is produced by automobiles. CO is toxic to animals that use hemoglobin to transport oxygen because it binds with hemoglobin and prevents oxygen transport (Bell and Samet 2010).

- **Volatile organic compounds (VOCs)**. VOCs are chemicals, such as benzene, chloroform, and formaldehyde, which evaporate easily at room temperature. Anthropogenic sources of VOCs include motor vehicles, aircraft, construction machinery, chemical processing, and electric power generation. Most of the VOCs in the atmosphere are produced by vegetation. VOCs are chemical precursors to ozone (discussed as follows) and can cause respiratory irritation, headaches, and cancer. Benzene is a known carcinogen (Bell and Samet 2010).

- **Chlorofluorocarbons (CFCs)**. CFCs, discussed in Chapter 2, can damage the protective ozone layer when released into the atmosphere. CFCs are man-made compounds that are inert and liquid at room temperature and normal atmospheric pressures. They have been used as coolants for refrigerators and air conditioning systems, solvents for electronics, and propellants for aerosol sprays. Decreases in stratospheric ozone levels result in increases in UV radiation reaching the surface of the Earth. Excessive exposure to UV radiation is harmful to all life forms because it causes genetic damage (Rowland 2006). CFCs are also greenhouse gases.

- **Tropospheric ozone (O_3)**. O_3 is formed when light energy interacts with oxygen and nitrogen oxides or VOCs. As mentioned previously, the layer of ozone in the stratosphere (about six to ten miles in elevation) helps to protect living things from excessive amounts of UV radiation. O_3 also occurs in the lowest level of the atmosphere, the troposphere. Tropospheric ozone exposure can decrease lung function, constrict airways, and produce respiratory irritation. Asthmatics are particular susceptible to the effects of ozone (Bell and Samet 2010; Laumbach 2010).

- **Heavy metals**. Lead can enter the atmosphere as a result of industrial processes, such as smelting, waste incineration, and battery production. For many years, lead was added to gasoline to improve engine function, but most countries have outlawed leaded gasoline, as a result of increased knowledge about the dangers of lead exposure. Children are especially susceptible to the effects of lead, which can cause neurological, cognitive, and developmental problems. Coal combustion is the primary source of atmospheric mercury, which enters the ecosystems when microorganisms convert it into methyl mercury. As mentioned in Chapter 2, mercury can accumulate and concentrate in the food chain. Excessive exposures to mercury can result in damage to the nervous system and kidneys, and produce memory loss and problems with coordination and vision. Children are also especially susceptible to the adverse effects of mercury (Bell and Samat 2010). Inhalation of manganese can also produce adverse respiratory effects (Davis 1999).

- **Toxic air pollutants**. Toxic air pollutants include a variety of compounds that can cause acute toxicity if inhaled, such as asbestos, hydrochloric acid, naphthalene, methyl bromide, heavy metals, and PCBs. Exposure to these pollutants often occurs in occupational settings, such as factory work, auto repair, and home construction. Acute and chronic exposures to these pollutants can adversely impact the neurological, reproduction, respiratory, and immune systems. Long-term exposure can lead to cancer (Samet et al. 2009; Bell and Samat 2010). One of the worst environmental disasters involved exposure to toxic air pollutants. On December 3, 1984, forty tons of methyl isocyanate gas leaked from Union Carbide's pesticide plant in Bhopal, India. The accident killed 3,800 people and severely injured many more. Thousands of people also developed long-term, chronic health problems as a result of their exposure. The company agreed to pay $470 million to the Indian government as part of a legal settlement (Broughton 2005).

- **Radioactive pollutant**s. Radon gas is emitted naturally from the soil in some areas and may collect in homes, where it can pose a health risk. For example, long-term exposure to radon gas can cause lung cancer. Proper ventilation of homes can reduce this risk. Radioactive gases may also be released during testing of nuclear weapons or accidents at nuclear power plants (Bell and Samat 2010).

Most developed nations have laws that regulate outdoor and indoor air pollution levels. In the United States, the Clean Air Act (CAA) authorizes the EPA to establish ambient air quality standards to protect human health and the environment. The CAA was passed in 1963, and was amended in 1970, 1977, and 1990. Pollutants regulated under the CAA include particulate matter, tropospheric ozone, sulfur oxides, nitrogen oxides, carbon monoxide, lead, and hazardous air pollutants, such as VOCs, and atmospheric pesticides. The EPA regulates pollutants from automobile emissions, electric power plants, and factories (Environmental Protection Agency 2010f). Implementation of the CAA has significantly improved the air quality in the United States according to EPA surveys of 255 sites across the country (Environmental Protection Agency 2011b) (see Figures 7.1 and 7.2). In the 1990s, many state and local governments adopted laws banning indoor smoking in public places after epidemiological data demonstrated that exposure to second-hand smoke is a significant health risk (Frumkin 2010b). OSHA regulations set standards for exposures to airborne toxins in the workplace (Perry and Hu 2010).

Although most developed nations have adopted laws that have significantly improved air quality, air pollution is a serious problem in some developing nations. For example, China's rapid industrialization and economic growth have led to air pollution problems. Major sources of pollutants include coal combustion in electric power plants, automobile emissions, industrial processes, and building construction. Indoor air pollution from cooking and heating is also a major concern. Since the 1990s, levels of PM, ozone, nitrogen oxides, sulfur oxides, and other pollutants in China have risen dramatically. China has overtaken the United States and is now the world's largest producer of greenhouse gases. Urban areas have been affected most by these changes. As one would expect, the rise in air pollution has led to increases in respiratory illnesses and cardiovascular disease. One reason why developing nations, such as China, have significant air pollution problems is that they have lenient air pollution laws and lax enforcement. In the last five years, however, China has become

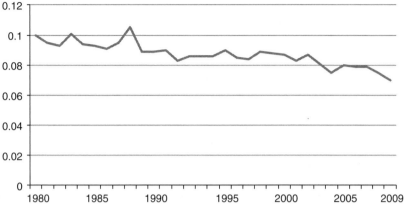

Figure 7.1. U.S. Ozone Air Quality, 1980–2009 (based on EPA data).

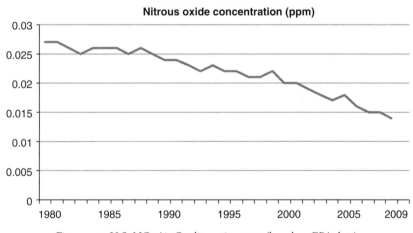

Figure 7.2. U.S. NO$_2$ Air Quality, 1980–2009 (based on EPA data).

much more environmentally minded, and has strengthened its pollution regulations and beefed up enforcement. It has also invested a great deal of money in developing sources of energy other than fossil fuels, such as solar, wind, and hydrothermal power (Zhang et al. 2010).

One of the controversial issues related to air pollution control is whether to regulate CO_2 emissions. CO_2 is a natural product of animal respiration or other organic processes, such as fermentation. CO_2 is not considered to be a highly toxic or dangerous gas. The main health risk of CO_2 exposure comes from the displacement of oxygen in an enclosed space. Climate change produced by global warming is the most important environmental and public health risk related to anthropogenic CO_2 production. Many industrialized nations have begun regulating greenhouse gases in response to this risk, although the United States does not have any regulations on greenhouse gases. However, as a result of a lawsuit against the EPA in 2007, the U.S. Supreme Court ruled the agency must determine whether greenhouse gases harm the environment and public health. In 2009, the EPA announced that it would begin developing regulations pertaining to CO_2, methane, and four other greenhouse gases. Environmental groups welcomed the announcement, but business interests argued that regulations on CO_2 would harm the economy, because they would increase the cost of transportation and electricity production (Broder 2009). While the Obama administration has supported EPA regulation of greenhouse gases, this policy could change if a Republican administration comes into power.

On December 11, 1997, eighty-four nations signed the Kyoto Protocol, an international treaty that sets greenhouse gas emission targets for thirty-seven industrialized nations and the European community. To date, 190 nations have signed the treaty. Industrialized nations and European countries would be obligated to reduce emissions to 5 percent below 1990 levels. One of the main mechanisms for reducing emissions would be to establish a market in greenhouse gas emissions. According to the idea, known as cap and trade, nations would cap their total level of greenhouse gas emissions and a market for emissions would be established. Under a cap and trade system for CO_2, large producers, such as power plants or factories, would purchase emission permits from the government. Permits could also be bought and sold on the market. For example, a company that plans to increase its emissions beyond its allotted amount could purchase permits from another company that has is emitting less than its allotted amount. This system would encourage companies to develop novel ways of reducing their emissions, because they would have incentives to reduce the amount of money they spend on permits or increase the amount of money they receive from selling permits. The cap could be gradually lowered over time to reduce overall emission levels (Environmental Defense Fund 2011). Cap and trade differs from traditional environmental regulations because it regulates a pollution market rather than specific sources of pollution, such as factories, electric power plants, and so on. The treaty would also include provisions for verifying compliance with emissions targets (United Nations Framework Convention on Climate Change 2010).

The United States never ratified the Kyoto Protocol, due to concerns about the economic impacts of setting limits on greenhouse gas emissions and China and India's decision to not participate in the accord (Rosenthal 2009). In December 2009, dozens of countries, including China, India, and the United States, worked toward a new climate change agreement in Copenhagen, Denmark, but no accord was reached (Friedman 2009; Stone 2010; Broder 2010b). In December 2011, the same group met in Durban, South Africa, and were able to reach an agreement in principle, not a treaty, known as the Durban Platform. The agreement requires all parties, including developing nations, to take steps to control greenhouse gas emissions. It also calls for developed nations to provide aid to developing nations to help them adapt to climate change. Following this agreement in principle, a new climate change treaty will be negotiated in 2015 (Eilperin 2011a).

ETHICS OF AIR POLLUTION

Air pollution raises a number of issues involving conflicts among ethical principles. One of the most important dilemmas related to air pollution is how best to balance economic development and protection of human health and the environment. Economic development is essential to promoting human health, reducing poverty, and avoiding famine (Bloom and Canning 2000; Marmot and Wilkinson 2005). However, activities related to economic development, such as electric power generation, transportation, mining, construction, industry, and agriculture, produce air pollution. Whether the setting is nineteenth-century England or twenty-first-century China, the story is the same: Harmful levels of air pollution accompany rapid industrialization and economic growth. The key is to find the right balance of environmental and public health protection and economic growth.

Consider the controversies surrounding the Kyoto Protocol. As noted earlier, the United States and other industrialized nations were concerned about the economic impacts of the agreement due to the increased energy costs resulting from regulations designed to reduce the use of fossil fuels. According to the Congressional Budget Office, climate change legislation that complies with the Kyoto Protocol would reduce the United States' gross domestic product by up to 0.75 percent in 2020 and up to 3.5 percent in 2050. It would also reduce household income and labor productivity. Though there will be economic benefits of reducing greenhouse gas emissions, including a shift to an economy that relies less on fossil fuels for energy, the adverse economic impacts of reducing greenhouse gas emissions would be real and substantial (Congressional Budget Office 2009). Because estimates of the economic impacts of pollution control policies are based on mathematical models informed by various assumptions, responsible scientists may disagree about the economic costs and benefits of these policies (Friedman 2009). Assumptions pertaining to the development of nonfossil fuel energy sources and greenhouse gas removal methods can be problematic because they depend on uncertain forecasts of technological advances. Most people agree that it is important to protect the environment and public health – but at what cost? Reasonable people may disagree about appropriate target levels for greenhouse gas emissions and the best way to achieve these levels (e.g., cap and trade, source regulation, or other methods).

The principle of utility has direct applications to debates about air pollution regulation because activities that produce air pollution, such as economic development, transportation, agriculture, and industry have beneficial effects, but pollution has harmful effects on public health. To estimate the benefits and risks of air pollution regulations it is important to have a good understanding of their impact on economic development, industry, agriculture, and other human activities, as well as the potential benefits and risks for public health. The principle of utility would recommend air pollution regulations that yield a favorable balance of social benefits and risks.

Justice is another ethical issue related to air pollution. People living near coal-burning electric plants have greater exposures to sulfur oxides. Urban residents are exposed to higher levels of ozone than residents of rural areas. People who work in a steel mill have higher exposures to heavy metals and toxic pollutants than people who do not work in the mill. The ethical question that needs to be considered is whether these differences are fair, and, if not, what should be done to address them. Air pollution regulations can help to address some of these environmental inequalities by limiting the amounts of pollution produced from various sources. However, some differences in exposure will inevitably remain. One of the criticisms of cap and trade policies is that they control the aggregate level of air pollution, not the distribution of pollution. Some polluters could purchase a large number of pollution permits to greatly increase their output, which would have adverse impacts on communities living near those polluters (Sagoff 1984). If it turns out the cap and trade schemes are the most effective way of minimizing some types of air pollution, this could create a conflict between pollution control and justice.

International justice issues have been a major concern in climate change treaty negotiations. The Kyoto Protocol focused on controlling the greenhouse gas emissions of industrialized and European nations, and exempted developing nations. While it makes sense to concentrate on controlling the output of the largest polluters, one could argue that developing nations should be required to take some action to control their emissions because all nations should do their part to help reduce greenhouse gas emissions. Developing nations may argue, however, that their economies are too fragile to bear even the slightest burden of greenhouse gas restrictions. They need to be allowed to develop economically before facing pollution restrictions similar to those that apply to developed nations. The Durban Platform represents a shift from Kyoto, because it requires developing nations to control their emissions. (Environmental justice issues will be discussed in greater depth in Chapter 10.)

Air pollution can also raise issues concerning individual rights. Consider the debate over second-hand smoke. Before the 1980s, smoking was common in public areas in the United States and many other countries. Some restaurants and bars had nonsmoking sections for customers who did not like to breathe tobacco smoke, but second-hand smoke was not considered to be a major public health issue. The issue was framed in terms of smokers' rights vs. nonsmokers' rights, and the smokers won this contest, with some minimal concessions to nonsmokers. Evidence concerning the health risks related to second-hand smoke that emerged in the 1980s tilted the balance of ethical considerations toward nonsmokers. As long as smoking was considered merely an irritation to nonsmokers, and not a significant health concern, the smokers prevailed because irritation is not a sufficient reason for restricting individual rights. If smoking is likely to harm a nonsmoker's health, however, this would be a good reason to restrict smokers' rights (Goodin 1990). The structure of this argument parallels Mill's harm principle, discussed in Chapter 3.

Although most people would now agree that smoking should be restricted in public places to safeguard health, smoking raises other, controversial ethical issues. For example, a parent who smokes around a child can negatively impact the child's health, especially if the child has asthma or some other respiratory disease. Some have argued, following the logic of the harm principle, that parental smoking rights can be restricted to protect the health of children (Jarvie and Malone 2008). In *Lizzio v. Lizzio* (1994), the New York City Family

Court determined that a parent's refusal to stop smoking around an asthmatic child is a valid reason for awarding custody to the nonsmoking parent. In *Johnita v. David* (2002), the New York City Family Court ruled that parental smoking can be a reason for awarding custody to a nonsmoking parent, even if the child does not have a respiratory disease, because exposure to second-hand smoke is not in the child's best interests.

While it is hard to argue against protecting the health of children, restricting the rights of smoking parents sets a troubling precedent for those who value individual rights and family privacy. Parents allow their children to engage in many activities that are unhealthy or potentially dangerous, such as horseback riding, skateboarding, farming, driving, and hunting. If it is acceptable to take away custody from a smoking parent, then why not take away custody from a parent who allows a child to ride a skateboard without a helmet or hunt? The potential for a slippery slope toward unwarranted government restrictions on parental rights and intrusions into home life looms large here. To protect parental rights and the privacy of the family, most jurisdictions have a legal presumption in favor of parental rights (Dare 2009). However, government action related to parental smoking may erode this presumption.

I will not propose solutions to these different controversies concerning air pollution in this book, but I will suggest that the method for ethical decision making, described in Chapter 4, can provide some insight for moving forward. The method offers a way of developing a reasonable balance between competing values and principles, such as individual rights, economic development, and public health. Though people may disagree about the proper balance of these competing values and principles, the method can help opposing parties pinpoint the source of their disagreement and work toward acceptable policies. Local and national public forums addressing air quality issues can also help promote open, meaningful dialogue among different stakeholders.

WATER CONTAMINATION AND SCARCITY

Environmental health issues related to water fall into two categories: contamination and scarcity. Because water is necessary for all forms of life on this planet, water contamination can pose a significant threat to species, ecosystems, and human health. Water contamination can come from point sources, such as factories or power plants, or nonpoint sources, such as runoff from agriculture or domestic waste. All of the water resources on the Earth – seawater, groundwater, and surface water (i.e., lakes, streams, and rivers) – can be affected by various contaminants. There are two types of water contamination: anthropogenic contaminants (i.e., pollutants) such as industrial chemicals and wastewater treatment discharge, and natural contaminants such as microorganisms and chemicals present in the soil or water. Some types of anthropogenic water contaminants include (Ford 2010):

- **Disinfection products**, such as bromate, chloroform, and trichloroacetic acids.
- **Industrial wastes**, such as acids, anticorrosion chemicals, ash, desalination brines, and fluoride.

- **Metals**, such as arsenic, cadmium, copper, lead, and mercury.
- **Municipal and agricultural wastes**, such as antibiotics, carbon, chemical fertilizers, chlorine, cosmetics, disinfectants, fluoride, fragrances, nitrogen, pharmaceuticals, and phosphates.
- **Petroleum and coal hydrocarbons**, such as gasoline, diesel fuel, aromatics, and polycyclic aromatic hydrocarbons.
- **Radionuclides**, such as plutonium, cesium-137, cobalt-60, strontium-90, and zinc-65.
- **Synthetic organics**, such as PCBs, pesticides, and solvents.
- **Wastewater treatment products** such as nitrogen, chlorine, and fluoride as well as various pathogens that infect human waste, such as cholera, *E. coli*, salmonella, shigella, legionella, campylobacter, and various types of viruses and protozoa.
- **Phosphates, nitrates, and other fertilizers,** which run off from fields and overwhelm water supplies with organic nutrients that cause the growth of pathogenic microorganisms, such as algae and bacteria.
- **Pesticides** (discussed in Chapter 5).

Many types of chemical pollutants become more toxic as a result of chemical or biological transformations that occur when they enter the environment. For example, chlorine added to drinking water can produce chlorinated byproducts, such as chloroform and halomethane, which are potentially toxic (Ford 2010). Trichloroethylene becomes the carcinogenic compound vinyl chloride. Atmospheric gases can also contaminate water via transformations. Ozone is transformed into bromates, which are toxic (Ford 2010). When CO_2 dissolves in ocean water, it increases the acidity of the solution and reduces the availability of calcium carbonate, which many marine animals use to form shells. Increases in atmospheric CO_2 can therefore alter the chemistry of seawater and adversely impact fish, marine animals, and marine ecosystems. Coral reefs may be especially susceptible to the unprecedented changes in seawater chemistry brought about by human activity (Doney 2010).

The common assumption that chemical wastes will be diluted as they spread throughout the water system does not always hold. As discussed in Chapter 2, some chemicals (e.g., DDT, PCB, and mercury) are persistent organic pollutants (Ford 2010). Special attention must therefore be paid to how these chemicals affect water.

Natural sources of water contamination include (Ford 2010):

- **Arsenic**. Arsenic occurs in dangerous concentrations in groundwater in countries such as Bangladesh and West Bengal, but even lower concentrations of arsenic are worrisome. It also occurs in the groundwater in the United States and other developed nations. Arsenic increases the risk of skin disease and cancer. It is number one on the Agency for Toxic Substance and Disease Registry (2009) list of hazardous substances. Arsenic occurs in inorganic and organic forms. Organic arsenic, which is found in seaweed and seafood, is much less dangerous than inorganic (Lewis 2007).
- **Microorganisms.** The release of chemicals into the environment, such as fertilizers, nitrogen, and phosphates, can increase the availability of nutrients in the water and

stimulate the growth of microorganisms, such as cyanobacteria and algae. These organisms produce toxins that are harmful to human beings, fish, livestock, and other species, and can turn the water green, blue-green, or brown. In some cases the water may be covered by a slimy film. Sometimes toxins from microorganisms can also accumulate in shellfish and lead to human poisonings. Natural events can also stimulate the overgrowth of microorganisms.

- **Nitrogen**. Though most of the nitrogen in the water comes from fertilizers or wastewater treatment, bacteria in the soil produce nitrogen that dissolves in the water.

Water contamination can have significant, adverse impacts on human health and the environment in addition to those mentioned earlier. Pathogenic microorganisms in the water supply constitute the most serious source of water contamination. Pathogenic microorganisms in drinking water can cause a variety of infectious diseases, including cholera, typhoid, salmonellosis, diarrhea, *E. coli* infection, gastritis, gastric ulcers, gastric cancer, dysentery, shigellosis, skin infections, hepatitis, hemolytic-uremic syndrome, giardiasis, meningitis, toxoplasmosis, and meliodosis (Ford 2010). About 1.1 billion people, mostly in the developing world, lack access to safe drinking water. Each year, 1.6 million people, mostly children in developing countries, die from diarrheal diseases caused by unsafe drinking water and lack of adequate sanitation (World Health Organization 2010g). Over a hundred thousand people became severely ill and over two thousand died during a cholera epidemic in Haiti in the fall of 2010. The epidemic resulted from contaminated flood waters. Haiti's poor sanitation system was also a major factor in the spread of the disease (Archibold 2010; Robles 2010).

Chemical pollutants in drinking water have been linked to many different adverse health outcomes, including leukemia, lymphoma, bladder cancer, breast cancer, and reproductive problems (Ford 2010). Chemical pollutants remain a problem in countries that have taken adequate steps to prevent contamination from microorganisms.

Many diseases are caused by water-borne vectors, such as mosquitoes. In addition to malaria (discussed in Chapters 1 and 5), other water-borne vector diseases with a major adverse health impact include schistosomiasis, onchocerciasis (river blindness), West Nile encephalitis, and dracunuliasis. River blindness affects about 17.7 million people, mostly in Africa. The disease is caused by a parasitic worm carried by the black fly (Centers for Disease Control and Prevention 2008b). Dracunuliasis is caused by worms carried by copepods. As a result of the WHO's dracunuliasis eradication program, the disease now only infects about 10,000 people a year, when twenty years ago it infected millions of people annually (Ford 2010).

Much of our knowledge of the adverse health impacts of water contamination comes from disease outbreaks and environmental disasters. For example, 400,000 people were infected with cryptosporidiosis and fifty died in 1993, after heavy rainfall flooded Milwaukee's water supply with human sewage. Similar disasters occurred in Milwaukee in 1916, 1936, and 1938. Six hundred and fifty people became ill with salmonella and seven died in Gideon, Missouri, in 1993, after bird feces contaminated a water storage tank. In Walkerton, Ontario, in 2000, 268 people became ill and seven died as a result of *E. coli* and campylobacter in the water supply. The bacteria entered the water because a shallow well that supplied the town was too close to a cattle field (Hrudey et al. 2006). In 1986, a chemical factory caught on fire in Basel, Switzerland. Chemicals from the plant dissolved in water that was used to put out the fire, which drained into the Rhine River, killing thousands of fish and eels. The human health impacts have been difficult to assess (World Health Organization 2010g).

Because many diseases are caused by unsafe drinking water, basic sanitation and water treatment are cost-effective ways of improving public health (Ford 2010). Thirty-eight percent of the human population lacks access to improved sanitation (Water.org 2011). A key principle of sanitation is that drinking water supplies should be sequestered from sewage, industrial and agricultural waste, and other sources of contamination. In developed nations, water contamination is often due to industrial waste, runoff from urban development, and agriculture. In developing nations, human and animal feces frequently contaminate drinking water (World Health Organization 2010g). Lack of basic sanitation is the biggest cause of infection in developing countries (Water.org 2011). Most cities in industrialized nations have water treatment plants that provide safe drinking water for the local population. When people obtain their water from wells, simple treatment methods, such as filtration and disinfection, can significantly improve water quality.

Most industrialized nations have regulations to prevent or minimize water contamination and pollution. These regulations have significantly improved water quality in many urban areas. In the United States, the Safe Drinking Water Act (SDWA), passed in 1974, authorizes the EPA to establish water quality standards and regulate contaminants in drinking water. The SDWA applies only to public utilities, not private wells or private water systems serving fewer than twenty-five people. The EPA sets maximum levels for various contaminants. The acceptable level is a level below which there is not likely to be a risk to health. For some contaminants, such as carcinogens and lead, the acceptable level is zero. The EPA requires water utilities to monitor drinking water supplies and report violations of EPA standards. State and local governments have established their own laws and regulatory agencies that help to enforce the EPA rules and minimize contamination of watersheds from industry, landfills, or runoff. The EPA and state and local governments also have established safety standards for recreational water sources, such as swimming pools and lakes (Ford 2010; Environmental Protection Agency 2010g). Though some developing nations have enacted laws to promote safe drinking water, many have not (Zhang et al. 2010).

Water shortages are an increasingly significant public health concern. In many parts of the world there is not enough drinking water to meet human needs. Water scarcity threatens human health, agriculture, economic development, and national security. In the past, people have engaged in violent confrontations over water sources, and it is likely that access to water will be a source of conflict and controversy in the future. In the last ten years, hundreds of people in Africa have died in disputes over water (Global Policy Forum 2010).

By 2025, 11 percent of nations will face water scarcity (Ford 2010). A number of different factors contribute to water shortages, including population growth, increasing agricultural and industrial uses of water, inefficient or wasteful water use, drought, and climate change (Ford 2010).

Climate change (discussed in Chapter 9) is expected to have a major impact on water shortages. As average global temperatures rise, ice caps and glaciers will melt, which will release more water into the ocean and atmosphere. The increase in temperature and atmospheric water vapor will produce uneven effects. Flooding will affect low-lying and coastal areas, while droughts will impact other areas (Ford 2010). Decreased snowfall resulting from climate change is likely to exacerbate water shortages in areas that obtain much of their water from spring and summer snowmelt, such as regions of India and China, and the western United States (Adler 1010; Immerzeel 2010).

Agricultural practices have a profound impact on water use. Seventy percent of water drawn from aquifers and water reservoirs is used to grow crops. According to some estimates, it takes 1,600 gallons of water to grow a day's worth of food for one person. Improvements in the use of water in agriculture, such as efficient irrigation methods, mulching, and the development of drought-tolerant crops (discussed in Chapter 6), can help to reduce agriculture's impact on water scarcity (Ford 2010).

Many of the methods of increasing the water supply available for human use have significant environmental impacts. By altering the flow of water through a region, dams can cause decline or extinction of fish and other aquatic species. Dams destroy habitats and can eliminate floodplains, fisheries, and wetlands, which leads to ecosystem disruption and species loss (International Rivers 2007). China's Three Gorges Dam, a $24 billion project completed in 2006 with a reservoir length of 373 miles, has caused erosion and mudslides, and displaced 1.3 million people and countless animals (Hvistendahl 2008). The dam has also increased the prevalence of water-borne diseases, such as schistosomiasis infection among people living near disrupted areas. Schistosomiasis infections have increased because the dam has expanded the habitat of a snail that carries this disease. China has begun a ten-year, $26 billion effort to mitigate the environmental and public health impacts of the dam (Stone 2011).

Desalination of ocean water offers a limitless supply of water but current methods use considerable energy and capital and generate waste. Desalination also involves high transportation costs for moving water to areas far away from the ocean (Shannon et al. 2008). Depending on desalination to address the world's water shortage could contribute significantly to pollution and global warming. Until better methods of desalination are developed, desalination is not a sustainable policy for providing a supply of drinking water.

Reusing wastewater from municipal, industrial, and agricultural sources is a promising alternative to dam construction and desalination. However, because wastewater is often highly contaminated, wastewater treatment can be energy-intensive and expensive using current technologies (Shannon et al. 2008).

ETHICAL ISSUES RELATED TO WATER

Water contamination and scarcity can create conflicts between environmental and public health protection and development. Many human activities related to development, such as agriculture, industry, and population growth, contaminate water supplies or contribute to water shortages. Urban development, for example, places tremendous strains on the water supply. Clearing of land for housing often destroys wetlands and forests, which help to purify water. Loss of wetlands and forests can also disrupt habitats and ecosystems and lead to species loss or decline. Urban development also increases runoff into streams, rivers, and lakes, which can increase chemical and biological contaminants in the water supply. Urban development increases the human population in the area, placing more demands on the water supply. To provide more water, communities often decide to build dams and reservoirs, which have detrimental environmental impacts. As noted earlier, agriculture contributes to water scarcity and contamination. Farming uses a great deal of water, and pesticides, chemical fertilizers, and animal waste can contaminate the water supply. Industrial activities, such as mining, smelting, chemical production, and electric power generation, produce wastes that may contaminate the water supply. Increased population growth is a major factor in all water problems because population growth increases the demand for agriculture, industry, energy production, and housing (Worldwatch Institute 2009). People often drink from unsafe sources when water is scarce, with adverse health consequences.

The principle of utility has applications to water contamination issues because sources of water contamination, such as industry and economic development, benefit society, but water contamination also has adverse effects on public health. To apply the principle of utility to debates about clean water regulations, it is important to have a thorough understanding of the economic and public health effects of different policies. The principle of utility would recommend regulations that produce a favorable balance of social benefits and risks.

Water contamination also raises issues of justice because contamination is often unequally distributed. People living near a source of contamination, such as a chemical plant, mine, or hog farm, may have more contaminants in their water than people who are not living near these sources. Justice requires that the benefits and burdens of water contamination be distributed fairly, and that people impacted by dangerous substances in their water can participate in decisions concerning control and mitigation of contamination. To address these issues, it is important for policy makers to understand environmental and health impacts of contaminants and to take steps to minimize risks to people living near a source of contamination. Community members should also be able to participate in decisions that affect them. Environmental justice issues will be discussed in more depth in Chapter 10.

Because water contamination adversely affects sentient animals, other species, habitats, and ecosystems, the principles of animal welfare, stewardship, and sustainability also have applications for clean water regulations. These three principles would recommend regulations that provide adequate protections for sentient animals, species, habitats, and ecosystems. In some cases, the principle of utility may conflict with these three principles because water policies that are favorable to human populations (e.g., dumping waste into a river) may have adverse impacts on other species.

Water scarcity can create conflicts between utility and animal welfare, stewardship, and sustainability. Having a plentiful supply of drinkable water is vital to human health, agriculture, and economic development, but measures taken to reduce scarcity, with the exception of conservation, can have adverse environmental impacts. Damming of rivers and streams is perhaps the most striking example of this type of conflict. Constructing a new dam can increase the water supply but may also destroy wetlands and forests, and reduce water flow in streams and rivers. Dams can destroy habitats, fundamentally alter ecosystems, and contribute to species decline and extinction. As human populations expand, it is almost inevitable that the demand for water will adversely impacts species, habitats, and ecosystems. Population control could help to alleviate some of the pressures on the environment created by the demand for more water. While there is a natural tendency to place human concerns above environmental protection, impacts on species, habitats, biodiversity, and ecosystems should not be ignored when making decisions related to the development of water supplies.

Property rights also impact water scarcity issues. Since ancient times, people have had conflicts over the ownership of water (Global Policy Forum 2010). To help settle these disputes, most countries have developed water rights laws. There are two traditional ways of acquiring water rights: 1) by owning the land on which the water is located; 2) by making beneficial use of the water before someone else does. Even though individuals may claim ownership over water, governments usually restrict the exercise of these rights, because water is a common resource with wide-ranging impacts (Metcalf 1997). Water regulations may lead to conflicts between individual rights and the common good. For example, should the government require a farmer to obtain permission to drill a well on his land when he runs out of water? On the one hand, one could argue that government permission should be required because the farmer's well could drain the local water table and impact his neighbors. On the other hand, one could argue that government permission should not be required because it is his land and by the time he obtains a permit, his crops or animals may be damaged. Mill's harm principle may offer some insight here. The rule implies that governments may restrict water rights to prevent harm to other people, such as water contamination or depletion.

Matters become even more complex – and controversial – when governments dispute water rights. In the early twentieth century, six states in the western United States had a bitter dispute over access to water from the Colorado River. Upper Basin states – Colorado, Wyoming, and Utah – were concerned that Lower Basin States – Arizona, New Mexico, and especially California – would take an unfair share of the water. The six states signed the Colorado River Compact in 1922, an agreement that apportioned different water rights to Upper Basin and Lower Basin states (Gelt 1997). Outside the United States, water access has played a major role in disputes between Tibet and China, Kenya and Ethiopia, Somalia and

Ethiopia, India and Pakistan, Israel and Lebanon, Kyrgyzstan and Kazakhstan, Singapore and Malaysia, and Lusaka and Zambia (Global Policy Forum 2010).

There are no simple and easy answers to ethical questions concerning water contamination and scarcity because these dilemmas involve conflicting interests and values. Laws and regulations designed to protect the water supply can help to reduce some of the adverse public health and environmental consequences related to development, but they cannot eliminate all problems and concerns. Damming of rivers and streams, reusing wastewater, and desalination of seawater can increase the supply of drinkable water, but they also have adverse environmental and public health impacts. Conservation can ease pressures on the water supply without producing adverse consequences for the environment or human health, but conservation alone cannot solve water scarcity problems because the human population is increasing. Public forums can help ensure that different stakeholders can participate in decision making, but they cannot eliminate all disputes and controversies. The method of ethical decision making, described in Chapter 4, can help participants in these forums to identify the important questions that need to be addressed in seeking a fair and reasonable balance of competing values and principles, but it cannot guarantee that all affected parties will accept the outcome of this process. Because population growth has a profound impact on water contamination and scarcity, it may not be possible to adequately address issues related to water without taking steps to limit population growth to sustainable levels. Population control will be examined in more depth in Chapter 9 (Worldwatch Institute 2009).

SOLID WASTE

Solid waste, like air pollution and water contamination, also poses a threat to human health and the environment. People have generated various types of solid waste since the beginning of civilization (Rodenbeck et al. 2010). Some of the types of solid waste include:

- **Agricultural waste** includes solid waste generated from farming, such as animal feces, fertilizer, and materials containing microorganisms and antibiotics. Some of these forms of waste have been discussed in Chapter 6. Solid agricultural waste can contaminate the water supply. Some forms of animal manure and sludge can be reused to fertilize crops. The EPA has special rules pertaining to the disposal of agricultural waste (Rodenbeck et al. 2010).

- **Construction waste** includes waste generated from building construction and demolition, such as wood, concrete, bricks, drywall, glass, wires, nails, shingles, porcelain, vinyl, insulation, and metal and plastic pipes. Special rules and regulations apply to the disposal of asbestos, a type of material used in building construction at one time. Most asbestos has been banned from building construction in the United States due to its adverse health impacts, discussed in Chapter 2 (Rodenbeck et al. 2010).

- **Electronic waste** (or **e-waste**) includes discarded electronic equipment, such as personal computers, computer games, televisions, DVD players or VCRs, phones, and stereo systems. Advances in electronics and information technology are increasing the amount of electronic waste. E-waste is a significant environmental and public health concern because it contains dangerous metals, such as cadmium, lead, and mercury, as well as bromated flame retardants. Some states have banned the disposal of e-waste in landfills (Rodenbeck et al. 2010).

- **Hazardous waste** includes substances that pose a significant threat to human health or the environment, due to their toxicity, flammability, corrosiveness, or reactivity. Solvents, highly corrosive acids, wood preservatives and other chemicals from industrial activities are classified as hazardous wastes. Most industrialized nations regulate the disposal of hazardous waste separately from solid waste. The EPA, for example, has special rules pertaining to the disposal of hazardous waste (Rodenbeck 2010). Hazardous waste may be a solid, liquid, or gas.

- **Medical waste** includes waste generated from health care and veterinary facilities, such as blood and other fluids, tissues, bandages, gloves, gowns, scalpels and other surgical tools, culture dishes, and glassware. There are also special rules and regulations for the disposal of medical waste to protect sanitation workers from exposure to pathogens (Rodenbeck et al. 2010). Pharmaceuticals are an important type of unregulated medical waste. Medications can enter the water supply through the sewer system or from pharmaceutical plants. A variety of drugs have been measured in very low levels in drinking water, including analgesics, blood pressure medications, antidepressants, cholesterol-lowering drugs, antipsychotics, antibiotics, and hormones. While it is not known how long-term, low-dose exposures to these chemicals may impact human beings or other species, this problem is growing concern that demands further study (Fent et al. 2006; Kessler 2010; Lubick 2010).

- **Mining waste** includes materials leftover from the extraction, beneficiation, and processing of minerals, such as aluminum, copper, coal, iron, and zinc. Mining waste is regulated by solid waste, water pollution, and land use laws (Fent et al. 2006).

- **Municipal solid waste** includes items generated in homes and offices, such as paper products, yard waste, food, plastics and rubber, metal, clothing, glass, and wood. The amount of solid waste generated per person in the United States has increased from 987 pounds per year in 1960 to 1680 pounds per year in 2006 (Rodenbeck et al. 2010). Landfills contain mostly municipal solid waste.

- **Radioactive waste** includes leftover highly radioactive materials from nuclear reactors (spent nuclear fuel) and nuclear processing, as well as clothing and other items contaminated with lower levels of radioactivity. Strict rules govern the disposal of radioactive waste. Nuclear waste is stored in special facilities around the United States (Rodenbeck et al. 2010). In 1987, Congress selected a site in Yucca Mountain, Utah, as a central area to store the United States' highly radioactive waste. Scientists had determined that the site would be a safe place to store nuclear waste, but environmentalists and local community leaders successfully blocked efforts to ship nuclear materials there (Winograd and Roseboom 2008). Additionally, some problems with the sight emerged that were not apparent when it was selected. In 2010, the Obama administration decided to abandon plans to store radioactive waste in Yucca Mountain (Kerr 2011).

- **Sewage sludge** is a byproduct of wastewater treatment. It consists of organic solids that have been treated with chemical and biological materials to remove dangerous components. Disinfected sewage sludge may be safe enough to use as fertilizer on crops (Rodenbeck et al. 2010).

Two strategies for managing solid waste are prevention and treatment/disposal. Waste prevention is the most desirable form of control because it poses the fewest risks to human health and the environment. Prevention includes recycling, reuse, and reduction of waste. Many different types of waste are now recycled or reused, including aluminum, steel, plastics, rubber, paper, cardboard, electronics, glass, clothing, furniture, wood, tires, and batteries. The percentage of municipal solid waste that is recycled in the United States increased from 6.4 percent in 1960 to 32.5 percent in 2006. Although this is a significant improvement, the United States is not one of the top recycling countries. Other industrialized nations, such as Japan, Germany, and France, recycle a higher percentage of many types of waste. For example, Japan recycles 95 percent of its glass, while the United States only recycles 20 percent (Rodenbeck et al. 2010). Many states, towns, and counties have adopted mandatory recycling programs. Another important part of prevention is to reduce the amount of waste that is generated. For example, manufacturers can use less packaging or use recycled materials in their products and packaging. Consumers can throw away less food, paper, shopping bags, and other items. Each year, U.S. residents throw away billions of pounds of food. Food constitutes 12.4 percent of U.S. municipal waste (Rodenbeck et al. 2010).

Incineration was a popular method of waste disposal for many years. However, most industrialized nations have greatly reduced the amount of waste they incinerate due to the adverse environmental and public health impacts (i.e., air pollution) of this activity. Most solid municipal waste is now placed in sanitary landfills. Sanitary landfills should be carefully designed to provide adequate room for waste disposal, protect regional groundwater from contamination, and shield local populations from health impacts. Local communities are usually consulted about the placement of landfills, but they seldom accept them without protest. The NIMBY principle ("not in my backyard") usually impacts all debates concerning the placement of landfills and other waste disposal sites. All landfills generate leachate, a liquid produced from waste decomposition, as well as gases, such as methane, ammonia, and hydrogen sulfide. Landfills usually contain barriers below the ground to control the amount of leachate entering the environment. Landfills often have systems to collect and control leachate. Deep well injection is another method of waste disposal that is sometimes used to dispose of radioactive wastes, hydrocarbons, and other wastes that are too dangerous to place in landfills. In this process, liquid waste is injected into stable geological formations to prevent waste products from contaminating groundwater (Rodenbeck et al. 2010).

Solid waste disposal can have a number of different adverse impacts on human health and the environment. Some of the health impacts include exposure to infectious diseases from landfills and medical waste; exposure to disease vectors, such as rats, flies, and mosquitoes; contamination of drinking water; gas discharge from landfills; air pollution from incineration; food and water contamination from chemicals that enter the environment; and exposure to radiation from radioactive waste. Depending on the nature of the waste product and the level of exposure, solid waste disposal can increase the risk of infectious diseases, such as cholera; parasites, such as malaria; various types of cancer; kidney disease; poisoning from heavy metals, such as lead, mercury, and cadmium; respiratory ailments; cardiovascular problems; and severe burns, trauma, or death from the ignition of gases emitted from landfills. Environmental impacts include the destruction of habitats when land is cleared to make room for waste disposal, and loss or extinction of species due to water contamination from landfills or hazardous waste sites (Rodenbeck et al. 2010).

ETHICS OF SOLID WASTE MANAGEMENT

Many of the ethical issues pertaining to solid waste management are similar to those related to air pollution and water contamination. Solid waste management, like the regulation of air or water pollution, can lead to conflicts between utility and animal welfare, stewardship, and sustainability. Waste management policies that benefit human populations can have adverse impacts on habitats, species, biodiversity, and ecosystems. Waste production is an inevitable consequence of many different human activities, such as agriculture, industry, health care, and building construction. As the human population grows and develops economically, more waste is produced. Although reduction, recycling, reuse, and careful waste disposal can minimize the adverse impacts of population growth and development on the environment, these measures have limitations. Thus, to adequately deal with waste management issues it is necessary to address questions of environmentally sustainable population growth and economic development. These topics will be explored in greater depth in Chapter 9.

Because people who live near waste disposal areas may experience greater adverse health effects, solid waste disposal raises significant issues of social justice. Policy makers should address these concerns by minimizing health risks to people living near solid waste disposal sites, and allowing affected parties to participate in decisions concerning the location of waste sites. These and other environmental justice issues will be discussed in more depth in Chapter 10.

The exportation and importation of solid waste raises issues of international justice because some nations shift the risks of hazardous wastes onto other nations. The United States and European nations export thousands of tons of e-waste to Ghana, India, and China for recycling and reprocessing. China banned the importation of e-waste in 2000, but this trade still occurs illegally (Greenpeace 2010). In the late 1980s, 173 nations signed the Basel Convention to address the growing problem of exportation of hazardous waste to developing nations. The Basel Convention includes rules for controlling the exportation of hazardous waste, and encourages countries to carefully manage and minimize their own wastes (Basel Convention 2010). The United States has separate agreements with Canada and Mexico concerning the importation and exportation of hazardous waste (Environmental Protection Agency 2009b).

It is conceivable that some nations might view importation of solid wastes as an economic benefit rather than a burden. The United States government and private companies offered to pay Native American tribes millions of dollars for hazardous waste storage (Scientific American 2010). In 2007, the Skull Valley band of the Goshute Tribe in Utah abandoned their plan to allow spent nuclear fuel to be stored on their land in response to pressure from Native American advocacy groups and environmentalists (Scientific American 2010). Though Native America tribes are not recognized as nations, they have some sovereignty and independence, and can make their own laws. Would it be unethical for an impoverished tribe, a state, or a nation to import hazardous waste in order to promote economic development?

One could argue that it would be unethical for two nations to enter into an agreement in which a developed nation exports hazardous waste to an impoverished nation because the exporter would be exploiting the importer nation. Even though the importer would presumably benefit from this transaction and consent to it, this would still be exploitation because the exporter would be taking unfair advantage of the importer's socioeconomic circumstances (Wertheimer 1999). The importer would not agree to this arrangement if it were not in desperate need of income and jobs. This would be similar to a situation in which someone sells a glass of water to a person dying of dehydration for a price far above the fair market value of the water. Selling water at a fair market price is not exploitation, but taking advantage of someone's vulnerabilities to sell it at a greater than fair market price is exploitation (Wertheimer 1999). Exploitation will be discussed in more detail in Chapter 10.

NANOTECHNOLOGY

Nanotechnology is the final topic that will be discussed in this chapter. It can pose environmental hazards similar to those created by air pollution, water pollution, and solid waste production. Nanotechnology is the ability to manipulate, control, and engineer materials that are 1 to 100 nanometers in size (National Nanotechnology Initiative 2010a). A nanometer (nm) is one billionth of a meter. For comparison, a hydrogen atom is 0.1 nm in diameter, a strand of DNA is 2.5 nm in diameter, red bloods cell are 300 nm wide, and a strand of human hair is 100,000 nm in diameter. A carbon nanotube is 1 nm in diameter and manufactured nanoparticles are 1–4 nm in diameter (National Nanotechnology Initiative 2010a). Though most of the ethical and policy debate has focused on manufactured nanomaterials, many natural substances and objects, such as proteins, viruses, and particles of volcanic ash and smoke, are nanosized (Resnik and Tinkle 2007). Although scientists and engineers have developed new methods for manipulating and fabricating nanosized objects in the last decade or so, manufactured nanomaterials are not a twenty-first-century invention. Tire companies have used nanosized carbon particles to strengthen tires for 100 years, and artists have used nanosized gold particles in paints for years (Allhoff et al. 2010). Many commercial sunscreens contain zinc oxide or titanium dioxide nanoparticles. Research is being conducted on whether these particles are absorbed through the skin (Nohynek et al. 2007; Gulson et al. 2010).

Nanomaterials have generated considerable interest because they often have useful properties different from those found in larger scale objects made of the same material (National Nanotechnology Initiative 2010a). First, nanomaterials often have greater chemical and biological reactivity than larger sized materials due to their high surface area to mass ratio. Second, as a result of quantum mechanical effects, nanomaterials often have electrical, physical, optical, and magnetic properties different from the properties of larger sized objects. For example, the melting point and electrical conductivity of a nonsized particle may be different from the melting point and conductivity of a larger particular made of the same substance. Because the properties of nanomaterials may vary depending on their size, they can have unique and often unpredictable characteristics. A substance that is relatively nontoxic at a larger size may become toxic at the nanoscale or vice versa. Third, nanoparticles can aggregate to form larger sized objects or decompose into smaller sized ones, which can affect their properties. The tendency of nanomaterials to change their properties as they change in size means that it is often difficult to predict how nanomaterials will behave in different circumstances (Resnik and Tinkle 2007). Many different products developed in the last ten years utilize the unique properties of nanomaterials. For example, nanosized filters can block particles that are not screened out by larger filters, such as viruses and proteins.

Nanotechnology is one of the fastest growing sectors of the economy. Private companies and governments have invested billions of dollars in nanotechnology research and product development in the last decade. Hundreds of nanotechnology firms have been launched in the United States, China, Japan, India, Germany, England, France, Singapore, Canada, the Netherlands, and other countries. The United States has spent $14 billion since 2001 on the National Nanotechnology Initiative, a research and education project involving fifteen federal agencies. The 2011 budget for this effort is $1.4 billion (National Nanotechnology Initiative 2010b). Forecasters predict that nanotechnology will have significant impacts on manufacturing, medicine, cosmetics, food production, electronics, transportation, and other areas of the economy. Nanomaterials have been used to insulate wires, conduct electricity, lubricate machines, deliver drugs, filter liquids, detect chemicals, package foods, and strengthen and coat consumer products (Kessler 2011). In the future, researchers may develop nanorobots to perform various tasks, such as diagnosing and treating tumor cells and repairing damaged tissue (Allhoff et al. 2010).

Toxicologists and other scientists have conducted research on the environmental and health impacts of various nanomaterials. Although investigators have accumulated a wealth of data, much is not known at this point, and additional research is needed. One of the biggest obstacles to accurately assessing the risks of nanotechnology is that nanomaterials are not a single chemical or biological class: The only thing they have in common is their size (Allhoff et al. 2010). Consequently, some materials may be completely benign, while others may be toxic or even carcinogenic. Thus, it may be misleading and futile to attempt to assess the risks of nanotechnology in general. What may be more useful is to assess the risks of different types of nanomaterials (Resnik and Tinkle 2007). With this in mind, some of the potential environmental and public health impacts of various nanomaterials are as follows:

- Inhalation exposures to carbon nanoparticles can produce adverse respiratory and cardiovascular effects in rodents. These particles can cause respiratory inflammation and oxidative stress, and can migrate across the lung epithelia and enter the bloodstream. Epidemiological studies on humans have shown that exposure to airborne carbon nanoparticles contained in smoke increases the risks of respiratory and cardiovascular disease (Oberdörster et al. 2005; Savolainen et al. 2010).
- Olytetrafluoroethylene nanoparticles are highly toxic when inhaled, causing severe lung injury and death in rodents after only fifteen minutes of exposure (Oberdörster et al. 2005).
- Carbon nanotubes, which are used in many different products, can also produce adverse respiratory effects when inhaled. Rodents develop respiratory inflammation when exposed to carbon nanotubes. Carbon nanotubes have some similarities to asbestos (Oberdörster et al. 2005).
- Many different types of nanomaterials, including fullerenes and quantum dots, can produce reactive oxygen species, which are molecules that can produce oxidative stress in animals. Oxidative stress triggers inflammation and causes damage to various cells and tissues (Oberdörster et al. 2005). Oxidative stress increases the risk of a variety of illnesses, including cancer, atherosclerosis, arthritis, and neurodegenerative disease (Aruoma 1998).
- Studies have shown that some types of nanoparticles are able to cross different barriers in the body. For example, inhaled nanoparticles can enter the bloodstream and deposit in various organs and tissues, such as the kidneys or liver. Once in the body, nanoparticles can penetrate cell membranes, including the nuclear membrane. Nanoparticles can also cross the blood-brain barrier. Nanoparticles can therefore potentially impact many aspects of physiology beyond the exposure site (Hoet et al. 2004; Savolainen et al. 2010).
- It is not known whether nanoparticles can induce genetic damage, cause cancer, or exert toxic effects at very low doses. More research is needed on these topics (Savolainen et al. 2010).
- The environmental impacts of nanomaterials depend on how nanomaterials enter the environment, how fast they degrade, and whether they can accumulate and concentrate in tissues, organs, organisms, and ecosystems. Nanomaterials can enter the environment through various pathways, such as manufacturing, combustion, excretion in urine, solid waste disposal, and erosion from consumer products. Studies are currently underway to examine the potential for various types of nanoparticles to bioaccumulate (EPA 2009c).

The United States and European Union have taken different approaches to the regulation of nanotechnology and industrial chemicals. In the United States, companies are not required to conduct safety testing of industrial chemicals used in consumer products or manufacturing prior to marketing. Industrial chemicals are regarded as safe until proven otherwise. Only chemicals used in pesticides, pharmaceuticals, cosmetics, or food additives must undergo some type of safety testing before entering the market. There are an estimated 100,000 industrial chemicals used in the United States that have not undergone any safety testing, about 6,000 or which pose potential health concerns (Cranor 2011). If a chemical is later found to produce adverse environmental or health impacts after entering the market, then the government may take steps to regulate it (Schwarzman and Wilson 2010). For example, asbestos was introduced into the United States market without safety testing or regulatory oversight. Regulation occurred only after scientific studies demonstrated that asbestos causes respiratory diseases and cancer. The EU takes a more precautionary approach. According to a 2006 initiative known as Registration, Evaluation, Authorization, and Restrictions of Chemicals (REACH), chemical manufacturers and importers must provide the government with information about the properties of chemicals whose sales exceed one metric ton per year per producer. Additional information is required of chemicals sold in larger quantities. Some chemicals are classified as Substances of Very High Concern because they are known to cause cancer, genetic damage, or reproductive toxicity, or they persist in the environment and bioaccumulate (Schwartzman and Wilson 2010). To market these chemicals, manufacturers must provide the government with evidence of known environmental and public health risks, the safety of intended uses, availability of alternatives, and socioeconomic benefits. The government can weigh these factors to decide whether or how the chemical may be marketed (Schwartzman and Wilson 2010). The Toxic Chemicals Safety Act of 2010, proposed by Congressmen Bobby Rush and Henry Waxman, would amend the Toxic Substances Control Act (TSCA) to make United States oversight of chemicals similar to the EU's approach (H.R. 5820 2010). The legislation has not been adopted as of the writing of this book.

ETHICS OF NANOTECHNOLOGY

The most significant ethical issues involving nanotechnology have to do with managing risks to human health and the environment. People may be exposed to manufactured nanomaterials via drugs, foods, cosmetics, or consumer products. Exposures may occur at the workplace, school, or home. Mammals, birds, fish, insects, plants, and many other species may also be exposed to nanomaterials that enter the environment through the water supply, the atmosphere, or solid waste disposal. As noted earlier, scientists have studied some of the potential risks of nanotechnology to human health and the environment, but a great deal remains unknown at this point in time. Of particular concern is the potential for nanomaterials to cross membranes and barriers in the body, to cause genetic damage or cancer, and to bioaccumulate. It is not known whether exposures to very low levels of nanomaterials can produce adverse effects in human beings or other species.

Given the problems with assessing the risks of nanotechnology, a precautionary approach is warranted (Weckert and Moore 2006; Allhoff et al. 2010) because the threats posed by nanotechnology are credible but not well-understood presently, and the adverse consequences are potentially catastrophic. Although some types of nanomaterials may be completely benign, others could be similar to chemicals that are highly carcinogenic, such as asbestos and PCB, while others could be similar to chemicals that accumulate and concentrate in the ecosystem, such as DDT. Society should take reasonable measures to prevent, minimize, or mitigate plausible harms. Though writers, such as Michael Crichton (2002), have envisioned nightmarish sci-fi scenarios in which swarms of intelligent, self-replicating nanorobots take over the world, these risks need not be addressed at this point because they are far-fetched. It may be several decades before scientists and engineers can build commercially available, self-replicating, nanorobots.

Reasonable measures for dealing with nanotechnology should be proportional to the nature of the threats and be effective. They should achieve a fair balance between competing values, such as economic development, human health, and environmental protection. Banning nanotechnology would prevent adverse consequences to human health and the environment but would hamper economic development. Taking precautions to manage the risks of nanotechnology achieves the best balance among these competing values.

According to Allhoff et al. (2010), an important precaution would be to develop and implement rules for the management and oversight of nanotechnology similar to the EU's REACH policy. Agencies that oversee industrial chemicals and manufactured materials should develop criteria for regulating manufactured nanomaterials according to Allhoff et al. (2010). All manufactured nanomaterials would undergo some minimal safety assessment, such as a characterization of the chemical, physical, and biological properties of the product. Additional safety testing may be required of manufactured nanomaterials that have the potential to adversely affect human health or the environment. According to Davies (2006), the degree of premarket testing that is required beyond the minimal safety assessment should depend on the potential human health or environmental impacts of the product. Manufactured nanomaterials that will be used in medical treatments should undergo the type of testing that the FDA requires of new pharmaceuticals, biologics, or medical devices. Nanomaterials that will be used in pesticides should undergo the type of testing that the EPA requires of pesticides. Additional testing may also be required of materials that have the potential to produce genetic damage, cause cancer, induce toxicity, or bioaccumulate. According to Davies (2006), existing laws that apply to nanotechnology, such as the Toxic Substances Control Act (TOSCA), may need to be strengthened to enable agencies to effectively regulate nanotechnology. Cranor (2011) argues that existing laws need to be strengthened to provide adequate protection from all industrial chemicals, not just nanomaterials.

Further research on the risks of nanotechnology is warranted. Research should include in vitro and in vivo laboratory studies, environmental impact assessments, and epidemiological, clinical, and biomonitoring research involving human subjects. Research should take place prior to the introduction of a new technology and should continue after the product is on the market. It is important to study the long-term effects of nanomaterials on human health and the environment because some adverse impacts may take years to develop. Although governments should invest heavily in nanotechnology research, manufacturers should fund studies on the safety of their products. Agencies that oversee nanomaterials should assess new safety information as it becomes available and make appropriate regulatory changes.

Public engagement is another important area of ethical concern in the development of nanotechnology. One of the main lessons from widespread opposition to GM foods and crops in Europe is that it is important to educate the public about the potential benefits and risks of new technologies and to address significant worries and concerns prior to marketing. Companies attempted to introduce GM foods and crops in Europe without engaging in extensive dialogue and discussion with the public, which contributed to a backlash (Jones 2007). Scientists, industry leaders, and government officials should communicate honestly and openly with the public about nanotechnology (Nature 2003; Jones 2007). They should help the public to understand what nanotechnology is and how it may impact society, the economy, human health, and the environment (Allhoff et al. 2007). The public should also be involved in decisions concerning the regulation and oversight of nanotechnology. (Public engagement will be discussed in greater depth in Chapter 10.)

Nanotechnology raises ethical issues that will not be discussed here, such as concerns relating to the enhancement of human traits, invasion of privacy, military applications, and clinical trials. For further discussion, see Resnik and Tinkle (2007) and Allhoff et al. (2010).

SUMMARY

In this chapter, I have examined ethical and policy issues pertaining to air and water pollution, water scarcity, hazardous wastes, and nanotechnology. I have argued that issues concerning air and water pollution, water scarcity, and solid waste can be difficult to resolve because they involve conflicts between fundamental values, such as economic development, social utility, property rights, public health, justice, national sovereignty, international cooperation, stewardship, and sustainability. Responsible policies and practices should strike an appropriate balance among competing values. People who are significantly impacted by air, water, and solid waste should have input into decisions that will affect them. Because the growing human population is a major factor in pollution and waste production, many of these issues cannot be adequately addressed without developing population control policies. I have also considered the public health and environmental impacts of nanotechnology and argued that the precautionary principle should guide policy development. Current regulations concerning industrial chemicals may need to be strengthened in some countries to ensure that appropriate measures are taken to minimize, prevent, or mitigate the risks of nanotechnology. The next chapter will examine ethical and policy issues concerning the built environment.

8

THE BUILT ENVIRONMENT

As we have seen in previous chapters, location has a significant impact on exposure to environmental health risks. Where one lives or works can affect one's exposure to air and water pollutants, pesticides, solid waste, and industrial chemicals. In this chapter, we will focus on health risks related to the built environment, which includes all of the structures that people create to support different functions and activities, such as work, recreation, education, transportation, habitation, agriculture, and industry. The built environment includes houses, apartments, office buildings, factories, schools, malls, roads, levies, dams, mines, sidewalks, fields, waste disposal sites, and many more structures (Frumkin et al. 2004). In the last 10,000 years, human beings have radically transformed the landscape of the planet by clearing land, erecting buildings, creating cities, and damming rivers.

In thinking about the built environment, three trends are worth noting. First, the human population has grown from about 125,000 people at 1 million years BCE, to 5 million people in 10,000 BCE, to about 7 billion people today. The human population is expected to grow to 9 billion people by 2050 (United Nations 2009). As the population continues to increase, more houses, schools, roads, dams, and other structures will need to be built to accommodate more people, which will increase humanity's impacts on the environment.

Second, ever since the first cities emerged around 10,000 BCE, the human population has steadily shifted from rural to urban living. The percentage of people living in urban areas has increased from 13 percent in 1900 to 50 percent today. By 2030, it is expected that 60 percent of the world' population will be urban (United Nations 2005a). The European population is currently 75 percent urban and is expected to become 80 percent urban by 2020 (European Environment Agency 2006).

Third, land use in many metropolitan regions is increasingly spread out over large areas of low population density interconnected by highways and streets. This trend, known as urban sprawl, has occurred as development has taken place in the suburbs surrounding urban areas. People have left the densely populated inner city to have more space and escape traffic, crime, and other problems. Land use in the suburbs tends to emphasize single-family homes with ample space for lawns and parking. People tend to rely on automobiles for transportation to school, work, and shopping because distances are too vast for walking

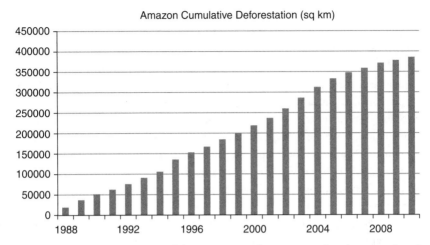

Figure 8.1. Cumulative Deforestation of the Amazon Jungle, 1988–2010 (based on data from Butler 2010).

or biking and alternative forms of travel, such as mass transit, have been underdeveloped (Frumkin et al. 2004).

ENVIRONMENTAL IMPACTS

For many years, ecologists have studied the environmental impacts of land use. Habitat loss or fragmentation is perhaps the single most important factor in species extinction and decline worldwide (Hughes et al. 1997). Habitat loss occurs when an area in which a population or species normally lives, such as a forest, is destroyed or radically changed. Habitat fragmentation occurs when a habitat is broken into discontinuous pieces. Many different human activities lead to habitat loss or fragmentation, including agriculture, industry, logging, mining, urban development, road construction, and water management. Water-rich areas that can support agriculture and human habitation, such as wetlands and rainforests, are frequent land development targets.

The clearing of rainforests for commercial logging and agriculture is a dramatic example of the effects of human activity on the land. Rainforests, an important source of biodiversity, once covered 14 percent of the Earth's land, but now cover only 6 percent. At this rate of destruction, there might be no remaining rainforests in forty years (Rain-tree.com 2010). Between 1980 and 1995, the world lost 12 million hectares (120,000 square kilometers) of forest per year (World Resources Institute 2011). Though the rate of deforestation has slowed since then, due to efforts to protect and replant forests, it still remains a significant concern, especially in tropical regions. Since 1970, the Amazon jungle has lost 60 million hectares (600,000 square kilometers) of rainforest (Butler 2010), an area larger than France (see Figure 8.1).

Though some species have been able to adapt to mankind's use of the land, many others have gone extinct, while others are on the brink of extinction. Some noteworthy species that have gone extinct in the United States in the last hundred years due to habitat loss and other causes (such as hunting) include the Carolina Parakeet (*Conuropsis carolinensis carolinensis*), Passenger Pigeon (*Ectopistes migratorius*), Bigleaf scurfpea (*Orbexilum macrophyllum*), and Round combshell (*Epioblasma personata*) (U.S. Fish and Wildlife Service 2010b). In the United States there are nearly 1,400 hundred known species endangered due to habitat loss or fragmentation, as well as other causes, including flowering plants (761), fish (139), birds (92), mammals (85), insects (60), reptiles (40), snails (35), ferns (29), amphibians (25), and arachnids (12) (U.S. Fish and Wildlife Service 2010c). The United States and other countries have developed laws, discussed as follows, to protect endangered species from habitat loss due to human development.

In addition to destroying habitat, land use can adversely impact water quality. Agriculture, industry, logging, and urban development increase the amount of runoff, which contaminates the water supply with farm waste, domestic waste, dirt, hydrocarbons, and phosphates. The loss of wetlands can also have negative effects on water quality because wetlands play an important role in purifying water and removing contaminants. Clean water is important for supporting human life as well as animal and plant species (Ford 2010).

As discussed in Chapter 7, dams can provide water and hydroelectric power for human beings, but can also dramatically alter the landscape and diminish the flow of water through rivers and streams, threatening aquatic species. Dams can destroy habitats and interfere with the migration patterns of salmon, which swim upstream from the ocean to return to their spawning grounds (Braatner et al. 2008).

HEALTH IMPACTS

The built environment also has significant impacts on human health. As people have shifted to an urban lifestyle, the impacts of the built environment on human health have become more important. People in industrialized nations spend about 90 percent of their time indoors (Frumkin 2010b). Some of the most important buildings that affect human health include homes, schools, places of employment (such as factories and offices), and health care facilities.

Poorly built or maintained homes pose significant risks to inhabitants. People may be injured as a result of falling down stairs with broken steps, coming into contact with broken glass, stepping on nails, falling off unsafe porches, or getting burned in fires from substandard wiring, gas, or heating. People may be exposed to various toxins in the home, such as lead (from paint), radon gas, formaldehyde (from plywood), cleaners and disinfectants, pesticides, smoke particles (from tobacco and stoves), and carbon monoxide (from stoves and heating systems), as well as allergens, such as dust, dust mites, pet dander, pollen, and mold spores, which exacerbate asthma, induce allergic responses, or irritate respiratory diseases. Pests, such as mice, rats, bedbugs, cockroaches, mosquitoes, fleas, and lice may be present in the home, as well as pathogenic bacteria and fungi. Pests can carry diseases (such as the plague or encephalitis), spoil food, or trigger allergies.

Socioeconomically disadvantaged people tend to face greater health risks due to substandard housing than well-to-do people because they may not be able to afford homes that are well-built or maintained. Although lead-based paint is no longer used in new home construction in the United States, millions of older homes in poor neighborhoods still have lead-based paint, which poses a significant risk to children. Families living in these older homes may not be able to afford lead abatement. Federal and state governments have sponsored lead-abatement programs to address the problem, but more work needs to be done. Older homes may also contain asbestos insulation, which poor families may not be able to afford to have removed or covered up. Socioeconomically disadvantaged people often live in homes with water damage, which causes mold, and they may not be able to afford mold remediation. Poor people may face greater exposures to radon gas than wealthy people because they may not be able to afford proper ventilation systems (Frumkin 2010b).

Sound design, construction, and maintenance are also important in schools. Children have been killed as a result of structurally defective or poorly maintained schools. In some cases, roofs have collapsed on children. Some schools have problems with ventilation, indoor air quality, cooling, and heating. Children may be exposed to volatile organic compounds, carbon monoxide, allergens, pesticides, and pests, in schools. Playground equipment, science laboratories, woodworking shops, and art studios can pose unique safety challenges for schools. At one time many schools in the United States had asbestos insulation, but this has been largely covered up or removed (Frumkin 2010b).

Sound design, construction, and maintenance are essential in health care facilities to protect patients and staff from injuries. Proper heating, cooling, and ventilation are also essential. In addition, health care facilities must be built to manage dangerous conditions and substances unique to medical care, such as toxic chemicals, radiation, medications, cleaning materials, medical equipment, and pathogens (Frumkin 2010b). As mentioned in Chapter 5, antibiotic-resistant bacteria, such as MRSA, are becoming a significant problem in many hospitals, rehabilitation centers, and nursing homes. Health care facilities must establish proper hygiene, disinfection, and sterilization techniques to protect patients from infections. Health care institutions have significant environmental impacts because they generate a great deal of medical and nonmedical waste and use considerable energy (Pierce and Jameton 2001).

The workplace poses a number of different risks to human health (Perry and Hu 2010). In Chapters 2 and 5, we discussed some of the risks of exposures to toxic substances in the workplace. Health risks are also associated with buildings and other structures that constitute the work environment. Building design, construction, and maintenance can increase or decrease the risks of workplace accidents, exposures to hazardous materials, and repetitive motion injuries (Frumkin 2010b). For example, underground coal miners face a number of occupational risks, such as injuries or fatalities due to cave-ins; respiratory illnesses, like black lung disease and pneumoconiosis due to inhaling toxic gases and coal dust; and hearing damage from loud noises. To minimize occupational hazards in an underground coal mine, it is necessary to build stable tunnels with proper ventilation and cooling, provide workers with protective equipment, and maintain facilities (Weeks 1991). Building design, construction, and maintenance are also important in relatively safe occupations, such as office work. Proper ventilation, well-functioning cooling and heating, adequate lighting, safe elevators and staircases, and ergonometric desks and chairs can help to protect the health of office workers (Frumkin 2010b).

People may be injured or killed when natural disasters impact buildings. Though it is virtually impossible to prevent death and injury from natural disasters, steps can be taken to minimize the damage. Poorly built homes, schools, or office buildings are not as able to withstand earthquakes, floods, hurricanes, or tornadoes as well-built structures. For example, inferior home construction was a major contributing factor to the death toll from the Haitian Earthquake of January 12, 2010. Over 250,000 people died and many more were seriously injured in this 7.0 magnitude quake (Romero 2010). Far fewer people were killed or injured in a much larger (8.8 magnitude) earthquake that hit Chile on February 27, 2010. Only 521 people died in this disaster. One of the main reasons why the human toll was much lower in the Chilean quake is that Chile had instituted stringent building codes after previous devastating quakes (Barrionuevo and Robbins 2010).

Location also plays an important role in the impact of natural disasters (Freudenberg et al. 2009). People who live in flood-prone areas are more likely to suffer from the impacts of torrential rains than people who live at higher elevations, and coastal residents are more likely to be affected by hurricanes, typhoons, or tsunamis than in-landers. One of the reasons why Hurricane Katrina had such a devastating impact on New Orleans is that 80 percent of the homes in the city were built below sea level. The levees that protected these homes from flooding could not withstand the influx of water. More than 1,800 people died as a result of the hurricane and floods in Louisiana and Mississippi (Travis 2005; Freudenberg et al. 2009). Heavy rain in Pakistan in July and August 2010 produced floodwaters that displaced more than 15 million people and killed more than 1,500. Many regions in Pakistan are subject to periodic flooding due to low elevation and heavy precipitation (Masood 2010).

People often have economic, cultural, and aesthetic motives for living in areas at high risk for natural disasters. An area that is prone to flooding may also be an ideal location for agriculture due to the nutrients in the soil or the availability of water. Many people desire to live near the seashore to enjoy the ocean, but coastal areas are often threatened by hurricanes or typhoons. Most of the world's major cities have been built near rivers or coastal inlets to take advantage of geography that is conducive to shipping. However, that same geography may also be flood-prone. Governments often compound these problems by subsidizing flood insurance, which encourages people to build houses in flood-prone areas (Black 2005).

Disaster preparedness and response can also play a key role in minimizing the human toll. Critics and commentators argued that the Federal Emergency Management Administration

(FEMA) as well as local government leaders did a poor job of preparing for and responding to Hurricane Katrina. Many have argued that FEMA did not respond quickly enough with the necessary aid and supplies, and local politicians did not take hurricane preparations seriously enough. Additionally, many have claimed that Army Corps of Engineers had not adequately maintained the levees that protected the New Orleans area (Cooper and Block 2006). Natural disasters provide a vivid illustration of health disparities related to the built environment. Hurricane Katrina also provided a vivid illustration of how natural disasters tend to impact the poor more than the wealthy because poor people are more likely to live in unsafe areas, have substandard housing, or lack the resources to prepare for and respond to floods, hurricanes, or earthquakes (Mutter 2010).

The location of houses, apartments, factories, and schools also has impacts on health. Socioeconomically disadvantaged people tend to live closer to sources of pollution and waste than people with higher incomes. Proximity to landfills, factories, freeways, construction sites, ports, and other sources of environmental risk is an important consideration in deciding where to locate schools, homes, and recreation areas (Frumkin 2010b). The ability for students to safely walk or bike to school is also an important consideration in school placement because walking and biking promotes fitness and health (Frumkin 2010b). As we saw in Chapter 6, location also plays an important role in access to healthy food because socioeconomically disadvantaged neighborhoods often have a higher concentration of fast food restaurants than neighborhoods with higher incomes. The location of shipping ports also has a significant impact on health because people who live near these areas have an increased exposure to diesel exhaust from trucks and locomotives (Impact Project 2009). These and other issues related to location will be discussed in more depth in Chapter 10 when we focus on environmental justice.

The planning, growth, construction, and location of cities can also impact human health. A development pattern that requires extensive use of automobiles for transportation, i.e., urban sprawl, produces more air pollution from car and truck exhaust than a pattern that provides for alternative forms of transportation, such as walking, biking, and riding buses or trains. As noted in Chapter 7, air pollution increases the risks of respiratory and cardiovascular disease. By making it more difficult to walk or bike to school, work, or other activities, urban sprawl can decrease opportunities for exercise, which is important for weight control, cardiovascular function, stress reduction, and various aspects of health. Sprawl can also adversely impact the water supply by increasing the amount of runoff and decreasing wetland areas. The significance of water quality for human health was also discussed in Chapter 7 (Frumkin 2002; Frumkin et al. 2004; Heaton et al. 2010). Urban development can also increase the local temperatures in and around a city, because asphalt roads and parking lots, metal and concrete buildings, and other structures absorb more heat than natural areas, such as forests and fields. Increases in temperature can adversely impact human health and imperil organisms and species (Frumkin et al. 2004).

Some of the most sprawling metropolitan areas in the United States are Riverside-San Bernardino, CA, Greensboro-Winston-Salem-High Point, NC, Raleigh-Durham, NC,

Atlanta, GA, Greenville-Spartanburg, SC, West Palm Beach-Boca Raton-Delray Beach, FL, Bridgeport-Stamford-Norwalk Danbury, CT, Knoxville, TN, Oxnard-Ventura, CA, and Fort Worth-Arlington, TX (Ewing et al. 2002). Sprawl also affects many different metropolitan areas in Europe, such as Paris, France; the Rhone River corridor, France; Madrid, Spain; northwest Germany; Belgium; Northern Italy; and Luxemburg (European Environment Agency 2006). Sprawl is also occurring in rapidly developing nations such as China and India (Deng and Huang 2004; Sudhira et al. 2004).

Many public health advocates and urban planners have recommended that cities counteract sprawl by promoting development that emphasizes high population density, walkable and bikeable neighborhoods, mixed-use development (residential and commercial), green spaces, mass transit, and limited road construction (Frumkin et al. 2004; Jackson and Kochtitzsky 2009). This type of urban development, known as smart growth, has the potential to control air pollution in urban areas, promote exercise, and reduce mortality and injury from motor vehicles accidents (Heaton et al. 2010). Pedestrian safety is also a major consideration in smart growth development because biking or walking can be counterproductive if one is not protected from traffic and other urban hazards. The first major city to implement smart growth urban planning was Portland, Oregon. In the 1970s, Portland limited urban growth to an area around the inner city. In the last two decades, many cities have encouraged real estate developers to create smart growth communities in which people can live, work, attend school, and shop in the same locale with minimal automobile use (Jackson and Kochtitzsky 2009).

REGULATION

National, state, and local governments have developed laws that apply to the built environment, and countries have implemented laws to minimize the impact of land use on species and ecosystems. For example, the Endangered Species Act (ESA), which the United States adopted in 1973, is designed to protect species from extinction due to economic growth and development. The ESA also serves to maintain populations and reduce threats to their survival. The ESA has blocked numerous industrial, commercial, logging, housing, and other projects that threatened imperiled species (Czech and Krausman 2001). The ESA also bans the killing of endangered animals, except in self-defense. The United States Fish and Wildlife Service (FWS) and the National Oceanic and Atmospheric Administration (NOAA) are charged with implementing the ESA (National Oceanic and Atmospheric Administration 2010). The ESA has generated considerable controversy because it pits environmental protection against economic development and private interests. There have been disputes about listing species under the ESA, taking economic considerations into account in implementing regulations, and the scope of government power under the law (Czech and Krausman 2001). For example, in 1990 environmental groups petitioned FWS to place the northern spotted owl (*Strix occidentalis caurina*) on the endangered species list, which required the logging industry to implement plans to protect the owl's habitat (Stokstad 2008).

OSHA has developed standards to protect individuals from workplace hazards, such as toxic exposures. OSHA standards also apply to building construction, design, and maintenance. OSHA standards apply to a number of different worksites, including factories, health care facilities, and offices (Perry and Hu 2010). Governments have also adopted safety standards for specific industries, such as mining (Weeks 1991). The Federal Mine Safety and Health Act (1977) protects workers who mine coal and other minerals.

Most states and counties also have adopted building codes that play an important role in promoting public health and safety. Building codes apply to many different aspects of design and construction, such as roofs, walls, foundations, building materials, and plumbing, heating, cooling, ventilation, and electrical systems (Heaton et al. 2010).

Zoning laws also play a key role in the development of the built environment. Zoning laws regulate particular uses of land, such as residential, commercial, industrial, agricultural, or recreational. Zoning laws can also help control population density, require access to roads, and limit development in flood-prone areas (Heaton et al. 2010). Subdivision regulations pertain to the subdividing of land into different lots to form residential communities. These rules can specify the size of lots, street layout, and access to sidewalks, bike paths, and open spaces.

Access to city water and sewer services can help to control growth and development around cities. If city leaders decide to stop expansion into a particular area, they can restrict city services to deter development. If leaders want to encourage expansion, they can extend services (Resnik 2010b).

Financial incentives from the government can influence development. As mentioned earlier, government subsidies of flood insurance can encourage people to build homes in flood-prone areas. Also, tax breaks can be used to encourage smart growth development (Resnik 2010b).

Many nations and states have decided to preserve thousands of square miles of land as national parks or national forests. National parks and forests provide regions where animals and plants can live in their natural habitats without being disturbed, and can help to preserve species, ecosystems, and biodiversity. The United States National Park Service, for example, oversees 392 national parks encompassing 131,000 square miles of land and 7,000 square miles of lakes, oceans, and reservoirs (National Park Service 2010).

ETHICAL ISSUES

There are a variety of ethical issues related to the built environment (Jamieson 1984, King 2000). Many of these involve conflicts between social utility on the one hand and animal welfare and stewardship on the other.

Homes, schools, hospitals, worksites, roads, and other aspects of the built environment promote health, economic growth, and other human interests. But, as we have seen, transforming the environment to accommodate human activities can threaten species, habitats, ecosystems, and, ultimately, biodiversity. While curtailing some types of development may be necessary to protect endangered species, habitats, or ecosystems, it may also have negative impacts on human populations. How can we find the right balance between development and environmental protection?

Though settling conflicts between these opposing values is no easy task, the principle of sustainability offers a useful approach to the issues (Norton 2005). To see the relevance of this principle, suppose all of the nations adopted a land use policy that placed no limitations on development. If people around the world adopted this policy, we would drastically deplete rain forests, wetlands, natural habitats, and undeveloped land. This outcome would not only devastate species, ecosystems, and biodiversity, but it would severely harm human interests because we need other species to perform many functions that are vital to human health and well-being. Even people who have little concern for the environment should be able to see the wisdom of placing some limits on development. An "anything goes" land use policy is ultimately self-defeating because it is not sustainable over the long run.

Sustainable land use policies permit enough development to meet human needs but also include safeguards to protect and preserve the environment. Determining the level of land use that is sustainable is a complex task because it may be affected by many factors, including technology, degree of urbanization, agriculture, infrastructure, manufacturing, as well as geology, topography, habitats, weather, and ecology. I will not explore this issue in depth here. (For further discussion, see Norton 2005.)

Some policies that promote sustainable land uses include:

- Laws, such as the ESA, which prevent or minimize development that threatens endangered species;
- Limitations on development on wetlands and other areas that support biodiversity and important ecological functions;
- Careful planning of dams to minimize or mitigate their environmental impacts;
- Zoning regulations or tax incentives, which encourage more efficient use of land and discourage low-density, urban sprawl;
- Forest and timber management regulations that require replanting and reclamation of forests that have been logged;
- Mining regulations that reduce the environmental impact of mining operations through judicious use of the land and reclamation of habitat;
- The use of public money and land to preserve wilderness areas, such as national parks;
- Tax incentives or other government support for private efforts to preserve land, such as the Nature Conservancy (2010).

While these sustainable development policies sound good in theory, they are often difficult to implement in practice for several reasons. First, some sustainable development policies, such as zoning laws, timber management regulations, and endangered species protections involve government control over private property. Property owners may object to laws that limit the use of their property. Second, because habitats, species, and ecosystems often transcend national boundaries, sustainable development often requires international cooperation (United Nations 1992). International cooperation on development issues can be difficult to achieve because nations often have opposing interests. The debate about controlling greenhouse gas emission illustrates some of these problems. Third, as the global population grows, pressures will continue to mount to clear land for housing, agriculture, industry, mining, and other purposes. It may be impractical to pursue sustainable development policies without some form of population control because gains in efficiency with respect to land use might be more than offset by increasing demands for development. (Population issues will be discussed in more depth in Chapter 9.)

LIMITS ON PROPERTY RIGHTS

Controversies concerning the limitations on property rights are key ethical issues related to land use, urban development, and the built environment. Disputes over property rights have undermined efforts to implement smart growth policies to counteract urban sprawl because property owners and real estate developers have opposed laws or regulations that limit development and adversely affect property values (Resnik 2010b). Property rights concerns have had an impact on efforts to implement the ESA because logging companies, farmers, real estate developers, and other property owners have been required to limit their development activities to protect endangered species (Czech and Krausman 2001). Property interests also play a prominent role in debates about policies that limit development of wetlands. Property owners have objected to laws that prevent them from developing land that has been designated as wetland (Hope 2003). Indeed, property rights will be implicated in most issues related to the built environment because individuals own most of the buildings and other structures affected by government policies.

To have a better understanding of these issues, it will be useful to consider several different views of property rights. Libertarians hold that liberty and private property are fundamental human rights that should be protected by the state. Indeed, the whole purpose of government is to protect liberty and property, not to redistribute wealth (Nozick 1974). Libertarians hold that these rights may be restricted only when exercising them interferes with someone else's rights. My right to shoot a gun (my property) does not give me the right to use it to shoot an innocent person. Libertarians oppose the ESA, zoning laws, and other government actions that place significant restrictions on property rights.

Most libertarians treat the right to private property as a basic axiom of their theory that requires no further justification. But one might challenge this assumption. Why is property a fundamental right? Is it as important as life, liberty, or the pursuit of happiness? The nineteenth century German philosopher Georg Hegel (1770–1831) argued that property was necessary for human dignity and psychological development. People need to be able to have some control over private property to shape their personal identity, social relationships, and place in society. People can use their property to express their wants, interests, choices, values, and other traits necessary for self-realization (Hegel 1967).

German political philosopher and economist Karl Marx (1818–1883) was a Hegelian at the beginning of his career, but he soon critiqued and rejected Hegel's views about history and proposed his own account of property. Marx argued that private property plays a key role in a capitalist society by enabling the upper classes (the capitalists and the bourgeoisie) to exploit working class people (the proletariat) and deny them the fruits of their labor. Private property leads to vast differences in income and wealth. In a communist society, differences in economic status are supposed to be minimal with only one social class. To bring about a transition from capitalism to communism, private property must be abolished. Under communism, the state owns all property and may decide how land will be used (Marx 1992).

In between the views represented by libertarianism and Marxism, various philosophies recognize a right to private property but also hold that property rights may be restricted to promote important social goals, such as public health, social justice, or environmental protection. Rawls (1971) held that property is not a fundamental human right but that it is a social institution that should conform to principles of justice. Property rights can be restricted to promote equality of opportunity and benefit the least advantaged members of society. Utilitarians hold that property is justified because it promotes the good of society by encouraging hard work, innovation, and inventiveness, which produce economic prosperity. Property rights can be restricted, however, to maximize benefits or minimize harms (Mill 2003).

I endorse the intermediate view of property rights because both extreme views have serious shortcomings. A key problem with the Marxist view is that it does not recognize the importance of private property for human well-being. People need to be able to have some control over their own property to express freedom and develop their sense of self. Private property also provides incentives for hard work, innovation, and inventiveness, which are essential for economic development and prosperity.

A key problem with libertarianism is that it overvalues property rights. Private property is an important right, to be sure, but it is not equivalent to the right to life, political participation, or freedom of speech or religion. There are legitimate reasons to restrict property rights, other than preventing harm. Property rights may be restricted to promote public health and safety, social justice, and environmental protection. The intermediate view attempts to forge a fair and reasonable balance between property rights and competing values.

SAFETY VERSUS COST-SAVINGS

The issue of safety versus cost-savings is an important concern related to building codes and occupational health standards. There are many different ways of improving the safety of man-made structures, such as using stronger building materials and sturdier designs.

However, housing safety often comes at a price. It costs more to build a house out of bricks and steel than wood. Stringent building codes can help to protect public health and safety but they can also drive up the cost of housing, which can have negative impacts on the economy and prevent socioeconomically disadvantaged people from owning or renting homes. Haiti is one of the world's poorest countries with a per capita income of less than $1,000 per year (World Bank 2010b). Although building codes similar to Chile's could have helped to reduce the mortality and property destruction caused by the Haitian earthquake of 2010, most residents of that country would not have been able to afford housing built according to tougher standards. Earthquake-resistant buildings can cost considerably more than standard buildings, depending on the materials used and building design (Schulze et al. 1987).

There are also many measures that can enhance the safety of workplace activities, such as safety training, limitations on work hours, protective clothing and equipment, and containment of dangerous materials. However, workplace safety also comes at a price. It would be prohibitively expensive to make some inherently risky occupations, such as logging or commercial fishing, as safe as low-risk occupations, such as librarian or educator. Imposing unrealistic and costly safety standards on some types of high-risk industries could cause employers to reduce hiring, go out of business, or move their operations to countries with lower safety standards.

Considerations of safety and cost-savings both fall under the principle of utility, except they focus on different types of social values. Safety promotes public health, whereas cost-savings promotes economic efficiency. Although safety is essential to sound building codes and occupational health standards, affordability must also be considered, especially because affordability has an impact on social justice (Dowling 2010). If a municipality adopts an overly stringent building code, housing may become unaffordable for many people. If a state government adopts very strict occupational health standards, then companies may go out of business, hire fewer workers, or outsource their operations. The key is to find a fair and reasonable balance between safety and cost-savings. To determine the appropriate balance of safety and cost-savings related to homes or workplaces, one must have detailed information on the issue at hand. Though I will not render an opinion on any particular housing or occupational health policies in this book, I point out the importance of taking safety and cost into account.

JUSTICE

Many different aspects of the built environment can impact the distribution of health in society. For example:

- Waste disposal sites, factories, and interstate highways can adversely impact the health of people living nearby;
- Upscale urban development projects can displace and disrupt low-income minority communities in a process known as gentrification (Dowling 2010);

- Housing standards can protect the health of low-income people but may also drive up the cost of housing, which affects affordability and access;
- Occupational health and safety standards can protect health of low-income people but can also adversely impact employment opportunities;
- Locating buildings and communities in areas prone to flooding (or other natural disasters) can have a negative impact on people living in those areas.

To apply the principle of justice to the built environment, it is important to consider how decisions related to urban development, housing, workplace safety, and other aspects of the built environment will affect the distribution of health and other socioeconomic goods. Additionally, stakeholders who are impacted by public policies related to the built environment should have a significant contribution to any decisions that affect them, such as zoning changes, safety regulations, and so on. Efforts should be made to include socioeconomically disadvantaged groups, who may lack the power to influence political decisions (Shrader-Frechette 2002, 2007a). Justice will be explored in more depth in Chapter 10.

SUMMARY

In this chapter we have examined some of the ethical and policy issues concerning the built environment. The built environment raises a number of important ethical issues, some of which we have already examined in this book: human health and well-being vs. environmental protection; property rights vs. social goods; safety vs. cost-savings; and justice. The principle of sustainability, discussed in Chapter 4, offers some useful guidance for balancing human interests and environmental protection with respect to economic development and land use. Property rights are important to human well-being and economic prosperity, but they can be restricted to promote human health and safety and protect habitats, ecosystems, and species. The next chapter will examine global issues with implications for the built environment and other aspects of environmental health.

9

CLIMATE CHANGE, ENERGY, AND POPULATION

This chapter will examine ethical and policy issues related to three global environmental health topics: climate change, energy use and production, and population. These issues are global in scope because they affect everyone on the planet and require international cooperation for their resolution. The issues are also fundamentally interconnected because increases in population lead to greater demands for energy, which can impact climate change.

CLIMATE CHANGE

We have already mentioned climate change due to global warming during the discussion of air pollution in Chapter 7, meat eating in Chapter 6, and urban sprawl in Chapter 8. In this chapter, we will explore the topic in greater depth. A primary mechanism for global warming is the greenhouse effect, which occurs when radiant heat entering an enclosed area through a transparent medium is trapped, which raises the temperature. A variety of gases present in the atmosphere, including carbon dioxide (CO_2), methane, ozone, water, and nitrous oxide, trap the sun's heat by absorbing infrared radiation reflected by the surface of the Earth and re-emitting it. Sources of greenhouse gases include volcanic activity, decaying vegetation, animal respiration and waste, combustion of biomass and fossils fuels, and industrial processes, such as cement manufacturing. Without any greenhouse gases, the Earth would be too cold to support life as we know it (National Aeronautics and Space Administration 2010a).

While greenhouse gases play an important role in warming the Earth, other factors help to cool it. Ice sheets and clouds reflect light back into space. Aerosols, particulate matter, and dust can prevent solar radiation from reaching the surface of the Earth and also contribute to cloud formation. Plants on the surface of the Earth and in the ocean draw CO_2 from the atmosphere and seawater and convert it into organic material. Water in the ocean and on the surface of the Earth can also absorb CO_2. Other important factors that affect the climate include ocean currents, the positions of the continents, and the strength of solar radiation (Solomon et al. 2007). Although the energy coming from the sun usually remains fairly stable, sometimes solar activity decreases or increases slightly. For example, decreases in solar radiation triggered an unusually cool period known as the Little Ice Age in Europe from 1650 to 1850 (National Aeronautics and Space Administration 2010a).

The Earth's climate has changed numerous times in its 4 billion year history. During the last 420,000 years, the Earth's climate has alternated between colder, glacial periods and warmer, interglacial periods four times. Temperatures remain relatively stable during these alternating periods. During the last glacial period, approximately 20,000 years ago, sheets of ice covered much of North America and Europe. Changing levels of two important greenhouse gases – CO_2 and methane – correlate with changes in the Earth's climate. As these gases increase, the climate warms; as they decrease, the climate cools. The climate is currently in an interglacial period, but another glacial period is expected to occur within 50,000 years (Augustin et al. 2004). Recent global temperatures are based on measurements from meteorological stations around the world. Evidence for past variations in the Earth's climate comes from analyses of Antarctic ice cores. The depth of the ice serves as a measurement of time, and air trapped in the ice indicates the composition of the atmosphere at that time. The concentration of different isotopes of oxygen (e.g., ^{16}O) and hydrogen (e.g., ^2H, ^3H) in the water that formed the ice provides an indication of global temperatures. Heavier water (e.g., water containing a higher proportion of ^{16}O, ^2H, and ^3H) forms ice in warmer temperatures than lighter water. Air bubbles trapped in the ice provide an indication of the composition of the atmosphere (Augustin et al. 2004).

Considerable evidence supports the hypothesis that human activities are largely responsible for changes in the Earth's climate since 1900. Global temperatures have increased 0.74°C since 1900, and the twenty warmest years have occurred since 1981 (see Figure 9.1). Ocean temperatures have risen about 0.16°C since 1969. The ice sheets covering Antarctica, Greenland, and the Arctic Sea have shrunk in the last three decades and glaciers on many continents have retreated. Global sea levels have risen 6.7 inches in the last hundred years as a result of melting ice (National Aeronautics and Space Administration 2010a). Levels of atmospheric CO_2 have risen steadily since the mid-1700s, when people began using more fossil fuels, and are much higher today than they have been in the last 400,000 years (Solomon et al. 2007) (see Figure 9.2). Because greenhouse gases have played an important role in warming the Earth throughout its history, it is reasonable to conclude that the observed changes in global temperatures are due to increases in greenhouse gases produced by human activity. Unless steps are taken to reverse or stabilize levels of greenhouse gases in the atmosphere, global temperatures are expected to rise between 1.8°C and 4.0°C by 2100 (Solomon et al. 2007).

Although an overwhelming majority of scientists accept the idea that human activities are causing global warming, a small minority of researchers are skeptics. Skeptics acknowledge that global warming has occurred in the last hundred years but argue that human activities are not primarily responsible for this change. Some claim that the recent warming trend is a normal variation in temperatures, while others argue that nonhuman causes, such as changes in solar radiation and volcanic activity, are largely responsible for global warming (Spencer 2010). Skeptics also challenge predictions concerning future changes in climate or the impacts of global warming on human health and the environment (Tollefson 2011).

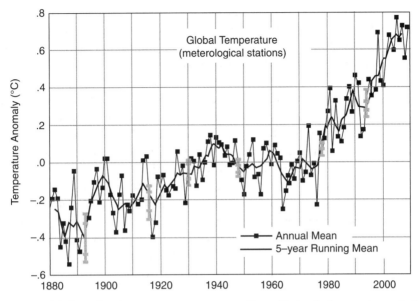

Figure 9.1. Global Surface Temperatures since 1880 (from National Aeronautics and Space Administration 2010b).

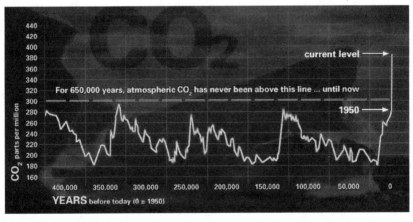

Figure 9.2. Atmospheric Carbon Dioxide Concentrations since 400,000 BCE (from National Aeronautics and Space Administration 2011).

Skepticism about climate change has been significantly impacted by politics. The administration of President George W. Bush was very skeptical of anthropogenic global warming. Administration officials censored several government-funded reports on climate change in an effort to minimize the impacts of climate change and to downplay humanity's role in global warming (Mooney 2005). Government agencies under the Bush administration also restricted government scientists' communications with the media about climate change (Revkin 2006). The Bush administration's skepticism about anthropocentric climate change stemmed from its alignment with business interests who opposed government policies designed to mitigate or prevent climate change (Mooney 2005).

In the fall of 2009, someone hacked into the email server at the University of East Anglia's Climatic Research Unit (CRU) and posted on the internet thousands of emails exchanged between climate change researchers at the CRU and researchers around the world. Most of the email involved exchanges between Phil Jones (CRU director), Ken Briffa, Tim Osborn, and Mike Hulme. Many of the studies from the CRU had been cited in the in influential reports from the Intergovernmental Panel on Climate Change (IPCC). The hacking has been investigated as a criminal matter, but so far no suspect has been named. Many of the emails show CRU researchers refusing to share data or computer codes with global warming skeptics or trying to discredit the work of skeptics. In one of the emails, Phil Jones and Pennsylvania State Researcher Michael Mann discuss how Mann used a statistical "trick" to hide the decline in global temperatures since 1950 indicated by tree ring data, in a graph depicting global temperatures over the past 1,000 years. The graph combined actual measurements of temperatures, which began in 1850, with proxies for actual temperatures, including data from tree rings, ice cores, and corals. Actual measurements of global temperatures since 1950 conflict with tree ring data and show a sharp rise in temperatures (Revkin 2009). Global warming skeptics argued that the emails demonstrated that researchers were manipulating data, suppressing evidence that conflicted with their theories, and undermining peer review. They labeled the alleged conspiracy "Climategate" (Revkin 2009).

Several independent reviews of the emails exonerated the researchers of any misconduct, and concluded that the email exchanges in no way undermined the scientific consensus on global warming (Revkin 2009). However, a National Science Foundation investigation that cleared Mann of misconduct raised concerns about the statistical techniques he used to generate the graph depicting global warming trends in the last thousand years (Campbell 2011). Also, many commentators criticized the researchers for stonewalling skeptics and not sharing data available under the United Kingdom's Freedom of Information Act. The IPCC took the matter seriously and has affirmed the importance of openness and transparency in climate change research (Revkin 2009).

Climate change has emerged as an issue in the 2012 U.S. presidential campaign. While President Obama, the likely Democratic nominee, accepts the scientific consensus on global warming, some Republican candidates, such Texas Governor Rick Perry and Minnesota Congresswoman Michelle Bachman, have challenged it. Perry has claimed global warming is an unproven theory based on manipulated data. Under the Obama administration, the EPA has taken some steps to begin regulating CO_2, but this could change if a president skeptical of global warming is elected (Achenbach and Eilperin 2011; Reston 2011).

While human-caused global warming is still fraught with political controversy, I will assume that the scientific consensus concerning climate change is basically correct (Union of Concerned Scientists 2011), although many uncertainties remain, such as the amount of global warming that will occur in the next hundred years if current greenhouse gas emissions remain the same or increase. (For further discussion of the scientific and political issues related to global warming, see Dessler and Parson 2006.)

Global warming is expected to have numerous adverse effects on the environment and human health, such as:

- **Heat waves.** A rise in global temperatures will lead to more extremely hot days in the summer months. Extremely warm temperatures overcome the body's ability to thermoregulate and can increase morbidity and mortality (Interagency Working Group on Climate Change and Health 2010). Forty thousand people died in a heat wave in Europe in the summer of 2003 (Patz 2010).

- **Rising sea levels.** As polar ice caps and glaciers melt, they will add water to the oceans, which will increase sea levels. Estimates of sea level rise vary considerably, from 0.5 to 1.4 meters above 1990 levels, depending on expected increase in global temperatures, changes in ocean currents, and the fate of the Greenland ice sheet (Rahmstorf 2007; Patz 2010). The flooding resulting from rising sea levels will have potentially devastating impacts on coastal cities and island nations (Patz 2010).

- **Floods and droughts.** Global warming will increase the amount of water vapor in the atmosphere, which will increase the total amount of precipitation on the planet. This precipitation will not be distributed evenly, however. Regions at higher latitudes are expected to receive more precipitation, and regions at subtropical latitudes are expected to receive less rain. As a result, floods will impact some areas, while droughts will affect others. Coastal regions are also at an increased risk of flooding due to the expected sea level rise (National Aeronautics and Space Administration 2010a, Schiermeier 2011).

- **Problems with food production.** Droughts in central Asia and southern Africa will decrease agricultural output, which may lead to famine and malnutrition. Although agricultural technologies, such as irrigation and genetic engineering, can help farmers to deal with droughts, food production still depends a great deal on precipitation (Patz 2010).

- **Problems with drinking water.** Droughts will decrease the amount of drinking water available. Floods may contaminate drinking water supplies. In both situations, global warming will reduce access to drinking water (Patz 2010).

- **Wildfires.** Droughts will also increase wildfires in some regions, such as the western United States (Patz 2010).

- **Reduced fisheries.** The oceans have increased in acidity since 1750 due to absorption of CO_2 from the atmosphere (National Aeronautics and Space Administration 2010a). A rise in the acidity of ocean water threatens organisms that form shells from calcium carbonate, such as corals, mollusks, and some types of plankton. Reductions in coral and mollusk populations will have wide-ranging adverse effects in ocean species and ecosystems because many fish depend on coral reefs for shelter and feed on mollusks or plankton. Reductions in fisheries will threaten human populations that depend on fish as a main source of food (Patz 2010).

- **Increased tropical storm activity.** Warmer sea surface temperatures are expected to increase the frequency and strength of tropical storms, such as hurricanes and typhoons. Hurricane activity in the North Atlantic doubled in the last fifty years as a result of warmer sea surface temperatures. As noted in Chapter 8, tropical storms can have devastating impacts on the environment and human health (Patz 2010).

- **Increased tropospheric ozone.** Higher air temperatures increase the formation of ozone in the troposphere and also increase the emission of volatile organic compounds, which are ozone precursors, from some species of trees (Patz 2010).

- **Increased allergens.** Higher levels of CO_2 in the atmosphere increase the growth of plants that produce pollen, such as ragweeds. Increased levels of pollen in the atmosphere will trigger allergic reactions among susceptible individuals. CO_2 also promotes the growth of poison ivy and stinging nettles, which cause contact dermatitis, an allergic response (Patz 2010). Droughts may lead to increased levels of dust, which is an allergen. Individuals with airway diseases, such as asthma, will be especially vulnerable to the effects of increased levels of allergens in the atmosphere (Interagency Working Group on Climate Change and Health 2010).

- **Increased infectious diseases.** Many different types of infectious diseases are likely to increase as a result of warmer temperatures (Interagency Working Group on Climate Change and Health 2010). Waterborne infectious diseases, such as cryptosporidiosis, will increase as a result of flooding into drinking water systems. Warmer water temperatures will lead to more harmful algal blooms in marine ecosystems, which will impact fish populations. People who eat infected fish may be harmed by toxins contained in fish that are exposed to algal blooms. Higher temperatures will increase the prevalence of some foodborne diseases, such as salmonella. Mosquito-borne diseases, such as malaria, are also likely to increase in response to higher temperatures and flooding. Rodent-borne diseases, such as hantavirus, are also expected to increase (Patz 2010). Other vector-borne and zoonotic diseases may increase as a result of changes in geographic distribution of species that transmit diseases to humans (Mills et al. 2010).

- **Impacts on species, habitats, ecosystems, and biodiversity.** Many different species will respond to increased temperatures. Some species may become extinct or decline dramatically as a result of global warming, while others may adapt or thrive. Species that thrive in warmer climates, such as fire ants, may be able to extend their range as regions with moderate temperatures become warmer. Species that require colder climates, such as polar bears, may find it difficult to survive due to loss of habitat. Some species may live at higher elevations in response to temperature changes. As noted earlier, corals and mollusks may be adversely impacted. Changes in species and habitats will have impacts on ecosystems and biodiversity, which are difficult to assess at this point (Patz 2010; Rosenthal 2011).

There are two basic responses to the prospects of climate change: mitigation and adaptation (Patz 2010). Mitigation includes efforts to reduce or minimize global warming by reducing greenhouse gas emissions. The Kyoto Protocol, which establishes greenhouse emission targets for industrialized nations, is an example of an attempt to mitigate climate change. The Kyoto goals could be achieved by regulating greenhouse gas emissions from various sources, instituting a cap and trade system for emissions, or imposing special taxes on fossil fuels to discourage consumption. Some European countries have already adopted cap and trade systems for CO_2 emissions within their borders and heavily tax gasoline (Maslin and Scott 2011). As noted in Chapter 7, the Kyoto Protocol has been controversial, in part because it may have adverse economic impacts, and countries are continuing to work on climate change agreements, such as the Durban Platform (Broder 2010b; Eilperin 2011a). Other mitigation strategies that have received considerable attention include developing alternative energy sources, such as solar, wind, hydroelectric, geothermal, and nuclear power (Metz et al. 2007).

Adaptation includes strategies for responding to climate change. Some of these include making preparations for natural disasters, such as floods, tropical storms, and heat waves; growing drought-resistant crops; increasing irrigation; protecting water systems from floods and securing additional sources of water; increasing the public health response to infectious diseases; protecting coastal areas from higher ocean levels; careful management of fisheries impacted by changes in the marine ecosystems; and educating the public about the effects of climate change (Wiley and Gostin 2009; Patz 2010).

There has been little disagreement concerning the importance of taking appropriate steps to adapt to climate change, but some mitigation strategies, such as a cap and trade system for CO_2 emissions or a carbon tax, are controversial because they may have negative impacts on the economy. As noted in Chapter 7, a cap and trade system is likely to negatively impact gross domestic product, household income, and labor productivity in the United States (Congressional Budget Office 2009). One reason why energy legislation would have wide-ranging economic impacts is that energy costs impact virtually every sector of the economy. Higher energy prices lead to higher prices for food, manufactured goods, transportation, healthcare, and housing (Samuelson and Nordhaus 2009). The oil crisis of the 1970s, for example, played a major role in inflation, recession, and slowdowns in economic growth in the United States and other countries (Barsky and Kilian 2004). A cap and trade system or carbon tax would increase the price of energy and could drag down economies that rely heavily on fossil fuels (Lieberman 2010). Because economic development plays an essential role in overcoming poverty, famine, and disease (Bloom and Canning 2000; Sen 2000; Samuelson and Nordhaus 2009), nations should be wary of climate change legislation that is likely to have adverse economic impacts.

A proponent of climate change legislation could reply to this economic argument by claiming that the costs of not doing anything to address global warming would also be substantial. Natural disasters linked to global warming would cause economic devastation in affected areas. Global warming would also increase health care costs related to infectious diseases, airway diseases, and heat exhaustion. Other effects of global warming, such as rising sea levels, shortages of drinking water, loss of species, and habitat change would also impact the economy. When these expenses are taken into account, legislation to stabilize greenhouse gas emissions may actually save more money than it costs (Metz et al. 2007).

The economic implications of legislation to mitigate climate change are complex and uncertain, and further study is warranted. While it is important to mitigate climate change to protect the environment and human health, economic considerations must be taken into account (Posner and Weisbach 2010). The precautionary principle advises us to take reasonable measures to mitigate potential harms caused by global warming. Reasonable measures would balance the competing values at stake, that is, economic development versus environmental and health protection, in a way that is fair and consistent. Methods and strategies for mitigating global warming that do not send the world economy into a tailspin would include (Patz 2010):

- Public funding for climate change mitigation research;
- Public funding and economic incentives for the development of alternatives to fossil fuels;
- Higher fuel economy standards for automobiles;
- Using vehicles powered by electricity, natural gas, or biofuels;
- Increasing the energy efficiency of automobiles, appliances, industrial processes, electric power generation and transmission, lighting, and cooling and heating systems;
- Building and using mass transportation;
- Biking and walking for transportation;
- Carpooling;
- Telecommuting, teleconferencing, and videoconferencing;
- Growing trees and other plants to remove CO_2 from the atmosphere;
- Genetically engineering trees and other plants to enhance their ability to remove CO_2 from the atmosphere;
- Protection of forests that remove CO_2 from the atmosphere;
- Containing methane emitted from landfills and other sources;
- Reducing reliance on meat as a source of food;
- Population control (discussed later).

If these methods and strategies are not likely to have a significant impact on greenhouse gas levels, it may also be necessary to implement forms of energy taxation and regulation that impose more substantial impacts on the economy. A cap and trade system for CO_2 emissions or a carbon tax may be necessary to achieve acceptable levels of greenhouse gases. However, these policies should be carefully designed to minimize economic impacts. The long-term goal of climate change policies should be to lead the world away from dependence on fossil fuels and toward greater reliance on sources of energy that are environmentally and socioeconomically sustainable (Rockström et al. 2009; Patz 2010).

Some scientists and engineers have argued that geoengineering may be a desirable way of mitigating climate change because other methods may not succeed. Geoengineering would be an attempt, on a global scale, to alter the climate by removing CO_2 from the atmosphere or blocking solar radiation (Jamieson 2010; Keith et al. 2010; Kintisch 2010a). Methods that have been proposed for removing carbon dioxide from the atmosphere include building machines that draw CO_2 from the air and pump it underground for long-term storage, and fertilizing the oceans with iron to promote the growth of algae, which remove CO_2 from the water and air (Kintisch 2010a). Methods for blocking solar radiation include spraying SO_2 into the stratosphere, which would form aerosols that enhance cloud albedo and block the sun's rays (Crutzen 2006). Proponents of geoengineering note that the eruption of Mount Pinatubo in 1991 released enough sulfur dioxide into the stratosphere to obscure solar energy input significantly. The eruption is credited with cooling the Earth by 0.5°C by releasing sulfur dioxide into the stratosphere (Keith et al. 2010). Other methods of blocking solar radiation that have been proposed include spraying specially designed nanoparticles into the stratosphere to enhance cloud albedo, and constructing giant solar reflectors that orbit the Earth (Keith 2010; Kintisch 2010a).

While geoengineering may be a promising method for mitigating climate change, it has been controversial. Opponents of geoengineering point out that it has significant risks, some of which are not well understood at this point (Jamieson 1996, 2010; Gardiner 2010). For example, in a world cooled by blocking solar radiation, there might be less precipitation, which could lead to droughts. Blocking solar radiation also would not address the problem of ocean acidification because atmospheric CO_2 would remain at present levels or increase (Keith et al. 2010). Spraying SO_2 into the stratosphere could lead to increased acid rain and respiratory problems. Carbon sequestration and storage removes greenhouse gases but also uses considerable energy. Increased growth of algae in the oceans could have disastrous effects on fishes and marine ecosystems. Additionally, geoengineering could lead to excessive global cooling and trigger an ice age if we block too much sunlight (Jamieson 2010; Kintisch 2010a). Geoengineering opponents also argue that it would potentially divert research, education, and policy efforts from strategies to reduce greenhouse gas emissions. People would be even less likely to reduce CO_2 emissions or protect forests if they think that geoengineering can solve our climate change problems. Our time, money, and effort would be better spent pursuing other forms of climate change mitigation (Gardiner 2010; Jamieson 2010).

Although geoengineering has some significant problems, it should not be rejected out-of-hand. Climate change is a serious problem that must be addressed by the effective means at our disposal. Other efforts to mitigate climate change have not been very successful thus far, and they may never be. There are a few reasons why this is the case. First, climate change is an abstract problem that people have a hard time understanding or appreciating. The effects of climate change are not readily apparent to many people. When people don't understand a problem, they are less motivated to do something about it. Second, many climate change mitigation strategies require people to make sacrifices for the common good, such as using less fossil fuels, and people may be unwilling to do this, especially for an abstract problem that they scarcely understand. Third, climate change mitigation requires a high degree of global cooperation, which, as we have seen, is difficult to obtain (Gardiner 2006). Fourth, as noted earlier, climate change is fraught with political controversy. Politicians who do not accept the scientific consensus concerning global warming may be unwilling to seek an effective response to the problem.

Geoengineering is far from a perfect solution to climate change, but it should at least be considered because other efforts to mitigate climate change may fail. Because geoengineering may have significant risks that are not well understood, a precautionary approach is warranted (Elliott 2010; Tollefson 2010). A precautionary approach would involve moving forward with geoengineering but taking reasonable measures to prevent, avoid, or mitigate harms that may result. Scientists and engineers could study geoengineering and experiment with small-scale projects. Large-scale projects would not be implemented until there is adequate evidence concerning their risks and benefits. Plans to impede or reverse harmful effects of geoengineering would also need to be developed. Also, we should continue to implement other climate mitigation strategies (discussed earlier) while we are studying geoengineering. The promise of an engineering solution to climate change should not be used as an excuse to abandon or cut back current climate mitigation strategies.

Justice is an important ethical concern related to climate change because the adverse impacts of global warming are not likely to be distributed equally (Posner and Weisbach 2010). Poor countries in Africa, Asia, and Oceania are likely to experience more adverse consequences of climate change, such as droughts, floods, famine, and infectious diseases than richer nations in North America and Europe. Poorer countries also have fewer resources to adapt to the effects of climate change (Wiley and Gostin 2009; Patz 2010). One could argue that richer nations have a moral obligation to help poorer nations deal with climate change, especially because richer nations have produced most of the CO_2 emissions largely responsible for global warming (Patz 2010; Wiley and Gostin 2010). These issues will be explored in more depth in Chapter 10.

ENERGY PRODUCTION AND CONSUMPTION

Every form of human activity depends on some source of energy. We use energy for transportation, agriculture, industry, education, recreation, and communication. We need energy (in the form of food) to live. For many years, biomass, such as wood, dung, and peat, was humanity's primary source of energy other than food. People burned wood for heating, cooking, and lighting and used animals for transportation and labor. Waterwheels and windmills also provided some energy. During the 1700s, this pattern of energy use changed as people began to make greater use of coal (Hess 2010). Soon, the steam engine was invented and people used coal to power factories, steel mills, locomotives, and steam ships. Coal was also used for heating and cooking. As the industrial revolution progressed, the demand for energy (chiefly in the form of coal) increased. In the 1800s, oil wells were drilled, and people began to use petroleum products, such as kerosene and gasoline, as a source of energy. The reliance on petroleum increased greatly with the invention of the gasoline-powered, internal combustion engine, which was used in automobiles. Coal and oil also fueled electric power plants, which provided energy for a variety of uses including industry, lighting, and heating. Today, human beings obtain energy from a wide variety of sources, but still rely heavily on coal, oil, and other fossil fuels. The demand for energy continues to grow as a result of increases in population and developments in technology and industry (Hess 2010).

Energy use is currently distributed unequally around the world. The average use among the nations of the world in 2005 was 1,778 kilograms of oil equivalent (KGOE) per capita. The North American region had the highest KGOE per capita at 7,943, followed by Europe (3,773), the Middle East and North Africa (1,766), Central America and the Caribbean (1,366), South America (1,151) and Asia (1052) (World Resources Institute 2010; data not available for Oceania and sub-Saharan Africa). The main reason why energy use is distributed unequally is the different countries have different levels of economic and technological development. In 2005, developed countries used 4,720 KGOE per capita and developing countries used 976 (World Resources Institute 2010). As low-income countries continue to develop, they will use more energy, which will lead to more pollution and other environmental impacts. China and India have been rapidly developing in the last twenty years and will soon each use as much energy as the United States. Energy policies must take these changes in energy use into account (Hess 2010).

The production and use of energy has many different impacts on human health and the environment, some of which we have discussed earlier in this book, such as the adverse effects of automobile exhaust on human health and hydroelectric power on habitats, species, and ecosystems. Some of the major sources of energy used by humans and their environmental and health impacts are discussed as follows.

COAL

Coal is classified as a fossil fuel because it was formed millions of years ago from organic material deposited on the surface of the Earth, which became buried and subjected to high pressures and temperatures. Coal accounts for 27 percent of the world's energy consumption (International Energy Association 2010) (see Figure 9.3). Coal is also a nonrenewable resource because it will eventually run out. Coal production is expected to peak around 2034 and then steadily decline, though some scientists claim coal production may peak as early as 2011 (Mohr and Evans 2009; Heinberg and Fridley 2010). Coal is used primarily for electric power in developed nations. Forty percent of the world's electric power comes from coal (Hess 2010). In developing nations, coal is still used for heating and cooking.

As mentioned in Chapter 7, coal combustion produces air-born particulate matter, sulfur dioxide, nitrogen oxides, and CO_2, which have many different adverse effects on human health and the environment. Particulate matter and sulfur dioxide can cause cardiovascular

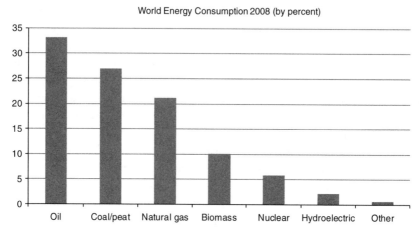

Figure 9.3. World Energy Consumption, 2008 (based on data from the International Energy Association 2010).

and respiratory problems. Nitrogen oxides help to form tropospheric ozone, which also causes cardiovascular and respiratory problems. As mentioned earlier, CO_2 is a greenhouse gas. Thirty-three percent of the CO_2 generated from human activity is produced by coal burning electric power plants (Kintisch 2007). SO_2 from coal burning can form acid rain, which has adverse impacts on vegetation and animal life. Coal mining can have detrimental consequences for the environment. In surface mining, vegetation, rock, and soil are removed to expose the underlying coal deposit. Surface mining destroys habitats and has detrimental impacts on local flora and fauna. Underground mining, discussed in Chapter 8, has fewer impacts on the environment but is a hazardous activity that can pose significant risks for human health and life. Coal mining and combustion also produce solid waste that can contaminate the water supply (Hess 2010).

Using "clean coal" technologies can help reduce the human health and environmental impacts of coal combustion. Most of these technologies involve removal of CO_2, SO_2, and particulate matter from smoke emitted from power plants. Clean coal technologies can increase the costs of electricity production significantly because the technologies are expensive to install and they reduce power plant output. Using current technologies to recapture 90 percentof the carbon emitted from a coal plant would reduce output by 30 percent. In the future, clean coal technologies are likely to become less expensive (Kintisch 2007).

PETROLEUM (OIL)

Most of the world's oil is used for transportation. Crude oil, another fossil fuel and nonrenewable resource, can be refined into gasoline, diesel fuel, and jet fuel. Currently, petroleum products provide energy for 95 percent of the world's transportation (Hess 2010). Oil also provides energy for home heating, agriculture, and industry, and is used to manufacture plastics. Oil accounts for 33.2 percent of the world's energy consumption (International Energy Agency 2010). As discussed in Chapter 7, combustion of petroleum products produces particulate matter, CO_2, and nitrogen oxides, which can cause cardiovascular and respiratory problems. Oil combustion also produces CO_2, which contributes to global warming. There have been many different estimates of the peak of global oil production. In the 1970s, experts predicted oil would peak around 2000, but that estimate has been revised as scientists have developed new methods of extracting oil (Hess 2010). According to current estimates, oil production is expected to peak sometime between 2020 and 2030 and then decline by about 3 percent per year (Sorrell et al. 2010).

Petroleum production can cause significant damage to the environment. Oil spills from malfunctioning wells, ruptured pipelines, or transportation accidents have caused environmental devastation numerous times. On March 24, 1989, the Exxon *Valdez* spilled 257,000 barrels (11 million gallons) of crude oil into the Prince William Sound off the coast of Alaska, when it struck a reef. The spill contaminated 1,300 miles of coastline and killed hundreds of thousands of seabirds, hundreds of otters and seals, and twenty-two killer whales. The spill also destroyed billions of salmon eggs and devastated the fishing and tourism industries. The impact of the spill was felt for many years and the region is only now returning to normal (Exxon Valdez Oil Spill Trustee Council 2010). On April 20, 2010, the Deepwater Horizon drilling rig, operated by British Petroleum, exploded, killing eleven people and injuring seventeen others. The explosion caused an oil leak from an exploratory well 5,000 feet beneath the sea. The well leaked 4.9 million barrels of oil into the Mississippi River Delta before it was finally capped on July 15, 2010 (Kerr 2010). The environmental impact of the oil spill has not been fully assessed as of the writing of this book, but it is expected to have significant adverse effects on shrimp, fish, turtles, marine birds, mammals, and marsh vegetation (Kaufman and Dewan 2010).

Fifty years of oil spills in Nigeria's Ogoniland coastal area have caused considerable environmental damage. A recently completed study found unsafe levels of hydrocarbons in communities near oil production sites. One community had benzene levels 900 times greater than those deemed safe by the World Health Organization. In some areas, oil is floating on top of groundwater, and in other areas the ground is soaked with oil five meters deep. The health impacts of these dangerous exposures have not yet been determined (Malakoff 2011).

Spills can also damage the health of cleanup workers who are exposed to the crude oil and oil dispersants. Crude oil contains volatile organic compounds, such as benzene, naphthalene, and toluene. Exposure to these chemicals can cause short-term problems, such as respiratory irritation, nausea, and headaches. Exposure to benzene and naphthalene increases the risk of cancer and toluene exposure is associated with birth defects. Oil also releases hydrogen sulfide gas, which can cause nerve damage. Exposure to oil dispersants can cause dermatitis, rashes, and secondary infections. Workers who cleaned up the Exxon *Valdez* spill filed workers compensation claims for acute injuries, respiratory problems, and dermatitis. The long-term effects of cleaning up oil spills are not well understood. Eating fish that have been exposed to oil may also pose a health risk (Solomon and Janssen 2010). In February 2011, the National Institute of Environmental Health Sciences launched a project to study the health of workers and volunteers involved in cleaning up the Deepwater Horizon oil spill. The project will enroll 55,000 participants who will be studied for at least ten years (National Institute of Environmental Health Sciences 2011).

Natural gas, also a fossil fuel and nonrenewable resource, occurs in oil deposits and near coal beds. Natural gas is composed of a variety of gases including methane, ethane, propane, nitrogen, helium, CO_2, and hydrogen sulfite (Hess 2010). Natural gas is used in electric power generation, home heating, cooking, transportation, and manufacturing. Natural gas accounts for 21.1 percent of the world's energy consumption (International Energy Association 2010). Global natural gas production is expected to peak by 2030 (Hess 2010). Natural gas combustion produces less particulate matter, carbon monoxide, and nitrogen oxides than oil or coal combustion. Natural gas combustion produces 30 percent less carbon dioxide per unit of heat produced than oil and 45 percent less than coal. Natural gas extraction, storage, and transport impose significant health risks. For example, leaks or ruptures in natural gas pipelines cause explosions that injure or kill people. People can die from asphyxiation from natural gas leaks in the home or workplace. Natural gas extraction workers also have an increased risk of some types of cancer (Hess 2010). Conventional natural gas extraction poses minimal risks to the environment, but a new method of extraction, known as hydraulic fracturing (or "fracking"), may pose significant risks to the environment and human health. Hydraulic fracturing uses water, sand, and chemicals to force natural gas out of underground rocks. Critics of this method argue that chemicals and natural gas can leach into underground water and contaminate wells and streams (Hogwarth and Ingraffea 2011). Supporters counter that hydraulic fracturing is safe because natural gas deposits occur several thousand feet below groundwater, so that chemicals and gas are not likely to impact groundwater, and that natural gas is a valuable and relatively clean energy resource that creates jobs (Engelder 2011). However, the safety of hydraulic fracturing may depend, in part, on geological factors that affect the containment of chemicals and gas. In areas where rock formations allow chemicals and gas to leach to the surface, fracking may not be safe. Because more research is needed, the EPA and other organizations are currently studying the risks of hydraulic fracturing (Zeller 2010).

Biomass includes wood, dung, peat, grass, leaves, and other plant materials burned to produce energy. Biomass is a renewable resource because plants continue to grow and produce organic materials. Biomass is used primarily in home heating, cooking, and electric power generation. Biomass accounts for 10 percent of the world's energy usage but 21.7 percent in developing nations (Hess 2010). Biomass produces particulate matter, CO_2, and other types of air pollution, which can have adverse impacts on human health, especially when burning occurs indoors in poorly ventilated homes or worksites. Burning of biomass in homes can increase the risk of respiratory infections and asthma in children, and can increase the risk of lung cancer and tuberculosis in adults (Hess 2010). The use of biomass as a fuel can have positive or negative impacts on the environment, depending on how it is cultivated and harvested. For example, using wood for fuel can devastate forest habitats and ecosystems, unless appropriate timber management practices are implemented, such as controlled cutting and replanting of trees. Biomass fuels may contribute less to global warming than fossil fuels, because fossil fuel combustion releases carbon into the atmosphere that has been buried for millions of years, while biomass combustion releases carbon that has been recently sequestered. In theory, wood burning might contribute no net carbon dioxide to the atmosphere if the wood that is burned is replaced by new forest growth (Hess 2010).

BIOFUEL

Biofuel, like biomass, is a renewable resource. The two most common ways of producing biofuel derive hydrocarbons from biomass. In the first method, ethanol is produced by fermentation of a food source high in sugar or starch, such as corn, sweet potatoes, or sugar cane. In the second, oil is extracted from plants with high oil content, such as oil palm, soybeans, or algae. Scientists have begun using genetic engineering techniques to design organisms that can improve the efficiency of these basic processes. Some researchers are designing yeast to produce ethanol and other hydrocarbons from agricultural waste products, such as cellulose mass, while others are attempting to develop algae and bacteria that will produce oil or other hydrocarbon fuels as an end-product of photosynthesis (Lynd et al. 2008; Robertson et al. 2008; Service 2008, 2010; Wijffels and Barbosa 2010). Biofuels today constitute less than 1 percent of the world's energy budget, but this percentage is expected to increase in the future (Hess 2010).

The health impacts of biofuels are similar to those of fossil fuels, except biofuels may produce less air pollution. Ethanol produces 12 percent less CO_2 when it burns than gasoline. However, ethanol has less energy per unit volume than gasoline, so an automobile may need to use more ethanol than gasoline to travel the same distance. Biodiesel fuel produces 41 percent less CO_2 than regular diesel fuel and less particulate matter. However, biofuels may still produce as much tropospheric ozone as fossil fuels (Hess 2010). Additionally, biofuels may contribute to famine and food shortages if crops, such as corn, are converted into fuels (Service 2008). As noted in Chapter 5, increases in food prices, due to the demand for corn to produce ethanol, exacerbated world hunger and led to food riots.

The environmental impacts of biofuels are uncertain at this point. Although biofuels produce less CO_2 than fossil fuels, the production of biofuels may increase deforestation because forests may be cleared to grow corn, sugar cane, or other materials used to produce biofuels. Also, gasoline and diesel oil are used in the production of biomass used to produce biofuels. Thus, any savings in CO_2 production from switching to biofuels could be negated by the reduction in carbon sequestration from the loss of forests and the use of fossil (or other) fuels in the production of biofuels.

As noted in Chapter 6, genetic engineering may be able to address some of the problems related to biofuels. See Chapter 6 for further discussion.

The most exciting development involves genetically engineering algae or bacteria to produce oil or other hydrocarbon fuels as an end-product of photosynthesis. These organisms would be grown in large tanks (i.e., bioreactors) and would not require arable land (Lynd et al. 2008; Service 2008). Major oil companies, such as ExxonMobile, have begun to invest hundreds of millions of dollars in this research. Craig Venter, who led a private effort to sequence the human genome, has formed a company, Synthetic Genomics, which has a goal of using genomics to develop synthetic organisms that manufacture oil from sunlight, water, and CO_2 (Service 2008). If it is possible to develop these microorganisms, this would be a carbon-neutral energy source because carbon added to the atmosphere would be removed by microorganisms. Also, production of these microorganisms would have minimal environmental impacts and would not increase deforestation.

NUCLEAR ENERGY

Nuclear energy is used primarily for electric power generation, though some submarines use nuclear engines. Nuclear energy accounts for 15.2 percent of the world's electricity and 5.8 percent of the world's energy usage (Hess 2010; International Energy Association 2010). Nuclear energy is produced from the fission of uranium 235, which decays into lighter, more stable elements and emits radiation and heat. The heat can be used to generate steam, which turns electric generators. For several decades, physicists have been attempting to generate nuclear energy from the fusion of light elements, such as hydrogen or helium, which would provide the world with clean energy. However, it may take many years before this vision becomes a reality. Fission-based nuclear energy is considered a nonrenewable resource because the world has a limited supply of uranium. Fusion-based nuclear energy is a virtually limitless resource because it requires only a small amount of hydrogen to produce an immense amount of energy, and the world has a plentiful supply of hydrogen in the ocean (Hess 2010).

Though nuclear energy does not produce any greenhouse gases, it poses significant risks to human health and the environment. Most of the risks of nuclear energy result from exposure to radioactive materials or byproducts, which emit ionizing radiation. Exposure to ionizing radiation can cause genetic damage, which can lead to cancer, sterility, and other health problems. Workers who mine and process radioactive materials have an increased risk of lung cancer, lymphoma, and leukemia. Nuclear power plant workers also have an increased risk of cancer (Hess 2010). The disposal of nuclear waste is a major environmental and public health hazard. Spent nuclear fuel remains radioactive for thousands of years. Waste disposal sites and containers must be secured safely to prevent leaks into the environment (Nuclear Regulatory Commission 2010). As mentioned in Chapter 7, communities have opposed nuclear waste sites in their areas, due to concerns about environmental and health risks. Transportation of nuclear fuel and waste also poses a significant environmental and public health risk. Although there have been no accidental releases of radioactive materials during transportation in the United States during the past thirty years, if it an accident were to occur it could have major environmental and public health impacts (Nuclear Regulatory Commission 2010).

The most dramatic risks associated with nuclear energy are accidents at nuclear power plants. An explosion triggered by a power surge at the nuclear power plant in Chernobyl, Russia on April 26, 1986 led to the release of a radioactive cloud that infected the water supply. Thirty workers died in the explosion and fire, and hundreds of residents became ill as a result of coming into contact with the cloud. Animals were also affected. Increases in radioisotopes in the water were detected as far away as Finland and Austria. Thyroid cancer in children has been linked to the Chernobyl disaster (World Health Organization 2010g). Other adverse outcomes may emerge in the future because it can take several decades to develop cancer from radiation exposure (Williams 2009). Chernobyl also caused adverse psychological effects, including depression and distress, among people directly impacted by the disaster and cleanup workers (Beehler et al. 2008). On March 28, 1979, the worst nuclear power accident in United States' history happened at the Three Mile Island plant near Harrisburg, PA. A partial meltdown of one of the reactors led to the release of radioactive gas. Epidemiologists have studied people living within a ten-mile radius of the plant. So far, the accident has not resulted in increased cancer risks (Levin 2008).

On March 11, 2011, an 8.9 magnitude earthquake off the east coast of Japan (and the accompanying tsunami) caused thousands of deaths and damaged the Fukushima Daini and Fukushima Daiichi nuclear power plants. The damage occurred because the plants lost cooling ability, which resulted in a build-up of steam and hydrogen gas. Two explosions and radiation leaks occurred at the Fukushima Daiichi plant. Plant operators flooded reactors and spent fuel rods with seawater to avoid a complete nuclear meltdown. Thousands of residents were evacuated who live within twenty miles of the plant to protect them from radiation (Onishi et al. 2011). It will take years to fully understand the health impacts of these accidents (Smith 2011).

Despite these major accidents, the nuclear power industry has made significant improvements since the 1980s, and accidents are rare. Newer plants using the latest technology are expected to be much safer than older plants, such as the Chernobyl plant and the Fukushima plants (Sailor et al. 2000). However, even the best-designed nuclear power plant will not be perfectly safe, and society must decide what level of risk is acceptable (Sailor et al. 2000).

An important environmental impact of nuclear power is the high demand for water. Nuclear power plants are built near lakes, rivers, or oceans because they require a large supply of water to absorb excess heat. Power plants also require additional water to cool reactors in case of an accident. If the water supply to a nuclear power plant is disrupted, the plant must shut down. Adult fish, fish larvae, turtles, frogs, and other forms of aquatic life may be killed when they are sucked into reactor cooling systems or become caught on filters or grates. Water discharged from nuclear power plants into lakes, rivers, or oceans is much hotter than surrounding water, which can adversely affect aquatic life and ecosystems (Union of Concerned Scientists 2010).

It is also important to mention that the processes used to enrich uranium for use in nuclear power plants can also be employed to generate materials for nuclear weapons. Also, nuclear reactors can produce materials that can be used in weaponry, such as isotopes of uranium and plutonium. Increasing the number of nuclear power plants in the world would therefore also increase the supply of materials for nuclear weapons, which could fall into the hands of terrorists or countries that are considering nuclear warfare. Many countries are concerned that Iran's plans to build nuclear power plants are a ruse for starting a nuclear weapons program (Sanger and Broad 2010).

HYDROELECTRIC POWER

Hydroelectric power is a form of renewable energy that accounts for 15 percent of the world's electricity and 2.2 percent of the total energy budget. Hydroelectric power plants convert the energy of water moving through dams into electricity. Many nations have begun building hydroelectric plants as a clean alternative to fossil fuel consumption. Although obtaining electricity from hydroelectric power plants is much more environmentally friendly than burning coal, hydropower has some disadvantages. As noted in Chapter 7, dams and reservoirs can cause major environmental and social disruption. Also, reservoirs can produce a significant amount of methane, a greenhouse gas with more warming potential than CO_2 (Hess 2010).

HYDROKINETIC POWER

Hydrokinetic power is another renewable energy resource that converts the energy of moving water (such as waves, streams, currents, or tides) into electricity. The environmental and health impacts of hydrokinetic power are thought to be minimal, but more research is needed to determine whether hydrokinetic power plants disrupt fish and other marine animals. Although some forms of hydrokinetic power, such as waterwheels, have been in use for thousands of years, hydrokinetic power constitutes less than 1 percent of the energy economy. However, hydrokinetic power's potential impact is large. According to some estimates, capturing the available hydrokinetic energy in rivers, streams, and coastlines in the United States could provide electricity for 67 million homes (Union of Concerned Scientists 2009).

GEOTHERMAL POWER

Geothermal power uses heat energy from the Earth to turn electric generators. Geothermal power has a minimal impact on human health and the environment and is a renewable resource. For the most part, geothermal power constitutes only a small part of the world's energy use (less than 1 percent). However, there are some notable exceptions. Iceland generates 50 percent of its electricity from geothermal power, and the Philippines and El Salvador produce more than 25 percent of their electricity from geothermal power. In the United States, California derives 5 percent of its electricity from geothermal power (Union of Concerned Scientists 2009).

SOLAR POWER

Solar power is a renewable resource with minimal human health or environmental impacts. Each day the Earth receives energy from the Sun equivalent to all of the world's stores of fossil fuels, though a third of that energy is reflected back into space. There are several different types of solar power. Many buildings are warmed when heat from the sun enters windows and is trapped inside. Other buildings have systems that collect and store solar heat in liquids composed of water and alcohol, which are circulated through the building. Solar water heaters can provide hot water for buildings. Because water heating constitutes 15 percent of the energy used by a typical home, using the sun to produce hot water can save a significant amount of energy. Solar thermal collecting systems use a series of mirrors to heat water, which can be used to generate electricity. Solar thermal collecting systems can also store the heat energy from the sun for use at night. Many communities have begun building solar thermal power plants to reduce the use of fossils fuels to generate electricity. Finally, photovoltaic cells convert the light from the sun into electric current. Photovoltaic cells have been used to power calculators, radios, lights, weather stations, and the international space station. Some households and business have installed panels of photovoltaic cells to reduce their use of energy from electric power grids. Though solar energy accounts for less than 1 percent of the world's energy usage, its impact is expected to increase substantially as people look for alternatives to fossil fuels (Union of Concerned Scientists 2009).

WIND POWER

Wind power is another renewable resource with minimal impacts on human health and the environment. Wind power has been rapidly increasing as a source of electricity. The United States has invested heavily in wind power. In 2008, the United States built enough wind power to supply the annual electricity needs of 2 million homes. Other leaders in wind power include Germany, Spain, China, and India. Recent improvements in efficiencies in wind turbines, tax incentives, and concerns about greenhouse gas emissions have increased interest in wind power. The costs of wind power continue to decline and may soon become competitive with fossil fuels. Though wind power currently constitutes less than 1 percent of the world's energy budget, it is expected to be one of the fastest growing sectors of the energy economy in the twenty-first century. The environmental and health impacts of wind power are minimal, but birds and bats can become caught in wind turbines (Union of Concerned Scientists 2009; Kintisch 2010b).

ETHICAL AND POLICY ISSUES

Mitigating climate change, discussed earlier, is one of the main issues related to energy use and production, but there are others. We have already examined many of these issues during discussions of air pollution and hazardous waste in Chapter 7, and urban sprawl in Chapter 8. In this chapter, we will consider some other controversies related to energy production and use.

Drilling for oil and natural gas in the United States has been controversial since the 1970s, and it became a major issue in the 2008 political campaign. Republican vice-presidential nominee Sarah Palin coined the slogan "Drill, baby, drill!" to signal her party's commitment to exploration and drilling, while the Democrats endorsed a more cautious approach. In March 2010, President Barack Obama announced a plan to open up petroleum and natural gas exploration and drilling off the U.S. eastern coast and parts of Florida and Alaska to help reduce dependence on foreign oil (Broder 2010a). Environmentalists condemned the move and warned that drilling for oil and natural gas off the eastern coast of the United States could destroy delicate marine ecosystems and spoil pristine beaches. Supporters of the plan said that it opens up an untapped resource and could create thousands of jobs. Estimates of the amount of resources available in these coastal regions vary, but some government reports claim it may contain enough oil and natural gas to fuel 2.4 million cars for sixty years and heat 8 million homes for sixty years (Broder and Krauss 2010a).

There has also been a heated debate for several decades about drilling for oil in the 1.5 million acre Arctic National Wildlife Refuge (ANWR) in Alaska. ANWR contains an estimated 10 billion barrels of oil, enough to meet the United States' oil needs for 7.7 years (Snyder 2008). It would take an investment of several hundred billion dollars to extract this oil, which would not be available for at least seven years after exploration and drilling have begun. Many people favor drilling in ANWR to reduce the United States' dependence on foreign oil and provide much needed energy. Drilling would also generate tax revenue for the federal government and economic development for the State of Alaska. The federal government could earn several hundred billion dollars from royalties and corporate income taxes, which would be shared with the State of Alaska. Environmentalists oppose drilling in ANWR because of the impact on species, habitats, and the arctic ecosystem. Even if the impact of drilling is minimal, there is still the possibility that oil spills would damage the area (Snyder 2008). Alaskans have mixed feeling about drilling in ANWR. Though many are concerned about the environmental damage caused by drilling, others would welcome the oil revenue and economic development (Wallace 2005).

Drilling for oil in vulnerable areas like ANWR and the United States east coast pits environmental concerns (e.g., protecting species, habitats, and ecosystems) against utilitarian ones (e.g., energy production and economic development). Increased oil and natural gas production can provide valuable energy to fuel the U.S. economy, which can lead to job creation, wealth, tax revenue, industrial production, and other positive economic outcomes. But oil and natural gas production can also threaten species, habitats, and ecosystems. Earlier in this chapter I argued that the long-term goal of climate change policies should be to shift from reliance on fossil fuels to utilization of energy sources that are environmentally and socioeconomically sustainable. The same goal also applies to energy production. Energy production should shift away from extraction of fossil fuels to the development of alternative sources of energy that cause less damage to the environment and human health and are sustainable over the long term, such as wind power, solar power, hydroelectric power, and biofuels. As noted earlier, fossil fuel production will peak in about twenty years, so a shift to alternative energy sources is inevitable. However, it may make take several decades to move away from dependence on fossil fuels because alternative energy technologies are still under development and the world currently obtains more than 80 percent of its energy from fossil fuels. Dramatically curtailing production of fossil fuels at this point in time could be economically disastrous. Prudence suggests that fossil fuel production should still go forward as the world makes a transition to a new energy economy.

Accepting the premise that new drilling and exploration should still take place need not imply that these activities should occur in ANWR or any particular area. The decision to drill in a specific place should be based on a careful assessment of the environmental risks of drilling and the expected socioeconomic benefits. An important part of this assessment should be a consideration of alternatives with minimal environmental impacts. For example, natural gas extraction that poses far fewer risks to the environment than oil extraction. A reasonable compromise between utility and stewardship of the environment would be to allow gas extraction in sensitive areas but not oil extraction. Another compromise position would be to allow off-shore oil extraction with additional safety features, such as blowout preventers and emergency shutoff equipment, which were not used in the Deepwater Horizon rig. H.R. 5634, a bill introduced by Representative Jay Inslee would amend the Outer Continental Shelf Lands Act to require the best technologies for offshore oil and gas drilling (Govtrack.us 2010). Legislation like H.R. 5634 could allow offshore extraction of oil and natural gas to move forward with up-to-date safety features to prevent environmental damage. In October 2010, the Obama administration lifted a temporary ban on off-shore drilling in the United States it had put in place following the Deepwater Horizon disaster. The administration also imposed new rules to promote safety (Baker 2010). However, only two months after lifting the ban, the administration changed its mind and imposed a ban on new offshore exploration and drilling along the eastern Gulf of Mexico coast and Atlantic coast (Broder and Krauss 2010b).

Building oil pipelines also raises environmental issues. Though pipelines can reduce transportation costs and risks, create jobs, and promote economic development, they can also disrupt habitats and ecosystems, and pollute the environment when leaks occur. As of the writing of this book, the Obama administration was considering whether to approve construction of the Keystone Pipeline Expansion Project, a 1,700-mile-long pipeline that would transport oil from Canada across the Great Plains to refineries in Texas. Environmentalists have objected to the pipeline because of its potential impacts on habitats, species, and ecosystems. They have also opposed the pipeline because the oil would come from extracting oil from tar sands in Canada, a process that requires the use of substantial resources (primarily energy and water) and can result in pollution of waterways and deforestation. Oil industry leaders and others have defended the pipeline on the grounds that it would provide a much needed source of oil, create jobs, stimulate economic development, help reduce the United States' dependence on oil from the Mideast, and have minimal environmental impacts. They also argue that Canada will sell its tar sands oil to other countries, such as China, India, and Japan, even if the United States does not build the pipeline (Eilperin 2011b).

Nuclear power presents another ethical dilemma related to energy production. Because nuclear power plants generate electricity without producing greenhouse gases, some environmentalists who opposed the development of nuclear energy in the 1980s and 1990s have changed their minds (Marshall 2005). Increasing reliance on nuclear power could help to mitigate climate change (Sailor et al. 2000). However, nuclear power still poses significant long-term environmental and public health hazards. While the industry has made significant safety improvements since the 1980s, the disposal of hazardous nuclear waste remains a difficult issue, because waste sites need to be designed to store nuclear material securely for hundreds of thousands of years. Also, local communities are likely to oppose plans to locate nuclear waste sites in their neighborhoods (Kerr 2011).

Additionally, nuclear power is a very expensive source of energy. Nuclear power plants require a huge investment of capital upfront. A new nuclear power plant can cost as much as $18 billion. Currently, most nuclear power plants are built with government funds or subsidies, and private investors have shied away from nuclear power (Grunwald 2008). Including construction expenses, electricity produced from nuclear power costs about $0.30 per kilowatt hour (Severance 2009), while the average price of electricity in the United States is $0.10 per kilowatt hour (Energy Information Administration 2010). Some argue that unless costs dramatically increase for other sources of energy, nuclear power does not make a great deal of economic sense (Grunwald 2008). However, others argue that costs can be reduced by extending the life of existing plants and improving efficiency (Grimes and Nuttall 2010).

Biofuels raise ethical issues as well. As noted in Chapter 5, the use of corn as a substrate for ethanol production has exacerbated world hunger by driving up the price of corn. Clearing new land to compensate for higher demands for fuel crops would help sustain food production, but also increase deforestation, which reduces biodiversity and contributes to global warming. Biofuel production may also increase the use of pesticides, fertilizers, and water (Buyx and Tait 2011). Using genetic engineering to develop microorganisms that manufacture biofuels may avoid these problems but also raise different ethical concerns. For example, environmental contamination could occur if GM organisms used to produce biofuels are released into the wild. According to Buyx and Tait (2011), biofuels should provide energy without worsening global hunger, reducing biodiversity, or increasing global warming.

Even clean technologies, such as wind power, can create ethical and political controversies. The mountainous and coastal regions of North Carolina have ideal conditions for wind power generation, due to high average wind speeds, and efforts are underway to establish wind farms in these regions. Wind power in North Carolina has the support of the federal and state governments and many community and industry leaders. In 2007, the state legislature passed a bill requiring that electric utilities derive 12.5 percent of their power from renewable sources, such as wind and solar power, by 2021 (Wall 2010). Utilities could develop their own renewable energy sources or purchase renewable energy from individuals or companies. The N.C. GreenPower Program provides tax incentives for individuals and companies to develop renewable energy, such as wind and solar power. County governments have also established incentives and regulations for wind power development (North Carolina Wind Energy 2010). However, some proposed wind power sites have been controversial. Concerned citizens have opposed placement of wind farms on top of North Carolina mountains because the turbines can harm birds and bats and spoil scenic views (Wall 2010). Similar opposition to wind farms has arisen in Texas and other states (Kintisch 2010b; Galbraith 2011). While it is important for people to be able to enjoy beautiful vistas free from artificial structures, such as wind turbines, other energy technologies, such as coal and oil power, can also spoil one's enjoyment of nature. Drilling for oil off the North Carolina coast could lead to oil spills, and coal combustion creates air and water pollution. A wind farm would seem to be preferable to these alternatives.

The controversy over wind power illustrates a fundamental point related to energy production: There is no "perfect" source of energy. Though energy production provides important economic and social benefits, all types of energy production involve some risks to human health or the environment. Some impose fewer risks than others, but all forms have some risks. A responsible energy policy is not one that avoids all risks, but one that carefully balances benefits and risks while providing enough energy to sustain the human population.

POPULATION GROWTH

As noted in the previous chapter, the human population currently stands at 7 billion and is expected to reach 9 billion by the middle of the twenty-first century, and then to level off (see Figure 9.4).

Although populations have leveled off or are declining in developed nations, population growth continues in developing nations (see Table 9.1). In the next four decades, more than 95 percent of the world's population growth will occur in the poorest regions of the world (Hinrichsen 2010). For example, Ethiopia and Uganda will triple in population, Congo will double, and Nigeria will nearly double. While the population in developing nations is expected to increase from 5.6 billion in 2009 to 7.9 billion in 2050, the population in

Table 9.1. *Top Ten Most Populous Countries in 2010 and 2050*

2010 Population	2050 Population
China, 1.33 billion	India, 1.66 billion
India, 1.17 billion	China, 1.30 billion
United States, 310 million	United States, 439 million
Indonesia, 243 million	Indonesia, 313 million
Brazil, 201 million	Pakistan, 291 million
Pakistan, 184 million	Ethiopia, 278 million
Bangladesh, 156 million	Nigeria, 264 million
Nigeria, 152 million	Brazil, 261 million
Russia, 139 million	Bangladesh, 250 million
Japan, 127 million	Congo, 189 million

Based on data from the U.S. Census Bureau 2010a.

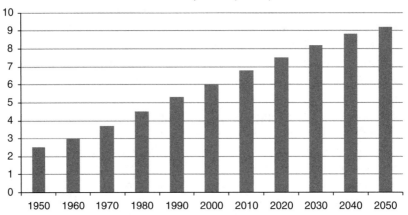

Figure 9.4. World Population, 1950–2050 (based on data from the U.S. Census Bureau 2010a).

developed nations is only expected to increase from 1.23 billion to 1.28 billion. The population of developed nations would be expected to decline without immigration from developing nations (United Nations 2009). Among developed nations, the United States significantly increases in population by 41 percent by 2050, but much of this growth will be due to immigration from Latin American countries. Japan, Russian, Germany, and Italy are expected to decline in population. By 2050, India will overtake China as the world's most populous nation (U.S. Census Bureau 2010).

Another important factor to consider in population growth is demographics (see Table 9.2). There will be a dramatic aging of the population. The fastest growing demographic groups will be 70–79 years of age, which will double as a percentage of the population; 80–89 years of age, which will nearly triple; and 90 years or older, which will more

Table 9.2. *Demographic Age Groups for the World Population in 2010 and 2050*

Age Range (years)	2010 Population (%)	2050 Population (%)
0–19	35.1	27.3
20–29	16.8	13.4
30–39	14.5	13.5
40–49	12.7	12.3
50–59	9.5	11.6
60–69	6.1	10.3
70–79	3.6	7.2
80 and older	1.6	4.7

Based on data from the U.S. Census Bureau 2010b.

than quadruple (U.S. Census Bureau 2010b). Currently, developed nations have much older populations than developing countries, due to lower fertility rates and higher longevity. By 2050, developing nations will start to age as well. The aging of the population will place tremendous financial and social pressures on many countries, who may find it difficult to provide adequate health care for their senior citizens. Many families will find it difficult to care for their older parents and children at the same time (Hinrichsen 2010). Increasing urbanization, discussed in Chapter 8, is another important demographic trend.

Population growth in a particular country is a function of three basic factors: fertility (the number of births per mother), mortality (the number of deaths in the population), and immigration from other countries. Since 1950, global population growth has resulted from reductions in mortality as a result of increased availability of food and drinkable water, better sanitation and hygiene, improved prevention of infectious diseases, reduction in poverty, and enhanced access to medical care (Fowler 2004). Historically, infectious diseases have taken a tremendous toll on human populations. For example, the bubonic plague, discussed in Chapter 2, killed an estimated 30 percent to 60 percent of Europe's population in the mid-1300s (Abee 2008). The 1918 Spanish flu pandemic killed 50 million–100 million people worldwide, or 3–6 percent of the human population (Taubenberger and Morens 2006). Famine and warfare have also been major contributors to human population declines. As many as 10 million people may have died in the Great Famine in the Ukraine (part of the former Soviet Union) in 1932–1933 (Shelton 2005), 30 million people died in a famine in China in 1962 (Fitzpatrick 2009), and 50 million soldiers and civilians were killed in World War II (Keegan 2005).

Although infectious diseases (such as malaria and HIV/AIDS) and warfare (particularly conflicts on the African continent) continue to take their toll on human populations, the burgeoning global population presents major problems for human health and well-being and the environment (Hinrichsen 2010). Poverty and famine are the main adverse outcomes of unchecked population growth. Approximately 20 percent of the people in the world live in extreme poverty, defined as available income of less than $1.25 a day (Hinrichsen 2010).

As families living in extreme poverty increase in size, they may not be able to afford to feed everyone an adequate diet, which leads to starvation and malnutrition. Malnutrition exacerbates infectious and chronic diseases. Thirty-five thousand children younger than age five die in developing nations each day as a result of starvation or malnutrition (Hinrichsen 2010). People who are living in extreme poverty may not be able to afford basic necessities, such as food, housing, clothing, education, or healthcare. Lack of these necessities can also contribute to disease and mortality. Finally, poverty is also a major factor in various social problems, such as crime, prostitution, and drug abuse (Hinrichsen 2010).

While unchecked population growth adversely affects human welfare, it has an even greater impact on the environment. As we have already seen numerous times in this book, population growth is a major factor in many different environmental problems, ranging from deforestation to air pollution. Some of the environmental impacts of population growth are as follows:

- **Increased land use**. As noted in Chapter 8, increases in population lead to more land used for housing, agriculture, industry, roads, and other activities. Forests, rainforests, wetlands, and other important habitats may be destroyed or damaged to accommodate population increases. Increased land use leads to loss of habitat, species extinction or decline, decreased biodiversity, and ecosystem disruption (Hinrichsen 2010).
- **Increased air and water pollution**. Population growth increases activities that create air and water pollution, such as automobile use, electricity generation, agriculture, urban development, industry, and mining (Hinrichsen 2010).
- **Increased solid waste**. Population growth also increases the generation of solid waste from industry, mining, health care, agriculture, energy production, and other sources (Hinrichsen 2010).
- **Increased demand for drinkable water.** As the population grows, more drinkable water is required. To provide this resource, governments may need to dam rivers and build reservoirs, which leads to adverse environmental consequences (Hinrichsen 2010).
- **Increased fishing.** Increases in population lead to increased fishing, which can lead to overfishing. Marine fish populations have declined in many areas as a result of excess fishing from commercial operations (Hinrichsen 2010).
- **Increased energy use.** An increase in population leads to increases in demand for energy, such as oil and petroleum products, coal, electricity, and so on. Energy production and use have a variety of adverse environmental impacts, including pollution and climate change (Hinrichsen 2010).

Efficient use of resources, pollution control, sustainable development, conservation of energy, recycling of waste, and other environmentally friendly practices can help to offset the effects of population increases on the environment. However, sound environmental policies must also address the importance of controlling population growth, because a burgeoning population may reverse any gains from environmentally friendly practices (Hinrichsen 2010). Without a serious effort to check population growth, the Earth may soon reach its carrying capacity for human life. The nations around the globe may need to take steps to make sure that the human population does not become so large that it overwhelms the environment (Ehrlich and Ehrlich 1990).

ETHICAL AND POLICY ISSUES

Population control raises ethical and policy issues. One set of issues concerns the actions that an individual might take to control population; another set of issues relates to the policies that societies might adopt to control population. Individuals need to consider whether to procreate, adopt children, or have no children at all. The decision to have or not have children is a very personal choice that we face at some point. Because this decision impacts society and the environment, the choice is also a moral one. Many of the world's religions advocate human procreation. Genesis 1:28 says "Be fruitful and multiply, and fill the earth" (Holy Bible 2004). The Catholic Church strongly favors natural human procreation and condemns artificial forms of contraception, such as condoms or the birth control pill. The only form of contraception the Catholic Church accepts is the rhythm method, in which couples voluntarily abstain from copulation when a woman is most fertile (Catholic Answers 2008). Many other religions, including various Protestant sects, Judaism, Islam, Hinduism, and Buddhism view new human life as a great blessing but do not specifically prohibit birth control (Maguire 2003).

Most ethical theories have little to say specifically about population control. Utilitarians would view reproduction as a moral obligation, provided that the benefits of reproduction to society outweigh the harms. Normally, the benefits of reproduction outweigh the harms because each new life brought into the world represents an increase in the total happiness (or utility). Additionally, people bring happiness to other people, such as their parents, family members and friends, and they make positive contributions to society through their vocations or employment, service work, literature, art, and so forth. In countries that face significant social and economic problems in the future due to a low birth rate, utilitarians would view procreation as a pressing social obligation. However, utilitarians would hold that people have an obligation to limit their reproduction when the harms of bringing too many new people into the world, such as increased poverty, resource use, and adverse environmental impacts, outweigh the benefits. Too many people in society can decrease the average happiness of everyone (Blackorby 1995). The ideal average number of children per couple favored by utilitarians would depend on the fertility replacement rate, that is, the number of children born per woman to replace the population. In countries with low rates of infant mortality, the replacement rate is 2.1, but in countries with higher levels of infant mortality the replacement rate would be higher. Fertility below 2 will result in a decrease in population (Morgan 2003).

Kantians would also view reproduction as a moral obligation, provided that it is consistent with the categorical imperative (CI). The CI would not endorse a rule like, "I will have no children," because if everyone followed this maxim then the human race would go extinct. Nor would the CI endorse a rule like, "I will have as many children as I can," because if everyone followed this maxim, there would be unabated reproduction and overpopulation. However, the CI might favor a rule like, "I will have children but not so many that this will cause significant social problems," because everyone could follow a rule like this one.

Virtue theorists, such as Aristotle, would recommend child rearing as a strategy for developing moral virtue. Parents must learn to practice patience, courage, kindness, justice, moderation, and many other virtues. Becoming a parent can make one a better person. Because one can be a parent without procreating, virtue theorists would view adoption as a sound strategy for developing moral virtue, and would place no special importance on being a biological parent.

The principle of sustainability (discussed in Chapter 4) offers some useful insights into population control. This principle implies that population levels, within and among nations, should be ecologically sustainable (Norton 2005). What level of human population is sustainable? 4 billion people? 5 billion? 7 billion? This is a difficult question to answer, because it depends on a variety of evolving factors, including agricultural productivity, land use, energy use, and technology. Increases in agricultural productivity and energy efficiency can make it easier to sustain larger populations on the same area of land. Population levels that are unsustainable, given the agriculture and technology of 1850, might be sustainable in 2050 (Hinrichsen 2010). Although scientists may disagree about estimates of the Earth's carrying capacity for the human population, it is clear that uncontrolled population growth is not sustainable. So, some measures need to be taken to control population growth (Hinrichsen 2010).

Societies have implemented a variety of strategies to control population, some of which are more controversial than others. Educating and empowering women, especially in developing nations, is one of the most important strategies for controlling population (Osotimehin 2011). The number of children that women give birth to declines as their educational attainment increases because they have other options to consider besides having babies and raising children. They may decide to limit their family size or not have children at all in order to pursue a vocation or career. Providing women in developing nations with at least a basic education and promoting their rights can help control population. However, in some Muslim and African countries women are denied education and basic human rights. Population may be difficult to control in these countries without changing these cultural conditions (World Commission on Environment and Development 1987; United Nations 2005b).

Providing education about forms of birth control and making contraception available are two other important strategies for controlling population. People in developing nations may lack access to condoms, oral contraception, or other effective methods of birth control. They may also lack a sound understanding of human reproduction and ways of preventing pregnancy. Reducing poverty and improving public health can also help to control population growth by reducing infant and child mortality. Historically, one of the reasons why people have had large families is to ensure that enough children survive to adulthood. When rates of infant and child mortality decline, people may become more comfortable with having fewer children (Commission on Environment and Development 1987).

In addition to providing education and access to resources, governments have used coercive methods to control population, such as China's One-Child Policy. China implemented the policy in 1979 to control population growth, despite the fact that a propaganda campaign to discourage couples from reproducing lowered the birth rate from 5.9 to 2.9 in only ten years (Hvistendahl 2010). The law prohibits couples from having more than one child without a permit if they are government employees or live in urban areas. People living in rural areas are generally allowed to have more than one child as long as they wait five years (Hesketh et al. 2005). Ethnic minorities and people who live in remote areas are allowed to have a third child. People who violate the law can be fined thousands of dollars. The law provides benefits to couples who delay child bearing, such as a longer maternity leave. Couples who have only one child are also awarded a certificate of honor.

Though the One-Child Policy has reduced China's fertility rate to 1.7 and helped to prevent famine, it has produced troubling social consequences. There have been various reports that Chinese authorities have forced women to have abortions to avoid giving birth to an additional child. Also, because boys are generally more popular than girls in China, many couples decide to abort female fetuses, and some have practiced female infanticide to ensure that their one child is a male (Fitzpatrick 2009). The sex ratio in some urban areas is 13:1 (boys to girls) (Hesketh et al. 2005). According to some reports, Chinese authorities have threatened to destroy the homes of people who failed to pay fines they were required to pay for violating the policy (Fitzpatrick 2009). The policy is also shifting the age demographics in China so that younger people bear a larger burden of caring for elderly parents (Hesketh et al. 2005).

Governments that are interested in increasing population have offered financial incentives for couples who have children. Poland, France, and Italy all offer cash incentives for women who give birth (BBC News 2006). France's birth incentives include three years of paid parental leave for new mothers and job protection, subsidized childcare, and fulltime preschool (Medical New Today 2006). Japan has also begun offering birth incentives. The Japanese government will pay parents $3,300 per year for every new child born until the child reaches the age of fifteen. Japan also provides free daycare (Wakabayashi and Inada 2009). For many years, the United States has given parents tax breaks. Taxpayers can exempt $3,650 per dependent child from their taxes and also receive a $1,000 tax credit per child (Personal Dividends 2010). Some governments also have used cash incentives to slow birthrates. In India, couples who wait at least two years before having children can receive $107 from the government (2point6billion.com 2010).

While most people would agree that governments should take an active role in slowing population growth (or encouraging it in some cases), coercive measures, such as China's One-Child Policy, are ethically suspect because they interfere with human rights. Government restrictions on reproduction pit the principle of utility against respect for human rights. Some ethical theorists argue that reproduction is a fundamental right that should not be restricted by the state (Robertson 1994). Even if one does not regard reproduction as a fundamental right, one could still view it as important for expressing other rights, such as freedom of religion and freedom of action. Thus, one could argue that utilitarian considerations should not outweigh human rights when it comes to population control.

Moreover, it is not always clear that restrictions on reproduction actually promote the greater social good, because these policies can have negative social consequences. Restrictions on reproduction can cause considerable unhappiness and frustration to couples who want to have children, lead to uneven sex ratios, and encourage abortion and infanticide. Although many people view abortion as morally acceptable in some circumstances, infanticide is widely regarded as immoral and is illegal in most countries (Warren 2000). Uneven sex ratios can lead to social problems, because members of the majority sex may have difficulty finding a mate.

Although it is important for governments to adopt policies that promote sustainable population levels (Norton 2005), they should not use coercive measures to control the birth rate. Restrictions on reproduction do not achieve a fair and reasonable balance among the competing values at stake – human rights, individual well-being, social utility, and environmental protection. Coercive measures emphasize social utility and environmental protection at the expense of human rights and individual well-being, and are justified only in dire circumstances. China's One-Child Policy, which may have been justified in 1979 to avoid another famine, is an anachronism that is no longer consistent with the country's current level of economic development (Hesketh et al. 2005; Hvistendahl 2010). Unless a nation is facing a genuine overpopulation crisis, governments should use noncoercive methods, such as education in birth control methods, empowerment of women, support for contraception and family planning, and financial incentives to pursue sustainable population levels.

Because population growth is a global problem, not just an intranational one, international organizations, such as the United Nations, the International Monetary Fund, and the World Bank, can take steps to raise awareness about social, economic, and environmental problems related to excess population growth. They can also assist countries with contraception and family planning, and educational campaigns (Osotimehin 2011). Nongovernmental organizations, such as the Gates Foundation, the Wellcome Trust, and CARE, can also play a role in helping countries achieve sustainable population levels. However, international efforts to control population should be sensitive to the cultural and religious beliefs and practices concerning reproduction and family life, as well as national sovereignty, otherwise well-meaning efforts could backfire. Developing countries may resent efforts by developed nations to control their population and interfere with their way of life and self-governance.

SUMMARY

In this chapter, I have examined ethical and policy aspects of three key global issues: climate change, energy use, and population growth. These issues have significant interconnections with each other and implications for other environmental health issues. The main theme that emerges from this chapter is the importance of socioeconomic and environmental sustainability as a policy objective (Norton 2005, Rockström 2009; Kerr 2010). Policies related to energy, climate change, and population should promote resource use and management that can be maintained over the long run. Tax incentives, cap and trade systems and other regulations, research funding, and other government policies should promote a transition away from dependence on fossil fuels toward the use of alternative, sustainable sources of energy to mitigate climate change and ensure that future generations have enough energy to prosper. International cooperation will be needed to develop policies relating to energy and climate. Governments should also use noncoercive measures, such as educational campaigns and economic incentives, to promote sustainable population levels. International organizations and nongovernmental organizations should also assist with population control efforts. The next chapter will explore issues of justice, which are an important concern in many controversies related to environmental health.

10

___

JUSTICE AND ENVIRONMENTAL HEALTH

As we have seen throughout this book, justice is an important concern in environmental health because health risks related to the environment are often distributed unequally. Risks are distributed unequally because people face different types of health hazards depending on where they live, work, attend school, shop, travel, or recreate (Shrader-Frechette 2002, 2007a). Though we have touched briefly on some justice concerns in earlier chapters, in this chapter we explore ethical and policy issues related to the distribution of health risks in the environment in greater depth.

HEALTH INEQUALITIES AND THE ENVIRONMENT

To better understand the relationship between the environment and justice, it will be useful to reflect upon how different aspects of the environment can contribute to health inequalities (often referred to as health disparities). A large body of literature has documented demographic differences in mortality, morbidity, and disease burden among people living in the same nation as well as differences among nations (Barr 2008). Life expectancy in the United States is higher for whites than for blacks (U.S. Census Bureau 2010b). Among these two groups, white females have the highest life expectancy (80.8 years), followed by black females (76.8 years), white males (75.9 years), and black males (70.0 years) (Xu et al. 2010). Latinos have a higher life expectancy than whites. Latino women have a life expectancy of 83.1 years, and Latino males have a life expectancy of 77.9 years (Arias 2010). Infant mortality rates vary considerably by race and ethnicity in the United States. Blacks have an infant mortality rate of 13.6 deaths per 1,000 live births, followed by Puerto Ricans (8.3), Native Americans (8.1), whites (5.8), Mexicans (5.5), Asians (4.9), and Cubans (4.4) (MacDorman and Mathews 2008).

Disease statistics also vary by race and ethnicity in the United States. Blacks have the highest incidence of cancer and the highest cancer mortality among all racial and ethnic groups, including whites, Asians, Latinos, and Native Americans (see Table 10.1). Asians have the lowest incidence of cancer and lowest cancer mortality (National Cancer Institute 2010). Black females have the highest incidence of breast cancer and breast cancer mortality, while Native American females have the lowest incidence of breast cancer

Table 10.1. *U.S. Cancer Incidence and Death Rates*

Cancer Incidence Rates per 100,000 Individuals from 1998 to 2007

All Races/Ethnicities		White	Black	Asian/Pacific	Native American	Hispanic
Both sexes	471.4	470.6	489.3	298.7	385.5	368.2
Male	552.5	544.9	623.1	332.3	424.6	426.1
Female	414.7	418.8	392.9	278.1	359.2	331.2

Cancer Death Rates per 100,000 Individuals from 1998 to 2007

All Races/Ethnicities		White	Black	Asian/Pacific	Native American	Hispanic
Both sexes	183.8	182.4	224.2	110.8	156.7	122.1
Male	225.4	222.5	296.5	134.2	183.7	150.6
Female	155.4	155	180.6	94.1	138	102.3

Based on data from Kohler et al. 2011.

and Asians have the lowest breast cancer mortality (National Cancer Institute 2010). Black males have the highest incidence of prostate cancer and prostate cancer mortality, while Native Americans have the lowest incidence of prostate cancer and Asians have the lowest prostate cancer mortality (National Cancer Institute 2010). Blacks, Native Americans, and Hispanics have higher rates of cardiovascular disease, diabetes, and HIV/AIDS than whites and Asians (National Partnership for Action 2010). Blacks have a higher rate of obesity (35.7 percent) than Hispanics (28.7 percent) or whites (23.7 percent). Black females have the highest obesity rate among these groups (39.2 percent) (Centers for Disease Control and Prevention 2009b).

There are also numerous health differences among different nations. The ten countries with the highest years of life expectancy from birth are: Japan (83), San Marino (83), Australia (82), Iceland (82), Switzerland (82), Canada (81), New Zealand (81), Singapore (81), Spain (81), and Sweden (81). The ten lowest are: Afghanistan (42), Zimbabwe (42), Angola (46), Lesotho (47), Somalia (48), Swaziland (48), Zambia (48), Mali (49), Nigeria (49), and Sierra Leone (49) (World Health Organization 2010h). The ten countries with the highest infant mortality per live 1,000 births are: Angola (180.2), Afghanistan (153.1), Liberia (138.2), Niger (116.7), Mali (115.9), Somalia (109.2), Mozambique (105.8), Zambia (101.2), Guinea-Bissau (99.8), and Chad (98.7). The ten countries with the lowest infant mortality are: Singapore (2.3), Bermuda (2.5), Sweden (2.8), Japan (2.8), Hong Kong (2.9), Macau (3.2), Iceland (3.2), France (3.3), Finland (.35), and Anguilla (3.5) (Central Intelligence Agency 2010).

Disease statistics also vary internationally. For example, the highest rates of HIV/AIDS occur in sub-Saharan Africa and the lowest rates occur in Europe and Asia (UNAIDS 2010) (see Table 10.2). As noted in Chapter 1, most of the new cases of malaria occur in sub-Saharan Africa and tropical regions (Centers for Disease Control and Prevention 2007). The

Table 10.2. *HIV/AIDS Prevalence among Adults in 2009*

Region	Percentage of Adult Population (15–49) Living with HIV/AIDS
Sub-Saharan Africa	5
Caribbean	1
East Europe/Central Asia	0.8
North America	0.5
Central and South America	0.5
South and Southeast Asia	0.3
Oceania	0.3
Western and Central Europe	0.2
North Africa and the Middle East	0.2
East Asia	0.1

Based on data from UNAIDS 2010.

obesity rate ranges from 30.6 percent in the United States to 3.2 percent in South Korea. Child malnutrition prevalence (the percentage of children under age 5 who are underweight) ranges from 48.3 percent in Nepal to 0.6 percent in Croatia (NationMaster.com 2010). Approximately 78 percent of all childhood deaths from diarrhea occur in developing countries (Boschi-Pinto et al. 2008).

We have examined numerous examples of how the environment can contribute to differences in health. Some of these are (in no particular order of importance):

- People living near coal-burning power plants have increased exposures to particulate matter and sulfur dioxide;
- City dwellers experience greater exposures to tropospheric ozone than people living in rural areas;
- People who live near solid waste disposal sites may have increased contaminants in their drinking water;
- People who live near hog farms have a higher incidence of diarrheal diseases and respiratory problems;
- People who live in substandard housing face increased health hazards;
- Agricultural workers have increased risks related to pesticide exposures;
- People living in sub-Saharan Africa have a greater risk of contracting malaria than people living in Europe due to endemic populations of mosquitoes that carry malaria;
- Developing countries in Africa, Asia, and Oceania are likely have more adverse health impacts related to climate change than developed nations in North America and Europe.

While ample evidence supports the hypothesis that the environment contributes to health inequalities, it is difficult to determine the precise relationship between the environment and differences in health because numerous aspects of the biological, physical, chemical, and social environment impact health (Gee and Payne-Sturges 2004; Lee 2010). Some of these include (in no particular order of importance):

- Income/wealth
- Education
- Race/ethnicity
- Culture
- Occupation
- Psychosocial stress
- Housing
- Geography
- Weather
- Access to drinkable water
- Access to health care
- Food/nutrition
- Tobacco smoke
- Exposures to pollutants and toxic chemicals
- Exposures to infectious diseases

These different environmental factors may interact in complex ways. For example, race can affect income, wealth, education, occupation, housing, access to healthcare, food and nutrition, access to clean water, exposure to pollutants and chemicals, and psychosocial stress (Marmot and Wilkinson 2005; Barr 2008; Lee 2010). Education can affect income, wealth, occupation, housing, access to health care, food/nutrition, smoking, and drug and alcohol use. Income and wealth can affect education, access to healthcare, occupation, psychosocial stress, and exposures to infectious diseases, pollutants, and toxic chemicals. (For further discussion of how these different environmental factors interact and impact health, see Fiscalla and Williams 2004; Marmot and Wilkinson 2005; Kawachi and Kennedy 2006; Morello-Frosch and Lopez 2006; Barr 2008; and Lee 2010.)

Even though it may be difficult to determine the precise role of any particular environmental factor in causing disease, it is clear that the environment plays a major role in health inequalities (Lee 2002; Barr 2008). Much of the political, scientific, and philosophical debate about health disparities in the United States and other countries has focused on inequalities related to access to healthcare (Daniels 2008). While inadequate access to care is, without a doubt, a major cause of health disparities, other aspects of the environment, such as air and water quality, safe and affordable housing, and occupational hazards, also deserve to be addressed in policy debates (Resnik and Roman 2007; Daniels 2008). It is important to ensure that people can benefit from healthcare services and medical treatments when they become ill or injured, but it is also important to take steps to prevent people from becoming sick or injured in the first place. Environmental health interventions, such as improvements in air and water quality, and the provision of safe and affordable food and housing, can help improve the overall health of the population and reduce health disparities (Shrader-Frechette 2002; Daniel 2008; Lee 2010).

THE ENVIRONMENTAL JUSTICE MOVEMENT

With this overview of the relationship between the environment and health inequalities in mind, we can better appreciate the motivation for the environmental justice movement, which began in the early 1980s, when minority communities objected to the placement of landfills and waste sites in their neighborhoods (Lee 2010). One of the first cases involving local protests against environmental injustice occurred in 1982, when the State of North Carolina decided to place a PCB disposal site in Shocco Township, located in Warren County (Shrader-Frechette 2002). Shocco is a low-income community that is 75 percent black. The EPA allowed the state to place the waste site only seven feet above groundwater level, even though fifty feet is the normal level for PCB sites (Shrader-Frechette 2002). Thousands of residents marched in protest of the disposal site and hundreds were arrested. Even though the residents did not succeed in preventing the disposal site from being placed in their neighborhood, their grass-roots efforts drew national attention and helped to launch the environmental justice movement (Shrader-Frechette 2002; Lee 2010).

Environmental justice soon became not only a public health concern but also a civil rights issue, and the term "environmental racism" was coined to describe the tendency to locate toxic waste sites and landfills near African American communities. In 1991, the first People of Color Environmental Leadership summit helped to launch the national environmental justice movement, and led to initiatives by the administration of President Bill Clinton, which established the Office of Environmental Justice at the EPA (Lee 2010). Under the Clinton administration, the Office of Environmental Justice focused on promoting justice for racial minorities and low-income populations, but the Bush administration expanded its scope to include justice for all people, regardless of race or income, which angered some leaders of the environmental justice movement (Marchant and Grodsky 2008). The EPA's current definition of environmental justice is "fair treatment and meaningful involvement of all people regardless of race, color, national origin, or income with respect to the development, implementation, and enforcement of environmental laws, regulations, and policies" (Environmental Protection Agency 2010h). The EPA's Environmental Justice Program awards grants to communities and states, and includes projects and programs to promote environmental justice (Environmental Protection Agency 2010h), such as:

- **GreenStreets** is a project to plant trees in low-income areas of Lawrence, MA, to increase urban tree canopy coverage and reduce summer heat, soil erosion, and runoff.
- **New Mainer Healthy Homes and Advocacy** helps new immigrant families in Lewiston, ME learn how to protect themselves from environmental hazards in low-cost housing, such as lead, allergens, mold, and pests.
- **Citizens Environmental Coalition** helps residents of Geneva, NY to understand and address environmental, public health, and climate change issues related to the Seneca Meadows Landfill. The project involves air and water quality monitoring near the landfill and educates community members on how to reduce solid waste.

- **Operation GRUB (gardens replace urban blight)** is a program that helps residents of Reading, PA to transform areas of trash accumulation into urban gardens. The program also educates residents about recycling and composting.
- **Green Building Education** is a program that educates residents living in affordable housing projects in Atlanta, GA about water efficiency, energy efficiency, indoor air quality, recycling, and alternative forms of transportation.
- **Cambio Climatico** promotes the health of migrant farm workers in Lafayette County, MO. The project educates farm workers about the dangers of sun and heat exposure, chemical poisoning, and lead poisoning. The project also addresses proper pesticide use.
- **Mountain Studies Institute** seeks to educate and empower people living in the Four Corners region of New Mexico and Colorado, who are impacted by air and water pollution and toxins emitted from oil and gas production facilities. The population of the Four Corners region is mostly low-income Native Americans.

The NIEHS launched its environmental justice program in 1994, which awards grants to communities to respond to environmental issues and sponsors community-based participatory research (CBPR) (National Institute of Environmental Health Sciences 2010b). CBPR involves community members in the development and implementation of research projects designed to gather information that is likely to benefit the community. CBPR can build trust and mutual understanding between investigators and community members, facilitate recruitment of research participants, and ensure that projects are culturally appropriate and useful to the community (O'Fallon and Dearry 2002). The NIEHS has partnered with NIOSH to address environmental justice issues related to occupational health and safety. Some of the NIEHS's environmental justice and CBPR projects have included (National Institute of Environmental Health Sciences 2010c):

- **Alaska Community Action on Toxics** links fifteen communities together in the Norton Sound region to determine how best to minimize the human health impacts of environmental contaminants. Most of the residents in this region are indigenous people who obtain most of their food from local sources, such as fishing and seal hunting. This project has studied the effects of environmental contaminants on the local food supply.
- **Cheyenne River Sioux Tribal Council** promotes appreciation and awareness of environmental health issues that affect the Cheyenne River Sioux Tribe, located in Eagle Butte, South Dakota. This projected has helped tribal leaders to develop an agenda for environmental health planning and policy.
- **Harlem Children's Zone, Inc.** promotes the health of children living in Central Harlem, New York City, with special attention to respiratory problems, such as asthma. This project has linked local public schools, health clinics, and hospitals to conduct research and develop environmental health initiatives.
- **Neighborhood House, Inc.** helps to promote environmental health among residents of Seattle's High Point public housing project. High Point is undergoing redevelopment to

make substantial improvements to the housing units, such as enhancement of physical safety, reduction of allergens, and more open spaces for recreation.

• **Oregon Law Center-Farmworker Program** addresses the occupational health needs of indigenous Oregon farmworkers and helps those who do not speak English or Spanish to better understand the hazards associated with agricultural work. The project has helped to increase farmworkers' access to economic, health, and social resources.

THE MORAL AND POLITICAL FOUNDATIONS
OF ENVIRONMENTAL JUSTICE

As discussed in Chapter 4, justice can be conceived in distributive or procedural terms. Distributive justice addresses the fair distribution of benefits and burdens in society, while procedural justice addresses the fairness of rules and processes used to make social policy (Rawls 1971). If we think of social justice as basically a problem of dividing up the proverbial pie, then distributive justice deals with the question of how much pie each person should get, and procedural justice addresses questions concerning how the pie is sliced. Distributive and procedural justice are both necessary to achieve social justice (Rawls 1971).

Many of the concerns relating to distributive justice are based on reflections on social inequality. If an important socioeconomic good, such as wealth or health, is distributed unequally in society, then one might question whether this distribution is just. One cannot infer that a distribution is unjust from the fact that it is unequal, however, because only distributions resulting from unfair treatment are unjust (Daniels 1984, 2008). For example, suppose there is an accident at a factory and dozens of workers are severely injured or killed. One could argue that this distribution of health, though unfortunate, is not unjust, if the owners had adequate safeguards in place to protect the workers, and if the workers chose to risk their health by working in the factory. If the owners did not have adequate safeguards in place, however, then this distribution could be considered to be unjust because the workers would have been treated unfairly.

Deciding what counts as fair treatment with respect to the distribution of environmental health risks is controversial because people may hold very different views about such issues based on diverse understandings of distributive justice. Consider how the three basic approaches to justice described in Chapter 3, libertarianism, utilitarianism, and egalitarianism, would approach a private company's request to build a chemical plant near a low-income, minority community in a socioeconomically and geographically diverse state. Libertarians would have no objections to placing the plant near this community, provided that company has purchased the property fairly because, in a free market, private companies should be allowed to make decisions concerning their operations and modes of production (Nozick 1974). Utilitarians would have no objections to placing the plant near this community, provided that the overall potential benefits of the plant to society (such as new jobs and economic growth) outweigh the risks (such as adverse impacts on health). Unlike libertarians, utilitarians would be concerned with how the chemical plant might impact the local community, but they would be willing to sacrifice the well-being of that community for a greater social good (Smart and Williams 1973). Egalitarians would be concerned about how the chemical plant would impact the local community's health and well-being. They would be opposed to placement of the plant near the community if this would reduce the welfare of community members relative to other members of the county. They would favor a site that distributes the risks of the plant more equally (Rawls 1971).

There is insufficient space in this book to critique all three of these different approaches to distributive justice, but I favor an egalitarian approach (for a review of theories of justice see Barry 1991; Roemer 1998). I have two objections to libertarianism. First, it is not concerned with socioeconomic inequalities. Vast differences in income, wealth, health, education, or other goods are acceptable, provided that they result from a free market process that respects property rights and rewards merit and personal responsibility (Nozick 1974). Many argue, however, that the government should provide a social safety net to protect the vulnerable members of society, such as people who are sick, poor, disabled, or otherwise disadvantaged. To do this, some redistribution of wealth is necessary (Rawls 1971; Shrader-Frechette 2002). Second, libertarians believe in minimal regulation of the free market. The main purpose of government is to protect property rights and liberty, not to promote a social agenda (Nozick 1974). Libertarians oppose a variety of laws that promote environmental health, such as occupational health and safety and rules, housing standards, and pollution controls, because these laws violate property rights and go beyond the legitimate scope of government (Shrader-Frechette 2002). Many argue that some form of government regulation of the free market is necessary to protect important values, such as public health, social justice, and environmental quality from the consequences of unfettered capitalism (Roemer 1998).

Utilitarians, unlike libertarians, can take a positive stance against unequal distributions of socioeconomic goods in society because differences in income, wealth, health, education, and other goods can have a negative impact on the overall good of society (Smart and Williams 1973). Providing disadvantaged individuals with healthcare, for example, promotes the overall good of society by promoting their health. Additionally, ensuring that all members of society have access to healthcare can promote the good of society by helping to prevent the spread of infectious diseases and by improving the productivity of the workforce. Thus, utilitarians have the conceptual tools to support government policies that provide a social safety net for vulnerable members of society. Utilitarians can also support laws that regulate the free market to promote goals that benefit society, such as public health and safety and environmental quality. For example, a utilitarian could argue that pollution controls and housing standards are necessary to promote the overall good of society.

However, utilitarianism's support for polices that help disadvantaged people or regulate the free market hinges on the likely consequences of these policies (Smart and Williams 1973). If the negative consequences of providing health care to poor people outweigh the positive ones, then utilitarians would not support a government program that provides healthcare for disadvantaged members of society. If the negative consequences of regulating air pollution outweigh the positive ones, then utilitarians would not favor regulation.

Utilitarians would also accept the placement of a hazardous waste site in a low-income, minority community if the potential benefits of locating the waste site in that community outweigh the risks (Shrader-Frechette 2002). Utilitarians' support for policies that help disadvantaged people or promote environmental health is a mile wide but an inch deep.

Egalitarians have a more robust approach to policies relating to the distribution of socioeconomic goods and the regulation of the free market. Egalitarians, unlike utilitarians, provide an account of the fair distribution of socioeconomic goods that is independent of the overall social consequences of that distribution. Some egalitarians, such as Marxists and socialists, favor a distribution of socioeconomic goods that is approximately equal (Marx 1992). One of the drawbacks of this extreme form of egalitarianism is that it takes away incentives for hard work, creativity, achievement, and personal responsibility (Rawls 1971). Rawls' egalitarian view provides incentives for hard work, innovation, responsibility, and achievement while maintaining a commitment to egalitarian ideals. Rawls emphasized equality of opportunity rather than equality of wealth, income, or other socioeconomic goods (Rawls 1971). As noted in Chapter 3, Rawls held that socioeconomic differences are acceptable provided that they do not undermine equality of opportunity and benefit the least-advantaged members of society (i.e., people who are poor, sick, uneducated, or disabled), compared to other social arrangements. For there to be equality of opportunity in society, decisions concerning employment and career advancement should be made on the basis of an individual's talents and abilities, not on the basis of race, ethnicity, gender, or social class (Rawls 1971). The government may use tax revenues to provide all members of society with some basic education and health care, so that people born into socially disadvantaged families still have the opportunity to develop the talents and abilities necessary for socioeconomic advancement (Daniels 1984, 2008). The government may also enact laws, including environmental or public health regulations, to promote equality of opportunity or other principles of justice (Daniels 2008).

Although I think Rawls has the best approach to environmental justice issues, other approaches also provide some valuable insights, which should be taken into account when making policy decisions. For example, policy makers should consider the rights of property owners when making decisions concerning zoning, urban development, and other choices that affect property interests. Recognizing the importance of property rights need not imply that property interests should trump distributive justice concerns, only that they should be given fair and reasonable consideration in public policy decisions. Likewise, policy makers should anticipate the potential impacts on social utility (such as loss of jobs or impeded economic growth) when making environmental health decisions. Giving consideration to utility need not imply that this principle should trump all other concerns, only that it should be taken into account.

Turning to procedural justice, the basic issue here is what constitutes fair methods for making policy decisions. Again, there are different positions on what would be considered to be fair procedures. Rather than review all of these different positions here (for review see Gutmann and Thompson 1998), I will explicate a view accepted by many theorists, including Gutmann and Thompson (1998), Shrader-Frechette (2002), and Daniels (2008), which draws on the work of Rawls (2005). The view makes the basic and largely uncontroversial assumption that members of society should have equal rights to participate in political decisions (Shrader-Frechette 2002). One common way of ensuring that people can participate in political decisions is to enact laws that give each person an equal right to vote on matters of public concern. In direct democracy, people vote on particular issues in referenda. In representative democracy, people vote for representatives, who make decisions on their behalf (Gutmann and Thompson 1998). It is also important to have laws that protect freedom of speech, especially on political issues, so that people can express their views and influence political debates (Gutmann and Thompson 1998). The U.S. Constitution (1787) guarantees citizens both the right to vote and freedom of speech, and establishes a form of representative democracy.

While the right to vote and freedom of speech are necessary for ensuring that members of society have an equal right to participate in political decisions, they may not be sufficient. In the United States and many other countries, powerful and wealthy interest groups exert enormous influence on political debates through lobbying, advertising, and donations to political campaigns (Cohen 2009). As a result, citizens who lack power and wealth can become disenfranchised, and their voices may not be heard. To help level the political playing field, many writers have proposed that direct democracy and representative democracy should be supplemented by an approach, known as deliberative democracy, which emphasizes meaningful public deliberation on controversial issues. Public deliberation includes methods such as town hall and planning board meetings, open forums, focus groups, and public debates, which allow individual citizens, especially disenfranchised ones, to participate in decision making (Thompson and Gutmann 1998; Shrader-Frechette 2002).

For deliberative democracy to be effective, several conditions must be met. First, the parties must view the deliberative process as a source of political legitimacy and be willing to accept whatever decision is reached. Second, the parties must respect each other's viewpoints and interests. Third, the parties should use publicly defensible arguments and publicly available evidence to support their positions. Arguments based on particular religious worldviews should be framed in terms of publicly defensible values, such as human rights, justice, the common good, public health, or environmental protection (Rawls 2005). Fourth, a special effort should be made to include people who lack political influence, due to their race, income, education, disability, or other factors (Guttmann and Thompson 1998; Resnik 2010b). Some have argued that because these conditions are often difficult to meet, deliberative democracy is an idealized form of decision making that is rarely implemented successfully (Fishkin and Laslett 2003). However, proponents argue that a deliberative approach merits consideration, especially when other forms of democracy fail to resolve controversial issues fairly (Gutmann and Thompson 1998).

Finally, no account of environmental justice would be complete without considering international justice because environmental health varies among nations. In Chapter 4, I defended a realistic approach to problems of international justice, arguing that procedural and distributive justice should apply to relationships among nations. International procedural justice requires that nations have equal rights to participate in international political decisions that affect them. Nations should be allowed to participate in negotiations concerning international treaties, and should have sovereignty and protection under international laws. International distributive justice implies that the benefits and burdens of international cooperation should be distributed fairly. Unfair sharing of benefits and burdens in relationships among individuals, groups, or nations can be regarded as a type of exploitation (Wertheimer 1999).

Exploitation has been – and continues to be – a major moral and political issue pertaining to relationships between developed and developing nations. Since the Age of Exploration in the 1400s, maritime powers, such as England, Spain, Portugal, France, and The Netherlands, as well as the United States, have exploited populations in Africa, South America, Asia, and the Pacific Islands by means of colonization, slavery, and political oppression. Governments and entrepreneurs from developed nations have extracted gold, minerals, rubber, and other natural resources from developing nations while offering local populations little in return (Shah 2006). Though developed nations have made great strides toward treating developing nations fairly and atoning for past injustices, interactions between developed and developing nations bear the scars of centuries of exploitation and injustice. Reflecting on this historical context is crucial to understanding international health issues, because it shapes attitudes, feelings, and expectations on both sides of many debates. To avoid exploitation, it is important for nations to reach fair agreements concerning their relationships (Wertheimer 1999).

APPLICATIONS

Having discussed the foundations of environmental justice, we can now explore some specific problems and concerns. We will start by considering some local issues and then move on to national and global ones.

COMMUNITY EXPOSURE TO RISKS

Increased community exposure to health risks is a major concern for the placement of solid waste disposal sites, waste transfer stations, nuclear waste sites, nuclear power plants, coal power plants, chemical factories, hog farms, prisons, freeways, and weapons testing sites (such as the Marshall Islands) (Shrader-Frechette 2002). These decisions pit the interests of the local community against the good of the larger community because the activity that generates the environmental health risks often benefits the larger community at the expense of the local community. Because the environmental health risks will not be distributed equally in society, justice is a major concern in these types of decisions (Shrader-Frechette 2002).

Two sorts of questions pertaining to justice must be considered when making these sorts of decisions: 1) is the proposed distribution of environmental health risks fair? and 2) is the decision-making process fair? To illustrate how these questions could be addressed, let us consider a hypothetical example of a decision to locate a new solid waste disposal site near a low-income, minority community in a rural part of a county. The old waste site is almost full and a new one is needed. The area where the site will be located has a much lower population density than the rest of the county. The county includes a metropolitan area (population 120,000, including suburbs), and two small towns (population less than 10,000). Three hundred thousand people live in the county. A river runs through the metropolitan area, which is in the center of the county. Geologists and civil engineers have determined that the proposed site is one among several that would be ideal for waste disposal due to its remoteness from population centers and sequestration from water supplies.

To address the fairness of the distribution, the risks imposed on the local community relative to the rest of the population must be assessed. Risks will need to be identified (what are the types of risks?), evaluated (how severe are the risks?), and quantified (what is the relative probability that certain types of harm will occur?) (Shrader-Frechette 1991). The distinction between evaluating and quantifying risks is important because some risks may be relatively benign (such as headache, nausea, or diarrhea), while others may be more severe (such as cancer or nervous system disorders). In addition to assessing risks, it is also important to explore methods of minimizing or mitigating those risks. For example, it may be possible to construct barriers that prevent harmful chemicals from leaching out of a waste site and contaminating the water. Other forms of containment may also reduce risks. Benefits, such as job creation, economic development, and centralized waste disposal must also be identified, evaluated, and quantified. Benefits may accrue to the local community, the larger population, or both. As noted earlier, considerations of social utility (i.e., benefits to the larger population) should not be ignored, even when focusing on issues of distributive justice. Finally, alternatives to the proposed site must be considered, and the risks and benefits of those alternatives must be assessed. Locating the waste site near the metropolitan area might minimize risks to the rural population but increase the risks for the whole population. Placing the site near a river might cause greater harm to the environment and the human population.

To address procedural justice concerns, it will be necessary to examine the decision-making process pertaining to the proposed placement, paying particular attention to the local community's involvement in any deliberations. While there is no systematic way of assessing the fairness of the decision-making process, it would be important to answer a number of different questions, such as: Have members of the community had an opportunity for meaningful participation in the decision-making process through town hall and planning board meetings, focus groups, public debates or other forums? Have efforts been made to reach out to socioeconomically disadvantaged groups or racial/ethnic minorities? Have powerful interests, such as corporations, industry associations, or political parties unduly influenced the decision-making process? Has the decision been put to a vote or been debated by people running for public office? Have local media outlets helped to inform people about the decision?

How would a Rawlsian view the decision to locate the waste site near this low-income minority community? Because Rawls' principles of justice were meant to apply to macro-level issues, such as the distribution of goods in society, it is difficult to determine what Rawls would have to say about this particular situation. However, three points seem clear. First, Rawls would hold that the decision should not be made on the basis of race, ethnicity, or social class, as this would violate equality of opportunity. The site should be selected because it is an ideal location for waste disposal, not because people who live near the site are from a low-income or minority group (Shrader-Frechette 2002). Second, Rawls would be concerned about the site's overall impacts on the community members' socioeconomic opportunities. If the site adversely impacts their health, this could compromise their opportunities and result in injustice (Daniel 1984). However, the site also might confer economic benefits on the local community, which might enhance their opportunities. Third, Rawls would want to ensure that people who live near the proposed site can participate meaningfully in public deliberations about placement of the site (Shrader-Frechette 2002).

Very often, there are no easy choices when it comes to imposing environmental risks on local populations. Projects that promote the overall good of the larger population frequently impose increased health risks on people living in a particular area. A county must have some place to put its solid waste, unless the residents try to export the waste and hand over their problem to someone else. When a county is selecting a site for its solid waste, it is likely that local citizens will stand in opposition because nobody wants a solid waste site in their backyard. When a particular place is chosen, nearby residents may view the decision as unfair, even though it may be preferable to the alternatives, such as placing the site near a river, a densely populated area, or a school. While it is important to try to seek a fair distribution of risks, utilitarian concerns (what is best for the population as whole) cannot be ignored. What may seem like environmental injustice may, in fact, be the lesser evil. I am in no way claiming that low-income, minority communities have not been treated unfairly when it comes to distribution of environmental risks. I am only asserting that the issues concerning the imposition of risks on local populations are complex, and that the good of the whole population must be considered in addition to the good of members of who will be exposed to increased risks.

OCCUPATIONAL HEALTH AND SAFETY

As noted in Chapter 8, occupational health and safety issues often pit the interests of workers against those of employers and society because interventions designed to promote occupational health and safety can increase the costs of production, which can reduce profit and affect the price of goods and services. Making an inherently risky job (such as coal mining) as safe as office work may so greatly increase the costs of production that hiring people to perform the work will no longer be economically competitive or feasible. Faced with high costs of protecting workers, employers may decide to reduce the labor force, automate production, or outsource jobs to other countries with lower occupational health standards (Viscusi 1983, 1992).

Since the time of Adam Smith (1723–1790), economists and libertarians have argued that the distribution of workplace risks is fair because wages compensate for the risks workers take on the job. According to economists, workers are free and informed rational agents who can decide whether to take high-risk or low-risk jobs. Because workers generally wish to avoid risks, employers must offer wages that account for risks: the higher the risks, the higher the wages. If a worker chooses to take a high-risk job, he (or she) will receive a fair wage in return. The free market provides a fair and just mechanism for allocating workplace risks (Viscusi 1983, 1993).

This economic/libertarian argument has some significant weaknesses, however. First, workers' freedom to choose among different jobs is often quite limited, due to their lack of skills, education, or experience, or a tight job market. People living in low-income, Appalachian counties in the United States may have few opportunities to make a decent wage other than working in coal mines. Second, workers are often not fully informed about the risks they will face on the job, how those risks will affect their health and well-being, or whether wages adequately compensate for those risks. Someone who accepts a job working in a coal mine may not understand the risks of lung cancer due to respiratory illnesses caused by breathing dust and gases, or death or severe injury due to cave-ins. He (or she) may also not understand the impacts of these health risks, and whether the wages offered by the mine will compensate for the risks. In an ideal world, that is, one in which workers make free and informed rational choices, wages could compensate for occupational risks. In the real world, however, these market conditions are rarely met (Shrader-Frechette 2002).

Because the free market does not adequately compensate workers for risks, occupational health and safety regulations are necessary to promote justice (Shrader-Frechette 2002; Daniels 2008). Crafting regulations that distribute occupational risks fairly can involve difficult tradeoffs between worker health and safety and practical and financial (i.e., utilitarian) considerations. Although the safety of many jobs can be significantly improved through affordable interventions, for other jobs there are limits on what occupational standards may reasonably achieve (Viscusi 1983). For example, reinforcement of tunnels and construction of escape routes can help to reduce or mitigate the risks related to cave-ins in underground coal mines, but no system can prevent tragic events from occurring. Firefighters, police officers, soldiers, lumberjacks, welders, carpenters, and many other workers face more occupational risks than the average office worker because their jobs have inherent risks. For other jobs, safety improvements may be achievable, but only by means of interventions that are costly or impractical. Requiring nurses to always wear disposable biohazard suits would prevent them from contracting or spreading infectious diseases, but it would be costly and highly impersonal and would interfere with their ability to do their job. Workers' compensation and disability programs, and health and pension plans can also help to promote fairness related to occupational health by covering the costs of occupational injuries, illnesses, or disabilities (Daniel 2008).

Rawlsians would favor occupational health and safety laws, workers' compensation and disability programs, and other arrangements that help promote equality of opportunity (Daniels 2008). Occupational illnesses and injuries can adversely impact individual well-being and socioeconomic opportunities because workers who become disabled as a result of job-related injuries or illnesses may have reduced abilities to earn income. Occupational illnesses and injuries can also cause pain and suffering and have adverse impacts on quality of life. Injured, diseased, or disabled workers may also incur increased healthcare costs. Rawlsians would also favor procedures that allow workers to participate meaningfully in decisions pertaining to the management of occupational risks. Worker participation in decision making is an important feature of the Rawlsian approach to occupational health and safety because employers can use their power, money, and political clout to significantly influence policies enacted by legislators and government bureaucrats. Unionization and other forms of collective bargaining can help workers defend their interests related to occupational health and safety issues (Daniels 2008).

HOUSING

Housing construction and maintenance also raises questions of justice, because substandard housing can adversely impact the health and well-being of occupants. Housing issues often pit the interests of residents against the interests of construction companies, landlords, realtors, and society as a whole because policies that promote safe and healthy building construction and maintenance can increase the costs of housing, which can have negative economic effects (Viscusi 1983).

One could develop an economic/libertarian argument against government regulation of housing similar to the argument against occupational safety and health laws. According to this view, there is no need to regulate housing because the free market will provide adequate housing standards. Home buyers or renters can make free and informed choices concerning housing. If a landlord has difficulty renting apartments due to health and safety issues, he (or she) will take steps to improve the apartments. Likewise, people who build and sell homes will also make health and safety improvements in response to market conditions. Over time, the market will improve housing standards because people will not pay to live in unsafe or unhealthy homes (Viscusi 1983).

This argument against government regulation of housing suffers from the same problems that undermine the economic/libertarian argument against occupational safety and health laws. First, people's housing choices may be limited, due to their low income. A socioeconomically disadvantaged person living in South Bronx, New York may have few choices for living arrangements, due to his/her poverty and the availability of housing in the area. Second, people often do not know about or understand the health and safety risks of their housing arrangements. Indeed, most states have adopted mandatory disclosure laws concerning lead, radon, termites, and other hazards known to exist in a home so that people will understand the risks they may be facing (Frumkin 2010b). Third, some people, such as children and mentally disabled adults, are not free to make their own choices concerning living arrangements.

Because the free market alone is not an adequate mechanism for producing safe housing, laws mandating housing standards (and disclosures) are necessary to promote justice. As mentioned in Chapter 8, the development of appropriate housing standards can involve difficult tradeoffs between health and safety and financial considerations. Health and safety improvements often increase the costs of housing, due to expenses related to building design, materials, and construction. Cost is a relevant consideration when it comes to developing housing standards, because it can affect the affordability of housing, which can impact the distribution of socioeconomic goods in society. If housing is too expensive for low-income people to afford, they will have difficulty participating in society, earning income, or maintaining health. Housing is a key socioeconomic good (Daniels 2008). This is not to say, of course, that housing standards are not a necessary part of a just society, only that economic factors can play a role in the development of housing standards. Considerations of utility (e.g., cost and safety) and justice (e.g., affordability of housing and distribution of health) need to be carefully balanced when making decisions about housing standards.

DISASTER PREPAREDNESS

As noted in Chapter 8, natural disasters raise issues of social justice because they tend to have greater impacts on low-income populations. Thus, government preparations for and responses to natural disasters can be evaluated in terms of their impact on the distribution of benefits and risks in society (Moreno 2005; Resnik and Roman 2007). Some uses of government resources to prepare for natural disasters include building and fortifying man-made structures; developing evacuation plans; stockpiling emergency supplies; developing systems to monitor weather; training disaster workers; coordinating different agencies; and educating the public (Federal Emergency Management Agency 2010; Newberry 2010). Some uses of government funds to respond to disasters include evacuating people and animals; providing additional support for law enforcement, emergency services, and public health; supplying food and shelter for displaced individuals; and making loans and other funds available to rebuild damaged property (Federal Emergency Management Agency 2010). Many different regulations can help minimize the impact of natural disasters, such as housing standards; zoning and other laws to prevent or control construction in unsafe areas; and regulations to prevent floodwaters from contaminating drinking water (Federal Emergency Management Agency 2010).

Because natural disasters can have a profound impact on health disparities, it is important to pay sufficient attention to policies designed to minimize the impact of natural disasters in health policy debates (Moreno 2005). Some have argued that bioethicists and other scholars have not paid sufficient attention to the ethical issues related to natural disasters, and that more discussion and debate is warranted (Moreno 2005). One of the key issues pertaining to natural disasters is how much money the government should spend on preparing for and responding to natural disasters. This is largely a debate about setting budgetary priorities because most people agree that the government should spend some money on mitigating natural disasters. Reports critical of the United States government's response to Hurricane Katrina claimed that funding for natural disaster mitigation had been insufficient (Hsu 2006).

Another key policy issue is the impact of government disaster mitigation regulations on property interests. When a county decides to prohibit new construction in the 100-year flood plain in order to minimize the impact of floods on the human population, land owners may object that this law unjustly interferes with their ability to use their property and reduces the value of their land. For example, a landowner who was planning to build and sell homes on the 100-year flood plain could object that the county's decision denies him of the economic benefits of his land. Although the interests of property owners should be considered when making policies that can affect them, as argued in Chapter 8, some types of government restrictions on property rights are justified to promote public health or protect the environment. In some cases, justice may require the government to compensate land owners for extensive restrictions on their property that amount to a taking of land for public use (Shrader-Frechette 1988; Caldwell and Shrader-Frechette1993). (For an interesting discussion of the "takings" issue, see Epstein 1985.)

VULNERABLE POPULATIONS

Some subpopulations have increased vulnerabilities to environmental health risks due to age, disease status, or genetic risk factors. For example, children are more susceptible to adverse effects of pesticides than adults because their bodies are still developing and going through critical periods; their hepatic, renal, and immune systems provide less protection against pesticides; and they may have increased exposures to pesticides due to their diet or behavior (Environmental Protection Agency 2002). Children are also more susceptible to detrimental effects of lead exposure than adults because they absorb more lead through ingestion and respiration and their bodies are still developing. Lead exposure in childhood is associated with learning disabilities, decreased school performance, and poor hand-eye coordination (Agency for Toxic Substances and Diseases Registry 2007). Asthmatics are more susceptible to the effects of air pollution than people with healthy respiratory systems (Wilson et al. 2005; Ho et al. 2007). People with peanut allergies are highly susceptible to dermal and oral exposures to peanuts. Allergic reactions to peanuts can lead to anaphylactic shock and death (Pansare and Kamat 2010). People with some types of genetic mutations may have an increased susceptibility to various chemical exposures (Marchant 2008a). Recent research suggests that genetic factors impact mercury and lead detoxification (Gundacker et al. 2010). Genetics can also impact susceptibility to air pollution (Kleeberger et al. 2000).

The increased vulnerabilities of some subpopulations to environmental risks raises issues of justice because environmental exposures that do not pose significant risks on the general population may adversely impact these groups (Cranor 2008). Citizens, regulators, and policy makers must decide whether to provide increased protection from environmental health risks for vulnerable subpopulations. One could argue, from a Rawlsian perspective, that society should provide additional protections for these vulnerable groups to promote equality of opportunity and a fair distribution of socioeconomic goods (Daniels 2008). Indeed, some environmental laws have been crafted to provide extra protection for vulnerable groups (Marchant 2008a). As noted in Chapter 5, the Food Quality Protection Act (FQPA) provides additional protection for infants and children from pesticide residue on food (Environmental Protection Agency 2010i). The courts have interpreted the Clean Air Act (CAA) as requiring the EPA to promulgate air pollution standards that protect not only the average individual but also sensitive (or vulnerable) individuals (*American Lung Association vs. EPA* 1998; Marchant 2008b).

However, protection of vulnerable groups may sometimes conflict with the principle of utility if it incurs significant social and economic costs (Carnor 2008). Consider the debate about banning peanuts from public schools in order to protect children with peanut allergies. About 1 percent of school-age children are allergic to peanuts (Finkelman 2010). To protect allergic children, some school systems have banned all peanuts and peanut products from campus (Young et al. 2009). The main argument for this policy is that it is the most effective way of protecting allergic children because children often share food and teachers cannot adequately monitor school lunches and snacks. Arguments against the policy are that it is difficult to enforce, places an unfair burden on children without allergies, gives a false sense of security, and could establish a precedent for banning other foods from school (Young et al. 2009). Some commentators recommend that schools pursue a comprehensive food allergy management policy that includes increased awareness of the problem and availability of medications to treat allergic reactions, such as epinephrine, but does not include a ban on specific food items (Young et al. 2009).

Cranor (2008) argues that protections for vulnerable subgroups must be balanced against utilitarian considerations, such as economic costs and practical limitations. Though vulnerable subpopulations have a right to protection from environmental risks, it may sometimes not be feasible or practical to provide them with every possible protection that could promote their health because the additional costs would be too much for society to afford. The optimal approach would involve fair and reasonable balancing of utilitarian and distributive justice concerns. Governments must decide what levels of protection for vulnerable groups are affordable.

GLOBAL CLIMATE CHANGE

As mentioned in Chapter 9, climate change has implications for international justice because populations in developing nations may be more adversely impacted by increased global temperatures than populations in developed nations (Patz 2010). One of the central international justice issues related to climate change is how to allocate the responsibility for mitigating climate change fairly (Posner and Weisbach 2010). Some commentators and humanitarian organizations have argued that developed nations should bear the brunt of socioeconomic costs related to climate change mitigation because they are better able to shoulder the economic burdens of policies designed to reduce greenhouse emissions (such as cap and trade systems) and they have contributed most of the gases that are responsible for global warming (Baer et al. 2008). According to Baer et al. (2008), nations below a development threshold ($7,500 average per capita income) do not need help to reduce greenhouse gas emissions. Their main goal should be socioeconomic development. Nations above this development threshold should be responsible for reducing greenhouse gas emissions and providing financial aid to developing nations to help them adapt to climate change. Responsibility for mitigating climate change above the development threshold should also be apportioned according to level of economic development: Richer nations should do more than poorer ones (Baer et al. 2008).

Posner and Weisbach (2010) develop three arguments against making rich nations shoulder a much larger burden of climate change mitigation than poor nations. First, using international climate change treaties to address the socioeconomic gap between developing and developed nations and historical injustices is politically unwise because it will cause resentment and sabotage negotiations (Posner and Weisbach 2010). As we saw in the discussion of Kyoto Protocol (Chapter 7), if developed nations are asked to take a disproportionate share of the burden of climate change mitigation, they may opt out of treaties. Second, assigning responsibility for climate change is difficult because many of the people who have produced greenhouse gas emissions are now dead, and a large percentage of emissions took place before scientists understood the impacts of human-produced greenhouse gases on climate (Posner and Weisbach 2010). Third, many developing nations are rapidly catching up with developed nations when it comes to greenhouse gas emissions. China, for example, now produces more total carbon dioxide than the United States (Posner and Weisbach 2010). India is also catching up with developed nations with respect to greenhouse gas emissions. Though China and India both contain large, underdeveloped rural areas, they also have many highly industrialized urban areas. In the Durban Platform, countries agreed, for the first time, that developing nations should also control their greenhouse gas emissions.

The realistic approach to international justice, discussed in Chapter 4, lends some support to Posner and Weisbach's view. According to this approach, justice requires that nations obey international laws, respect each other's sovereignty, follow fair procedures for settling disputes, and share in the benefits (and burdens) of international cooperation. Justice does not require the redistribution of wealth from rich to poor nations because this type of arrangement is unenforceable without a strong international government (Rawls 1999). International treaties, such as climate change agreements, should promote cooperation among nations on key issues, and distribute benefits and burdens fairly. As major contributors of greenhouse gas emissions, developed nations will need to shoulder most of the burden of climate change mitigation, but developing nations should also do their part. Developed nations can also set aside funds to help developing nations adapt to climate change. Nongovernmental organizations from developed nations can also play an important role in helping developing nations deal with the impacts of climate change.

SUMMARY

This chapter has explored a variety of issues related to justice, health, and the environment. Justice has been – and will continue to be – an important concern related to environmental health because environmental risks are often not distributed equally. Justice requires that benefits and risks related to environmental health be distributed fairly and that societies follow fair procedures when making environmental policy decisions. Environmental policy decisions should take into account how different choices impact the overall good of society, as well as equality of opportunity, property rights, and the welfare of the least advantaged members of society. To help insure that citizens have an equal right to participate in environmental policy choices, democratic decision-making procedures should include mechanisms for meaningful public deliberation on controversial issues. International treaties related to the environment should promote cooperation and a fair sharing of benefits and risks. The next chapter will examine ethical and policy issues related to environmental research involving human subjects.

II

ENVIRONMENTAL HEALTH RESEARCH INVOLVING HUMAN PARTICIPANTS

As noted in Chapter 2, research with human participants plays an essential role in understanding the health impacts of the environment. This chapter will focus on human participant issues that create unique or especially challenging problems in environmental health research. Before exploring these issues, it will be useful to review some of the important historical developments, ethics codes, regulations, and ethical principles pertaining to research with human participants. (Environmental health research with human and animal participants raises a number of ethical and policy issues that will not be discussed here. For a review, see Emanuel et al. 2008; Shamoo and Resnik 2009.)

BACKGROUND

Prior to World War II, there were no well-recognized international codes or guidelines concerning research with human participants. The American Medical Association had discussed drafts of potential guidelines, and a few countries, such as Germany, had developed some rules, but there was very little substantive guidance on the ethical conduct of research with human participants. Many experiments were conducted on vulnerable groups (i.e., individuals who have difficulty providing consent), such as mentally ill people, racial minorities, children, and prisoners (Lederer 1995). Informed consent was not a widely recognized principle of medical research, and doctors often experimented on their patients without their consent (Lederer 1995).

The policy landscape changed dramatically after World War II with the advent of the Nuremberg Code (1947), the first international guideline for research with human participants. The Nuremberg Code was developed in response to the need to have some type of international law for prosecuting Nazi physicians and scientists for war crimes committed against concentration camp prisoners. The Nazis had used these prisoners, mostly Jews, in many brutal and inhumane experiments, including wound healing studies, hypothermia research, infection studies, decompression research, and experiments to change eye color. Most of the human participants were severely injured or killed, and none of them gave consent (Lifton 2000). The Nuremberg Code (1947) states ten different directives for conducting human experimentation including the requirement that the free and informed consent of the participant be obtained, that risks be minimized, that experiments serve a socially valuable purpose and be well-designed, and that only appropriately qualified investigators conduct research.

In 1964, the World Medical Association (2008) published the Helsinki Declaration, a set of ethical principles for medical research involving human participants, which has been revised numerous times. The Helsinki Declaration discusses informed consent, scientific design, risk minimization, safeguarding confidentiality and privacy, special protections for vulnerable participants, clinical trial methodology, and other ethical aspects of biomedical research involving human participants, and continues to provide important international guidance. In 1966, the NIH adopted rules for the conduct of all NIH-funded research with human participants. In 1971, the FDA adopted its own human participant regulations (Shamoo and Resnik 2009).

Another major turning point occurred in 1972, when Peter Buxton, who worked for the Public Health Service, told his account of the Tuskegee Syphilis Study to the Associated Press. Although Henry Beecher (1966) had discussed the study in an article on ethical experiments published in the *New England Journal of Medicine* in 1966, the research did not receive significant national attention until the Associated Press covered it in depth (Jones 1981). The Tuskegee Study (1932–1972) was conducted by physicians in Tuskegee, AL, who received funding from the Public Health Service. The investigators followed 399 black men with untreated syphilis and 400 controls. The goal of the research was to study the etiology of syphilis in black men. The participants were not told that they were participating in research, and the patients with syphilis were not treated with penicillin, an effective treatment that became widely available in the 1940s. In fact, the researchers took steps to prevent syphilitic patients from receiving penicillin from other doctors. The United States government reached a legal settlement with the surviving research participants and families of participants in 1973 (Jones 1981). President Bill Clinton issued an official government apology in 1997.

The Tuskegee Study triggered a congressional investigation into ethical problems with biomedical research. As a result, Congress passed the National Research Act, which was signed into law in 1974. The law authorized federal agencies to develop regulations for research with human participants and created the National Commission for the Protection of Human Participants of Biomedical and Behavioral Research to study the ethical principles of research with human participants. The National Commission published the Belmont Report (National Commission 1979), which articulated three ethical principles for research – respect for persons, beneficence, and justice. Respect for persons, which is similar to the human rights principle discussed in Chapter 4, requires investigators to obtain informed consent from research participants (or their representatives) and to provide extra protections for participants who may have difficulty providing consent, due to illness, mental incapacity, age, institutionalization, or socioeconomic status. It also implies that investigators should protect privacy and confidentiality. Beneficence, which is similar to the principle of utility discussed in Chapter 4, requires researchers to maximize benefits to research participants and society and to minimize harms. Justice, which is similar to the principle of justice discussed in Chapter 4, requires fair distribution of the benefits and burdens of research and equitable selection of participants (National Commission 1979). The authors of the Belmont Report argued that these principles should be balanced when making ethical decisions, and they distinguished between clinical research, which aims to develop generalizable knowledge, and clinical practice, which has patient-centered goals (National Commission 1979).

The Belmont Report provided a conceptual foundation for a major revision of the federal research regulations that took place in 1981. Though the regulations have been revised since then, they have not changed significantly in nearly thirty years. Other countries have also enacted their own human research regulations, which are similar to federal regulations. The most influential set of federal regulations is known as the Common Rule (45 CFR 46), which has been adopted by seventeen federal agencies. The FDA has adopted regulations that are consistent with the Common Rule, and the EPA has adopted the Common Rule as well as special rules for intentional dosing studies and pesticide research, which will be discussed shortly (Shamoo and Resnik 2009). The Common Rule includes four different subparts with additional protections for pregnant women, fetuses, neonates, children, and prisoners (Department of Health and Human Services 2009). See Table 11.1 for key events in human research protections. The Common Rule requires research institutions to establish an Institutional Review Board (IRB) to review and oversee research with human subjects. Other countries have rules that mandate the formation of similar committees, known as Research Ethics Boards or Ethical Review Committees (Shamoo and Resnik 2009). The IRB may approve research only if it determines that the following conditions are met (Department of Health and Human Services 2009):

(1) Risks to the subject are minimized;
(2) Risks to the subjects are reasonable in relation to the benefits to the participant or society (i.e., the knowledge expected to be gained);
(3) Informed consent will be sought and properly documented;
(4) Confidentiality and privacy are protected;
(5) The selection of subjects is equitable;
(6) When appropriate, there are provisions in place to monitor the data to protect subjects from harm;
(7) When appropriate, additional safeguards are in place to protect vulnerable subjects.

The Common Rule also includes specific requirements for obtaining and documenting consent, reporting noncompliance and unanticipated problems, and institutional oversight. The Common Rule exempts some types of research, such as surveys and studies involving deidentified human biological samples or data, from IRB review, and includes procedures for expedited review of research (Department of Health and Human Services 2009). Other important sources of guidance include guidelines issued by the Council for International Organizations of Medical Sciences (2002) and the International Conference

Table 11.1. *U.S. Human Research Participant Protection Timeline*

1947	Nuremberg Code is adopted.
1964	First version of the Helsinki Declaration is adopted.
1966	Henry Beecher publishes an influential article describing unethical research in the United States.
1966	The NIH adopts human research regulations.
1971	The FDA adopts human research regulations.
1972	The Associated Press reports the story of the Tuskegee Syphilis Study.
1973	The United States government reaches a settlement with individuals and families impacted by the Tuskegee Study.
1974	The National Research Act is signed into law.
1979	The National Commission for the Protection of Human Participants of Biomedical and Behavioral Research releases the Belmont Report.
1981	Federal agencies implement a major revision of human research regulations.
1991	Seventeen federal agencies revise and unify human research regulations, which become the Common Rule.
1994	President Clinton creates the Advisory Committee on Human Radiation Experiments, which investigates previously classified radiation experiments conducted by the United States government on citizens and military personnel from the 1940s to the 1980s.
1997	The United States government issues an official apology for the Tuskegee Syphilis Study.
1998	The Government Accounting Office releases a report on institutional review boards, which calls for several steps to reform these committees and improve oversight.
1999	Jesse Gelsinger dies in a Phase I human gene therapy experiment at the University of Pennsylvania, a tragic event that leads to additional policies and guidelines designed to enhance the protection of human research participants.
2004	The EPA cancels the Children's Environmental Exposure Research Study in response to Congressional criticism.
2006	The EPA revises its human research regulations to conform to a congressional mandate to provide additional protections for pregnant and nursing women and children.
2011	The Department of Health and Human Services announces proposed revisions to the Common Rule designed to enhance human participant protections and reduce administrative burdens on investigators.

on Harmonization (2010), as well as guidance documents issued by the Office of Human Research Protections (2010) and the FDA (Food and Drug Administration 2010b). The Health Insurance Portability and Accountability Act (45 CFR 160) includes rules to protect the privacy and confidentiality of patients participating in (or who may participate in) research studies (Department of Health and Human Services 2010).

REPORTING RESEARCH RESULTS TO PARTICIPANTS

One of the important ethical challenges in environmental health research is deciding whether (and how) to report research results to human participants. Data collected during an environmental health study may be useful to the research participants. Investigators may collect clinical data, such as blood pressure, heart rate, blood glucose level, and blood hemoglobin or hematocrit levels; genetic/genomic data, such as genotypes or genetic polymorphisms; and environmental data, such as exposures to heavy metals, pesticides, toxic chemicals, air pollution, and allergens (Renegar et al. 2006; Brody et al. 2007; Wolf et al. 2008; Resnik 2009d; Sly et al. 2009). Research results may include information pertaining to the outcomes and variables under investigation as well as incidental findings (Wolf et al. 2008). For example, if a research team is collecting dust samples to test for the presence of lead in the home and inadvertently detects high levels of mold spores in the home, the information about mold would be an incidental finding (Resnik and Zeldin 2008). Results may be reported individually or collectively. Investigators usually report aggregate results even when they do not report individual results to participants (Renegar et al. 2006).

Reporting individual research results to human participants presents an ethical challenge for several reasons. First, because the implications of the information reported back to individuals may be uncertain and complex, sharing research results could cause harm because the participants may not understand how to use the information. For example, suppose that investigators are conducting a study on the health effects of exposures to different chemicals in the home, such as pesticides, flame retardants, and bisphenol A (BPA). Suppose that it is not known what level of BPA is safe (or unsafe) and that the source of the exposure is not well understood. If participants receive information about their exposure to BPA, they may not know what to do with this information. They may become anxious and stressed, and may decide to sell their homes, based on uncertain or misleading information. They may also develop a false sense of security if they have misleading negative BPA results (Brody et al. 2007; Resnik 2009d). Or suppose that investigators are analyzing genetic samples from participants and find that a particular genotype is associated with a 10 percent increased risk of developing Alzheimer's disease, but that more studies are needed to confirm this result. If they inform the participants about their increased disease risk, the participants may become excessively worried or make poor choices based on this information, such as spending their retirement investments or making plans to commit suicide before they become demented (Renegar et al. 2006).

In some situations, returning results to individuals could harm the community. Suppose that investigators are studying the effects of indoor spraying a particular pesticide to control malaria in an African community and that there are no established safe or unsafe levels for the pesticide in the blood (this is part of what the study is attempting to establish). Informing the research participants about their pesticides levels prematurely could lead them to convince the community to stop pesticide spraying, which could increase the incidence of malaria, which is known to be harmful. The entire community could make a poor choice based on an inaccurate understanding of the information (Resnik 2009d).

Information that is discovered as part of a study may impose legal liabilities on the participants. For example, if high levels of lead or mold are discovered in a home, the owners may be legally required to disclose this information to tenants or prospective buyers, or they may be statutorily bound to perform some kind of remediation. Participants may not have a good understanding of these legal risks when they agree to take part in a study (Institute of Medicine 2005; Brody et al. 2007).

Second, the testing methods used to obtain research results may not be accurate or reliable (Holtzman et al. 1997; Renegar et al. 2006) and could lead to poor decisions based on misinformation (Holtzman et al. 1997; Wolf et al. 2008). For example, a false positive HIV test result could lead a person to begin antiretroviral treatment and cause them needless worry. In 1988, the United States adopted regulations, known as the Clinical Laboratory Improvement Amendments (CLIA), to promote accurate and reliable clinical, laboratory testing (Holtzman et al. 1997). Laboratories that perform clinical testing must be CLIA certified, although research laboratories are not so required (Centers for Medicaid and Medicare Services 2010). If the tests used to obtain research data have been performed by laboratories that are not CLIA-certified, the results may not be accurate or reliable.

Third, the manner of reporting results creates ethical dilemmas. Investigators have an obligation to help participants understand the findings and make informed choices because receiving information without any follow-up or context can be harmful and distressing. For example, investigators can explain the potential significance of a result, and they could make a referral to a physician or clinic for counseling, treatment, or follow-up (Wolf et al. 2008). Because biomedical researchers are often not clinicians, it can be difficult to communicate results effectively. Participants may wrongly assume that a test conducted during a research study is the same as a test performed as part of a medical evaluation. They may not understand that the information they receive is not intended to diagnose, treat, or prevent a disease (Wolf et al. 2008). Investigators may want to enlist the aid of qualified medical professionals to help them communicate results to participants and assist the participants with obtaining treatment or a referral. They may also want to develop handouts and other materials to help participants understand their results (Brody et al. 2007; Wolf et al. 2008). All of these efforts can increase the cost and complexity of a study (Wolf et al. 2008).

There are several different responses to the ethical dilemmas related to providing research results (Brody et al. 2007). One response is to not report back any individual research results (Resnik 2009d). Individuals (and communities) may be informed of the aggregate results of the research project through publications, newsletters, or press releases, but they would not be informed about their particular results. The main argument for this approach is that data are being collected for research purposes only, and should not be used to guide individual decision making. The distinction between research and practice, emphasized in the Belmont Report, lends support to this view. Research is conducted to produce generalizable knowledge that can benefit society, not to produce benefits for individual human participants. Participants may happen to benefit from participating in research, but that is not the main goal. When researchers remove personal identifiers from the data for the purposes of protecting confidentiality and facilitating data sharing, it is impossible to recontact participants concerning research results (Brody et al. 2007).

A fundamental problem with the first approach is that research results can be highly beneficial to participants, and investigators have an obligation to share those results with participants (Resnik 2009d). Some results will be useful, accurate, and reliable and should be reported. For example, dangerous levels of lead discovered in a home should be reported to participants because scientists have established safe (and unsafe) levels of lead exposure, and many CLIA-certified labs perform these tests (Institute of Medicine 2005). Some genetic findings, such as BRCA1 breast cancer mutations, are also useful, accurate, and reliable (Renegar et al. 2006). Additionally, the results of clinical examinations and tests, such as blood pressure, heart rate, blood glucose levels and hemoglobin levels, and HIV status are useful, accurate, and reliable (Wolf et al. 2008). It would be highly unethical, one might argue, for an investigator to not inform a participant that he has dangerously high blood pressure (Wolf et al. 2008).

An important lawsuit in the United States addressed the investigator's legal duties to inform participants about research results. In the 1990s, the Kennedy Krieger Institute (KKI), which is associated with Johns Hopkins University, conducted a study of the effectiveness of different lead abatement techniques in homes with lead paint in Baltimore, MD. The study was funded by the EPA and the Maryland Department of Housing and Community Development (Mastroianni and Kahn 2002). One hundred and eight families with healthy, young children who were recruited to participate in the study were randomly assigned to one of five groups: one group that received maximum lead abatement, three groups that received different levels of lead abatement but not the maximum level, and a control group in which the occupants lived in a home with no lead paint. The investigators collected dust samples in the homes and blood samples from the children to monitor lead levels in the homes. The investigators told the parents they would monitor lead in their children's blood, but never told them that lead levels were the primary experimental outcome. The investigators collaborated with the landlords and helped them obtain grants for lead abatement (Lewin 2001; Mastroianni and Kahn 2002; Institute of Medicine 2005).

The parents of two of the children in the study sued KKI, alleging that the investigators neglected to inform them of dangerous lead levels in a timely fashion and adequately inform them of the risks of the study. Their cases were combined in the litigation (*Grimes v. Kennedy Krieger Institute, Inc.* 2001). In one case, the investigators did not inform the parents of dangerous lead levels detected in a child's blood until nine months after data collection (Mastroianni and Kahn 2002). The district court found in favor of the defendants and dismissed the case, but the Maryland Court of Appeals vacated this ruling and found that the investigators had a legal duty of due care to the participants, based on their special relationship with the participants evidenced by the federal research regulations and contractual obligations embodied in the informed consent document. The appellate court remanded the case back to the district court and the case was then settled out of court. Although the KKI lawsuit only establishes legal precedent in the State of Maryland, it supports the premise that investigators have legal and ethical duties to inform research participants about significant risks discovered during the course of a study (Mastroianni and Kahn 2002; Institute of Medicine 2005; Resnik and Zeldin 2008).

A second approach to returning research results is to provide only clinically significant results to individuals, such as blood pressure, blood glucose, HIV status, lead levels, mold levels, and genotypes that are clearly linked to significantly increased disease risk. The advantage of this approach is that it minimizes risks to participants and maximizes benefits without requiring participants to deal with uncertain and complex information (Brody et al. 2007). An important drawback of this approach is that participants are often interested in knowing their research results, even if clinical significance is not well-understood (Brody et al. 2007). Respect for autonomy implies that investigators should provide participants with information that they want to know (Brody et al. 2007). Indeed, investigators conducting a study of exposures to chemicals in the home found that 97 percent out of 120 participants wanted to receive their test results (McKelvey et al. 2003). Other investigators have reported similar findings (Altman et al. 2008).

The previous considerations suggest a third approach: full disclosure. The main argument for this approach is that the participants have a right to know their research results because the results are obtained from samples and data they have provided to the investigators. Additionally, this approach enhances the participants' autonomy. In some cases, participants may choose to not know their results (Brody et al. 2007), although research shows that most participants want to know their results (Altman et al. 2008). While this approach has considerable merit, it faces some difficulties because there is still the possibility that results reported back to participants may cause harm to the individuals or the community (Holtzman et al. 1997; Resnik 2009d). One might argue that the obligation to avoid causing harm trumps the obligation to honor a person's right to know, especially when the information is uncertain, difficult to understand, or obtained via methods that are inaccurate or unreliable (Holtzman et al. 1997). More information is not always better information.

To balance respect for autonomy and the obligation to avoid causing harm, return of research results should be handled carefully. Results should be returned only if 1) the testing methods are accurate and reliable; 2) the investigators have appropriate procedures in place to provide counseling or referrals; and 3) the results have definite practical or clinical significance, or the results do not have definite practical or clinical value but the participants want to know the results and they are able to deal with complex and uncertain information (Brody et al. 2007). Whatever approach that investigators take, they should become familiar with the population they are studying and work with the community to understand how best to approach returning research results (Brody et al. 2007).

PROTECTING PRIVACY AND CONFIDENTIALITY

As noted earlier, the U.S. federal research regulations, the Helsinki Declaration, and other ethical and legal rules require investigators to protect participants' privacy and confidentiality. Privacy and confidentiality are different, but related, concepts. Informational privacy is concerned with controlling access to private information about one's self; physical privacy is concerned with controlling access to one's body, biological specimens, or personal space.

Releasing a person's medical records, without permission, would be an invasion of informational privacy. Touching or observing a person's genitals, without permission, would be an invasion of physical privacy. Confidentiality is concerned with protecting informational privacy. Investigators can take different measures to protect confidentiality, such as limiting access to research records, removing personal identifiers from the data, and securing and encrypting data. Protecting privacy and confidentiality is important for preventing harm to research participants because violations of privacy or confidentiality may produce many adverse consequences for a person, ranging from embarrassment and stress to discrimination and loss of employment. Protecting privacy and confidentiality also respects participants' autonomous decision making concerning the disclosure of private information and the sharing of physical privacy (Hodge Jr. and Gostin 2008).

Protecting privacy and confidentiality presents some unique ethical challenges for investigators when they conduct research in homes, worksites, or other venues in which they inadvertently learn about private information when they are collecting samples or data (Institute of Medicine 2005; Resnik and Zeldin 2008). When investigators conduct research in a home or work environment, they may observe evidence of reportable illegal activities, such as child or elder abuse/neglect, illicit drug use, or violations of building codes, occupational safety and health laws, or environmental laws. In the United States most states have laws that obligate some types of professionals, such as healthcare workers, social workers, or educators to report child or elder abuse/neglect. Some states also have laws requiring anyone to report child or elder abuse/neglect (Resnik and Zeldin 2008). Legal rules protecting confidentiality and privacy usually include exceptions for reporting abuse/neglect and matters related to public health or environmental protection (Hodge Jr. and Gostin 2008).

Because legal issues pertaining to confidentiality/privacy and reporting requirements may be unclear and conflicting, we can set them aside for the purposes of discussing the ethical issues. Additionally, deciding whether to obey the law in a particular situation is itself an ethical issue. Investigators may therefore face ethical dilemmas that are not clearly settled by the law.

The ethical issues concerning reporting of private information discovered during research can be challenging, since investigators face a conflict between their obligation to safeguard privacy and confidentiality of individuals (a human rights concern), and their obligation to protect public health (a utilitarian concern) or the environment. While the federal research regulations, ethics codes, and other sources of guidance focus on the investigators' obligations to research participants, one might argue that they also have obligations to other people affected by the research, such as residents in the home or employees, based on a general duty of beneficence (Institute of Medicine 2005; Resnik and Sharp 2006). Beneficence implies, for example, that a bystander should not sit by idly while someone drowns in a pool. He (or she) should do something to help that person, such as calling a lifeguard (if one is around) or throwing the person a life preserver. Likewise, an investigator should not ignore a person in need of help that he (or she) encounters in a research setting. If an investigator observes evidence of child or elder abuse/neglect, then he (or she) should report the situation to the appropriate authorities, even if the investigator must violate confidentiality or privacy to make the report. An investigator should also report dangerous conditions observed at a workplace that threaten employees or others. Preventing imminent and significant harm to identifiable individuals can override the obligation to safeguard confidentiality and privacy in some cases (Hodge Jr. and Gostin 2008; Resnik and Zeldin 2008).

Even though investigators may need to breech confidentiality or privacy in some cases to protect individuals, confidentiality or privacy should only be violated to prevent imminent and significant harm to identifiable individuals (Resnik and Zeldin 2008). Not every illegal activity observed in a home or workplace would warrant breeching confidentiality or privacy. For example, an investigator who collects samples or data in a home might observe evidence of illicit drug use, gambling, or building code violations, but he (or she) should not report these activities unless they pose a significant threat to identifiable individuals. An investigator conducting research in the workplace may observe evidence of sexual harassment, discrimination, or violations of environmental laws, but he (or she) should not report these illegal activities unless they pose an imminent threat of significant harm to identifiable individuals.

Investigators should discuss these issues when they obtain informed consent from research participants, and explain the extent to which privacy/confidentiality will be protected. Investigators who intend to report suspected child abuse/neglect should inform the parents about this policy. Investigators who plan to conduct research in workplaces should discuss confidentiality/privacy issues with the management when they obtain permission to collect data or recruit research participants. They should also train research staff on confidentiality/privacy issues and mandatory reporting requirements, and the importance of avoiding unnecessary invasions of privacy when collecting data or samples in the home or workplace (Resnik and Zeldin 2008).

INTENTIONAL EXPOSURE STUDIES

As noted in Chapter 2, some environmental health investigators conduct research that intentionally exposes individuals to environmental agents, such as air pollution or pesticides (Resnik and Portier 2005; Resnik 2006). These studies can play an important role in improving our understanding of routes and mechanisms of exposure and physiological effects of environmental agents, such as metabolic reactions, inflammation, toxicity, and tissue damage. Although epidemiological research and animal studies can teach us a great deal about how environmental agents affect human health, it is also important to conduct human exposure research under carefully controlled conditions (Furtaw 2001). For example, the EPA conducts research on the effects of inhaling air pollution at its exposure research laboratory in Chapel Hill, NC. In a typical study, participants will enter a breathing chamber filled with air that has had impurities removed. The investigators will introduce a pollutant into the air (such as ozone or automobile exhaust), and the participant will breathe the air. The participant's physiological responses are monitored, and blood, sputum, and tissue samples are taken (Environmental Protection Agency 2010k). Investigators may perform a bronchoscopy on the participants to obtain cells from the trachea or bronchial tubes. Investigators administer antianxiety, analgesic, and anesthetic medications to the patient/participant. The procedure takes place in an area with equipment for managing airway emergencies, such as an operating room (Stenfors et al. 2010).

The most significant ethical challenge facing intentional exposure studies is justifying the risks imposed on human participants (Resnik 2006; Miller and Rosenstein 2008). Depending on the type of research being conducted, the risks to participants could range from relatively minor problems, such as respiratory irritation, bleeding, bruising, local infection, nausea or headache, to more serious ones, such as respiratory distress, heart arrhythmias, renal compromise, or cardiac arrest. Some studies may pose a risk of long-term adverse effects, such as cancer (National Research Council 2004). Federal regulations and ethical guidelines permit participants to be exposed to significant risks in research, provided that the net benefits to the participant and society outweigh the risks (Wendler and Miller 2008). Participants in Phase II and III clinical trials are often exposed to significant risks, but these participants also have a disease and may derive substantial benefits from participating in research that offers medical treatment. For example, a cancer patient participating in a clinical trial of a new chemotherapy combination may face the risk of severe injury or death, but the participant may also benefit from effective treatment of the disease or prolonged life (van Luijn et al. 2006).

When participants are not expected to significantly benefit from participating in research, as occurs in intentional exposure studies, the risks to the participants must be justified in terms of the benefits to society brought about by the advancement of knowledge. Ethical guidelines do not treat monetary compensation as a benefit, as this could be used to justify high-risk studies that would otherwise not be justified (Wendler and Miller 2008). There is little controversy about enrolling participants in studies that do not benefit them when the risks are minimal because the benefits to society will clearly outweigh the risks, as long as the study is well-designed and is expected to yield useful knowledge (Wendler and Miller 2008). ("Minimal risk" is defined by the federal research regulations as risks not greater than the risks ordinarily encountered in daily life or routine medical or psychological tests [Department of Health and Human Services 2009].)

There has been considerable controversy about enrolling individuals in studies that do not benefit them when the risks are more than minimal because people disagree about whether the social benefits of the research justify the imposition of risks on human participants (Resnik 2006; Miller 2008). For example, some Phase I (first in human) drug studies on healthy volunteers are designed to determine the maximum tolerable dose in human participants. To do this, the investigators gradually increase the dose to induce toxicity or intolerable side effects, such as severe nausea, vomiting, diarrhea, or headaches (Kimmelman 2009). Although healthy participants receive no benefits from Phase I drug studies, most people regard this research as ethical because it helps to promote an important social goal – the development of new medications (Kimmelman 2009). Phase I studies play an important role in drug development because the basic safety profile of a medication needs to be established before its efficacy can be studied (Kimmelman 2009).

Environmental exposure studies have been more controversial than Phase I drug studies because people question whether the social benefits of these experiments outweigh the risks they impose on human volunteers (Miller 2008). Some question whether there is a need to expose human volunteers intentionally to substances that are already known to be unsafe, such as ozone, automobile exhaust, or pesticides (Miller 2008). The most controversial environmental exposure studies have been pesticide experiments conducted by private companies on human volunteers to generate data to submit to the EPA for regulatory purposes (Resnik 2007b; Shrader-Frechette 2007b). Private companies sponsored these studies in the late 1990s and early 2000s to generate data to convince the EPA to loosen up restrictions imposed by the Food Quality Protection Act (discussed in Chapters 6 and 10). Companies hoped their data would convince the EPA to allow higher levels of pesticide residue on food (Resnik 2007b). Some experiments included: oral administration of dichlorvos to fifty-three participants, administration of orange juice laced with aldicard to forty-seven participants, and oral administration of chlorpyrifos to dozens of volunteers. Some of the participants were college students who were paid up to $460 for their participation, while others were company employees (Shrader-Frechette 2007b).

The Environmental Working Group (1998) exposed some of these studies in a report it published in 1998, which received wide media coverage (Resnik 2007b). Critics of the studies charged that they were scientifically and ethically flawed because:

- The studies were statistically underpowered. As a result, they gave a false impression that the pesticides produced no adverse health effects (Lockwood 2004; National Research Council 2004; Needleman et al. 2005).
- The studies were scientifically unnecessary because the adverse health effects of the compounds being tested were already well known (Environmental Working Group 1998; Needleman et al. 2005; Shrader-Frechette 2007b).
- The studies did not minimize risks to human participants (National Research Council 2004).
- The studies addressed the adverse health effects of pesticides in adults, not children, and therefore provided information that was irrelevant for the EPA's decision making related to protecting the health of children (Needleman et al. 2005).
- The studies were tainted or biased because they were sponsored by industry (Melnick and Huff 2004).
- The studies that used employees as test participants violated informed consent requirements, because the volunteers would feel compelled to participate (Environmental Working Group 1998).
- Even if the studies were well designed, they could not yield significant benefits for public health (Melnick and Huff 2004; Shrader-Frechette 2007b).

These charges deserve to be examined carefully. To guide the discussion, it will be useful to distinguish between 1) the actual studies that were conducted by industry, and 2) hypothetical studies that might be conducted. Lockwood (2004), the National Research Council (2004), Needleman et al. (2005), and Shrader-Frechette (2007b) have published incisive analyses of the studies that were actually conducted. They have argued, convincingly, that the studies contained significant scientific and ethical flaws, and I will not challenge their conclusions in this book. Instead, I would like to consider whether potential future studies that intentionally expose human participants to pesticides could meet scientific and ethical requirements. Could any controlled experiment that exposes human participants to pesticides be justified? To address this question, let's assume, for the sake of argument, that the proposed experiment is scientifically valid and necessary. That is, the experiment is adequately powered and designed to address an important scientific question concerning the health effects of pesticides on human beings that cannot be answered adequately through animal studies or human observational studies. Let's also assume that the volunteers are adult participants who will provide informed consent without any undue influence or coercion, that the investigators will take appropriate steps to minimize risks, and that the studies are not sponsored by industry. If these conditions are met, then the ethical debate would center on one key issue: Do the social benefits of the studies justify exposing human participants to pesticides (Resnik and Portier 2005)? This question embodies a conflict between the principle of utility and protection of human rights and well-being.

As noted earlier, critics of the industry studies argued that the benefits of pesticide research did not justify the risks because the experiments did not provide any useful information that could enhance public health (Melnick and Huff 2004). Indeed, the companies conducted the research in an attempt to convince the EPA to weaken restrictions on pesticides, which could have had an adverse impact on public health (Shrader-Frechette 2007b). But suppose that a nonindustry group, such as a government agency, proposes to conduct a pesticide study to obtain better information concerning a particular product. Suppose that the study could yield information that a regulatory agency would use to decide that restrictions on this product need to be strengthened to protect public health, or professional organizations would use in developing guidelines for safe use of the product. This type of study could conceivably be justified based on its potential positive impact on public health (Resnik and Portier 2005). After examining these issues, the National Research Council (2004) concluded that some pesticide experiments involving human participants could be justified, if they are likely to yield important knowledge for enhancing public health and they meet other scientific and ethical standards.

An example of pesticide research on human participants that can enhance public health and meet other scientific and ethical standards is research on insect repellents. As noted in Chapter 5, insect repellants are used to prevent bites or stings from various insect or arthropod pests, such as mosquitoes, ticks, fleas, and lice. Insect repellents can play an important role in preventing insect or arthropod-borne illnesses, such as malaria, yellow fever, encephalitis, Rocky Mountain spotted fever, and Lyme disease (Robson et al. 2010). The EPA has approved a variety of chemicals for use as insect repellants in adults and children (Katz et al. 2008). Although there is considerable evidence concerning the safety and effectiveness of many insect repellents, additional research is often needed to understand how different formulations and combinations of chemicals impact safety and efficacy: how repellents interact with human skin and are absorbed and eliminated by the body, how repellents interact with other chemicals applied to the skin (such as sunscreens), and how they are affected by variations in temperature and humidity. New repellents and new formulations of old repellants also need to be tested. The human volunteers in controlled experiments on insect repellants receive no direct medical benefits, but they are exposed to risks, such as insect bites, skin irritation, or rash (Fuentes and Sherman 2010; Logan et al. 2010). The EPA currently reviews insect repellent studies conducted by industry for regulatory purposes (Environmental Protection Agency 2010l).

If insect repellent studies can pass ethical and scientific muster, then other pesticide experiments could as well, if they serve an important public health purpose. Human testing of pesticides used on food crops could help investigators obtain a better understanding of how pesticides are absorbed, metabolized, and eliminated by the body, which could lead to beneficial changes in environmental regulations or public health practices (Resnik and Portier 2005). Human experiments involving other environmental agents, such as ozone, particulate matter, automobile exhaust, or BPA could also help to inform regulatory decisions and public health practices (Resnik 2006; Environmental Protection Agency 2010k).

Another major ethical challenge pertaining to intentional exposure studies is minimizing risks to human participants. These studies usually involve exposing people to some agents that can cause short-term damage to the person being studied. For example, exposure to ozone can cause respiratory inflammation, and bronchoscopy can cause bleeding, infection, fevers, sore threat, breathing problems, and heart problems (Stenfors et al. 2010). Investigators can use a number of techniques to minimize the risks of intentional exposure studies, such as clinical monitoring of participants, data and safety monitoring of the entire study, exclusion of participants who have medical conditions that place them at increased risk, reporting adverse events to the IRB and sponsor, use of data from previous animal or human studies to establish safe doses, and slow dose escalation (National Research Council 2004b; Resnik 2006; Miller and Rosenstein 2008). The National Research Council has recommended that intentional exposure studies be designed to avoid causing serious or irreversible harm to participants (National Research Council 2004). Chemicals that are carcinogenic, genotoxic, or neurotoxic may cause irreversible harm even in small doses, and should not be used in intentional exposure studies (National Research Council 2004; Resnik and Portier 2005).

It is worth mentioning that the dispute over pesticide testing and intentional exposure research led to changes in the EPA's human research regulations. In the 1990s, the EPA had adopted the Common Rule for EPA-funded human research, but it did not have any specific regulations for privately funded (i.e., third party) research. The EPA had accepted data from privately funded human studies on a case-by-case basis, applying relevant ethical and scientific standards (Resnik 2007b). In 1998, the EPA decided it would no longer accept privately funded human dosing studies for regulatory decisions and asked the National Research Council (NRC) to study the issue. The agency had planned to not develop any new regulations until the NRC had issued its report. However, several agricultural organizations sued the EPA, claiming that it had engaged in inappropriate rule making by refusing to accept the privately funded human dosing studies. The court agreed with the plaintiffs and ordered the EPA to engage in appropriate rule making, with a public notice and comment period (*Croplife America v. EPA* 2003).

In the fall of 2004, an ethical controversy arose concerning the Children's Environmental Exposure Research Study (CHEERS), an observational study on pesticides and other chemicals in homes in Jacksonville, Florida. CHEERS was sponsored by the EPA, CDC, and Duvall County, Florida Health Department to study how children are exposed to pesticides in homes. The investigators planned to recruit sixty families with young children who had a high pesticide use in the home and a control group of families with low or no pesticide use. There would be five home visits over a two-year period, during which investigators would collect blood and urine from the children and soil and dust samples from the homes. The families would also videotape their children's daily activities and keep a journal of pesticide and chemical use. Parents would be paid $970 to participate. The study was approved by peer review committees at the EPA and CDC and three IRBs (Resnik and Wing 2007).

CHEERS became controversial after environmental groups and the media portrayed it as an intentional exposure study that would treat children as guinea pigs. CHEERS was not an intentional exposure study, although many people interpreted it as one. In fact, the investigators had screening procedures in place to ensure that parents would not use pesticides heavily in order to be in the study. Parents were also permitted to remain in the study if they decided to reduce their use of pesticides. Critics were also concerned that the study was targeting a low-income minority population and that it was partly supported by a $2 million grant from the American Chemistry Council (Resnik and Wing 2007). In the spring of 2005, CHEERS became a political matter when Representative Barbara Boxer, a Democrat from California, and other politicians, threatened to derail Stephen Johnson's nomination for EPA Administrator unless the agency stopped the CHEERS study. The EPA complied with this demand, and the study was terminated in April 2005. Additionally, Congress passed legislation prohibiting the EPA from funding or relying upon intentional exposure research involving pregnant or nursing women or children and mandated that the EPA provide additional protections for women and children involved in research (Resnik 2007b).

In 2006, the EPA issued new rules intended to comply with congressional legislation (passed in response to CHEERS and human pesticide experiments) and recommendations from the NRC. The rules prohibit the EPA from funding intentional exposure studies involving pregnant or nursing women or children, and also do not allow the agency to use data from privately funded, intentional exposure studies involving pregnant or nursing women or children to make regulatory decisions. The rules prohibit the EPA from relying on unethical research conducted before 2006, and create a human studies review board to review privately funded intentional exposure human studies submitted to the EPA for regulatory purposes. The rules also provide additional protections for pregnant or nursing women or children involved in observational (nonexperimental) research (Environmental Protection Agency 2010l). The EPA's rules concerning pregnant or nursing women or children are more restrictive than the subparts of the Common Rule that protect fetuses and children. For example, under the Common Rule, children could participate in minimal risk experiments on the safety and efficacy of insect repellents applied to the skin, but not under the EPA's regulations (Resnik 2007c).

INTERVENTION STUDIES

Environmental intervention research, such as the KKI study (discussed earlier), also raises some challenging ethical issues. Environmental intervention studies are similar to clinical trials in that they aim to determine the effectiveness of health interventions, and they usually involve randomization to different groups, such as experimental versus control (Morgan et al. 2004). While clinical trials investigate the effectiveness of medical treatments, environmental intervention studies investigate the effectiveness of environmental interventions, such as lead abatement or mold remediation (Resnik 2008b). One of the perennial ethical issues in clinical trials is whether individuals can be assigned to groups that do not receive an active treatment, such as placebo control groups. Assigning patients to nontreatment groups is controversial because it appears to violate the physician's obligation to provide the best effective treatment to his (or her) patients, a fundamental principle of medical ethics (Fried 1974; Freedman 1987; Emanuel and Miller 2001; Resnik 2009c). Many commentators have argued that placebo control groups are ethical only when there is no effective therapy for the patient's condition, or the patient is not likely to suffer any significant harm as a result of denial of therapy (Freedman 1987; Miller and Weijer 2003). The Helsinki Declaration (mentioned earlier) states that placebos may be used in clinical trials only when no proven therapy exists or the patients receiving placebos will not suffer serious or irreversible harm (World Medical Association 2008). Some commentators argue that placebos may be used in research provided that commonly accepted ethical principles, such as valid study design, informed consent, risk minimization, and reasonableness of risks are satisfied (Miller and Brody 2002).

Though environmental intervention studies usually do not include placebo control groups, they sometimes include control groups in which participants are denied an intervention thought to be effective. Some commentators argued that the KKI study was unethical because participants in the experimental groups lived in homes that did not receive full lead abatement (Spriggs 2004). However, others have argued that this critique rests on a misunderstanding of the study because all participants lived in homes that received some level of lead abatement or they lived in lead-free homes (Buchanan and Miller 2006). For an example of a study in which a control group was denied an intervention, consider research conducted by Kercsmar et al. (2006) to determine the effectiveness of mold remediation at reducing the morbidity of childhood asthma. In this study, the families of sixty-two children with asthma, who were living in homes with indoor mold, were randomly assigned to receive mold remediation or information about cleaning mold from the home (the control group). The investigators took blood and urine samples from the children and dust samples from the homes. Dust samples were analyzed for the presence of mold spores, dust mites, cockroach parts, and other allergens. Blood/urine samples were analyzed for the presence of cotine (a nicotine metabolite, which is sign of smoking in the home), and chemicals indicative of immune responses. The investigators found that mold remediation significantly reduced the asthma exacerbations among the children in the study compared to the control group (Kercsmar et al. 2006).

Was the Kercsmar study ethical? On the one hand, one might argue that it was unethical because mold remediation is an effective method for reducing asthma exacerbations, and children in the control group did not receive this intervention. Denying children mold remediation would be analogous to denying children asthma medication in a clinical trial of a new asthma treatment. On the other hand, one might argue that the study was ethical because denying children mold remediation is morally different from denying children asthma medications. The investigators did not have a physician-patient relationship with the children living in the homes with mold (Resnik 2009c). They were environmental researchers studying the effectiveness of mold remediation, not physicians studying the effectiveness of a medical treatment. Because the investigators did not have a physician-patient relationship with the research participants, they were not obligated to provide them with mold remediation, even if it was thought to be effective. Moreover, the children in the experimental group did receive some benefits from participating in the study because their parents were informed about methods for cleaning mold from the home (Resnik 2008b).

Even if environmental health researchers do not have physician-patient relationships with their participants, intervention studies raise ethical issues and concerns that need to be addressed. Investigators still have ethical obligations to the participants even when they do not have a physician-patient relationship. Studies must be well-designed and expected to yield results that can benefit society. Investigators must do their best to minimize risks to participants and maximize benefits. They should inform participants about strategies they may implement to reduce their exposures to potentially harmful environmental agents, such as pesticides or mold, and share research results with participants that are reliable, accurate, and useful (Resnik and Wing 2007; Resnik 2008b).

COMMUNITY PARTICIPATION IN RESEARCH

The final cluster of ethical issues discussed in this chapter involves engaging communities in the design, review, and execution of research. During the 1990s, investigators and ethicists became increasingly aware of the importance of involving communities in research in order to protect them from harm and promote their interests (Israel et al. 1998; Minkler 2004; Dickert and Sugarman 2005; Gilbert 2006). Although human research regulations and policies focus on protecting the rights and welfare of individuals, many commentators argued that communities should also be protected (Weijer and Emanuel 2000). Investigators began to understand that community members and organizations can play an essential role in recruiting research participants, fostering public support, reviewing research, and in developing questionnaires, brochures, and research materials (Israel et al. 1998; O'Fallon and Dearry 2002). As a result, an approach known as community-based participatory research (CBPR) began to emerge. CBPR involves collaboration between investigators and community members at all stages of research, from study design and execution to the dissemination of results. CBPR addresses needs or problems identified by the community and aims to produce results that are useful to the community. Research procedures and interventions used in CBPR should be culturally appropriate (O'Fallon and Dearry 2002). Investigators can work with community members in different ways, such as hiring community liaisons as research staff, holding focus groups with community members, and forming community advisory boards or IRBs (Gilbert 2006; Watkins et al. 2009). CBPR is most appropriate when investigators are planning to study a readily identifiable, cohesive community, such as a tribe, an indigenous population, a group of workers, a county, or a town (Watkins et al. 2009).

Most of the ethical issues related to CBPR revolve around the conflict between the interests of investigators and the interests of the community (Minkler 2004; Resnik and Kennedy 2010). Most investigators are interested in publishing high quality research that promotes human knowledge, benefits their careers, and helps society (Haack 2003). They may also be interested in promoting the good of a particular community, but their primary interests focus on publication and research (Resnik and Kennedy 2010). Community members are mainly interested in protecting and promoting the interests of their community. They are likely to expect that information generated by research studies will be useful in dealing with problems that impact the community, such as infectious diseases, substance abuse, and environmental contaminants. They may also expect that the results of research will be useful in leveraging resources, such as government funding or expertise, to help the community (Israel et al. 1998). Community members may be interested in publication, but they may also be apprehensive about dissemination of findings that portray the community in a negative light (Minkler 2004; Dickert and Sugarman 2005; Resnik and Kennedy 2010).

Though the interests of scientists and community members often coincide in CBPR, sometimes they conflict (Minkler 2004). For example, community members may not want researchers to publish findings that could cause the community embarrassment, or lead to discrimination or stigma (Dickert and Sugarman 2005). Community members may also disagree with researchers about the interpretation of data, the goals of research, and the use and disposition of biological samples (Mello and Wolf 2010). If investigators and community members are unable to resolve disagreements amicably, this could negatively impact the research project and undermine the community's trust in science. Community members may decide they do not want to participate in any future studies as a result of bad experiences with investigators (Mello and Wolf 2010; Resnik and Kennedy 2010).

An example of a troubled relationship between investigators and a community involves researchers from Arizona State University and the Havasupai Native American tribe. In 1990, the investigators collected 200 blood samples from members of the tribe for a study on causes of behavioral and medical disorders (as stated in the consent form). However, communications with tribal leaders prior to the initiation of the study indicated it would focus on diabetes. The investigators used the samples to conduct several studies unrelated to diabetes, and shared the samples with other researchers. Members of the tribe objected to the use of their samples to study the genetics of schizophrenia, in-breeding, and the tribe's evolutionary–genetic origins (Mello and Wolf 2010). The tribe filed a $50 million lawsuit against the investigators and the university, alleging that the use of the biological samples for purposes other than diabetes research violated the informed consent provide by the participants. In April 2010, the university settled the lawsuit out of court. The university publicly apologized to the tribe and agreed to pay $700,000 (to be divided among forty-one participants in the study) and return the remaining biological samples (Mello and Wolf 2010).

The Havasupai case offers important lessons for investigators conducting CBPR. First, investigators and community members need to agree on key issues, such as the purposes of the research, the study design, publication plans, and the use of biological samples/data (Mello and Wolf 2010). To help prevent misunderstandings, it may be useful to develop a written agreement with community representatives or advisory boards prior to the initiation of a study. Investigators should also hold regular meetings with community advisory boards to keep them updated about important developments (Resnik and Kennedy 2010). Second, the informed consent document should clearly indicate how samples and data will be used, stored, protected, and shared. In some cases, it may be appropriate to offer participants different options for using their samples/data. For example, some individuals may want to participate in a study but not give permission for their samples/data to be shared with other researchers. Research participants should receive instructions on how to withdraw their samples if they decide to stop participating in the study (Mello and Wolf 2010).

SUMMARY

In this chapter, we have examined some ethical and policy issues that arise when environmental health investigators conduct research involving human participants. We have reviewed some of the ethical and legal rules and principles that pertain to research with human participants, and we have explored some of the moral dilemmas that environmental investigators face, such as reporting research results to individuals, protecting privacy and confidentiality, intentionally exposing human participants to environmental agents that are potentially harmful, conducting controlled trials of environmental interventions, and engaging in community-based participatory research. The ethical issues can be difficult to resolve because they involve conflicts between competing values, such as promoting autonomy versus protecting individuals from harm, safeguarding privacy versus protecting individuals from harm, and promoting the interests of science versus promoting the interests of individuals or communities. The method for ethical decision making, discussed in Chapter 4, can be useful in resolving these conflicts. The next chapter will summarize the book's important themes and recommendations.

12

————

CONCLUSION

Environmental health research and scholarship have come a long way since Rachel Carson published *Silent Spring* more than four decades ago, but the ethical and policy issues raised in her book still have relevance today. Questions about the appropriate use of pesticides reflect the ongoing tension between protecting the environment and promoting human interests. But, as we have seen in this book, environmental health controversies go beyond the one-dimensional humanity versus environment theme, and are shaped by a rich array of values and interests, such as public health, individual autonomy, property rights, justice, utility, economic development, animal welfare, biodiversity preservation, and ecological sustainability. Although people often equate protecting the environment with promoting human health, these two values are sometimes at odds, as illustrated by debates about whether to spray DDT indoors to control malaria, build dams to provide water for communities, or grow GM crops to feed a growing population.

The scope of this book has ranged from local concerns, such as toxic waste site placement, housing standards, urban development, water resource use, and occupational safety, to national and global concerns, such as climate change, energy use, pollution, population control, and agriculture. The book has examined perennial topics, such as air and water quality, pesticide use, and solid waste disposal, as well as new and emerging ones, such as GM crops, nanotechnology, geoengineering, environmental justice, and protection of human subjects in environmental health research. The book has described some of the laws, regulations, and treaties relevant to environmental health, as well as moral concepts, theories, and principles.

One of the book's chief concerns has been to develop a method for ethical decision making that can be applied to environmental health dilemmas. The method requires one to identify and compare competing values and interests in light of realistic options and the best available scientific evidence. After considering the facts, options, and relevant values and interests, one should reach a decision that provides a fair and reasonable balance of moral principles, such as human rights, social utility, justice, protection of animal welfare, stewardship of natural resources, and ecological sustainability. Ethical and policy decisions should also be consistent and able to withstand public criticism.

Because the method requires the balancing of competing values and interests, it often yields moral compromises. For example, with regard to an issue that involves conflicts between economic development and environmental protection, such as land use, the method may recommend protecting the environment in a way that does not unnecessarily impede economic development. This type of result is likely to displease people who hold strong views on opposite sides of these debates. Thus, environmentalists may object to my method (and much of my book) because it makes too many concessions to economic interests and human needs, while business and industry leaders may have the opposite complaint. While I appreciate that different sides in environmental health debates have sincerely held beliefs in support of their positions, it is often important to seek compromises on these issues so that practical solutions can be implemented. Dogmatic adherence to a particular principle or value may lead to a stalemate in which neither side is able to advance its agenda. The decisions we must make are too urgent and important for us to get bogged down in ideology. Pragmatism is the way forward (Katz and Light 1996; Norton 2005; Brand 2009).

The following is a brief summary of some the policy recommendations for specific issues discussed in this book.

PESTICIDES

Pesticides have useful applications in agriculture, the prevention of insect-borne diseases, and workplace and domestic hygiene. However, because they have the potential to threaten human health and can cause harm to other species, pesticides should be regulated and carefully controlled, and some dangerous pesticides should be banned. The environmental and public health impacts of pesticides should be studied and minimized. Integrated pest management (IPM) is a useful approach to pesticide use that appropriately balances environmental protection, economic development, agricultural productivity, and human health and well-being. The IPM approach can be applied to preventing insect-borne diseases, such as malaria, as well as controlling agricultural and household pests. IPM involves judicious use of pesticides as well as other pest control methods, such as manipulation of the environment, structural maintenance, solid waste management, physical and biological pest controls; active monitoring of pesticide use patterns and pesticide resistance; and public education.

ANTIBIOTIC RESISTANCE

Antibiotic resistance is a serious public health problem. Healthcare professionals, public health organizations, and government agencies should promote responsible use of antibiotics to treat or prevent diseases. Legislation may need to be enacted to provide companies with additional economic incentives to develop new antibiotics. Antibiotics should not be fed to farm animals unless there is a reasonable certainty that no harm to human health will occur as a result of antibiotic resistance.

GENETIC ENGINEERING

GM animals, plants, and microorganisms can play an important role in agriculture, bio-medical research, the manufacturing of medications, and energy production. However, GM life forms also pose potential threats to human health and the environment. The precautionary principle (PP) offers the best approach to the development of genetically modified foods, crops, and animals. The PP does not support a total ban on genetic engineering of plants and animals because GM organisms offer potential benefits to humanity and even the environment (such as reduced use of pesticides or chemical fertilizers). Instead, societies should take reasonable measures to prevent, minimize, or mitigate the environmental, social, and health risks posed by GM foods, crops, and animals, such as health and safety testing and monitoring, environmental impact assessment, control over GM organisms to avoid environmental contamination, and appropriate regulation and oversight. Current regulations may need to be expanded or clarified to cover all GM plants and animals, regardless of the mode of gene transfer.

FOOD POLICIES

Food and dietary policies should balance public health and environmental concerns, individual autonomy, and justice. For most issues, research combined with consumer education, not coercive laws, is the best way to promote public health and environmental protection. However some laws, such as food safety standards, are necessary to protect public health. Bans on particular food items should be avoided, unless the food poses a serious public health threat and consumers are not likely to understand the benefits and risks associated with eating the food. Food taxes should be avoided because they are regressive. Vegetarianism is an ethically sound choice for an individual to make, but it should not be legally enforced as a matter of social policy.

AIR, WATER, AND SOLID WASTE

Responsible policies and practices related to air and water pollution, water scarcity, and solid waste disposal must carefully balance competing values, such as economic development, social utility, human rights, public health, justice, national sovereignty, stewardship, and sustainability. Because the growing human population is a major factor in pollution, waste production, and water scarcity, these issues cannot be adequately addressed without formulating population control policies. Communities should have meaningful participation in decisions concerning the placement of solid waste sites, factories, coal power plants, and other local sources of pollution. Air pollution control policies should promote public health and social justice without crippling the economy.

CONCLUSION

NANOTECHNOLOGY

Nanotechnology has important applications in manufacturing, industry, medicine, and cosmetics. However, nanomaterials pose risks to human health and the environment that are not well-understood at the present time. The PP offers a valuable perspective on managing the risks of nanotechnology. Steps should be taken to minimize, prevent, or mitigate the risks of nanotechnology, including research, regulation, and oversight. Current regulations pertaining to the safety of industrial chemicals may need to be strengthened to manage the risks of nanotechnology.

THE BUILT ENVIRONMENT

Sustainability development is a useful approach to resolving some of the conflicts between human interests (such as agriculture and housing) and the environment. Sustainable land policies permit enough development to meet human interests but also include environmental safeguards, such as laws that protect endangered species, habitats, and ecosystems. Property rights should be considered when making policy decisions, but they can be restricted to promote human health and protect habitats, ecosystems, and species. Occupational safety and housing standards are necessary to promote public health and social justice, but they should not be so stringent that they seriously impede industry or make housing unaffordable. Workplace safety standards should be realistic and reasonable. Housing standards should ensure that buildings are safe but also affordable. Urban sprawl is a significant public health environmental problem. Zoning laws and urban planning can be effective tools for combating sprawl and promoting sustainable development.

DISASTER PREPAREDNESS

Natural disasters (such as hurricanes and earthquakes) pose a serious threat to public health. Governments should take appropriate measures to prepare for and respond to natural disasters to promote public health. Natural disasters raise issues of social justice because they tend to have greater impacts on low-income populations and people living in developing nations.

CLIMATE CHANGE

Considerable evidence supports the hypothesis that anthropogenic sources of greenhouse gases play a key role in causing global warming. Unless effective action is taken to counteract global warming, temperatures will continue to increase, which will alter the climate and produce many adverse effects on human health and the environment.

There are many different strategies for mitigating climate change, such as increased energy efficiency and fuel economy; greater utilization of mass transit, telecommuting, and walking or biking; planting trees and other plants to remove carbon from the atmosphere; reduced use of fossil fuels; reduced meat eating; and population control. A cap and trade system for CO_2 emissions or a carbon tax may be necessary to achieve acceptable levels of greenhouse gases, if these other methods are not likely to work. Because economic development plays an essential role in overcoming poverty, famine, and disease, policies should be carefully designed to minimize economic impacts. The long-term goal of climate change policies should be to lead the world away from dependence on fossil fuels and toward greater reliance on sources of energy that are environmentally and socioeconomically sustainable.

Though geoengineering may one day become an important tool for mitigating climate change, a precautionary approach to this method is warranted, because geoengineering could have adverse environmental impacts that are not well-understood at this time. Scientists and engineers can study geoengineering and experiment with small-scale, low-impact projects. Large-scale, high-impact projects should not be implemented until there is adequate evidence concerning their risks and benefits. Plans to impede or reverse harmful effects of geoengineering would also need to be developed.

Because climate change is a global problem, international cooperation is essential. Treaties should be negotiated fairly and should not be tilted heavily toward particular parties or groups of nations. While developed nations should shoulder the largest burden of climate change mitigation, developing nations should also do their part. Developed nations should also make funds available to help developing nations adapt to climate change.

ENERGY

Energy production and consumption have a variety of impacts on human beings and the environment. Though energy use is vital to economic development, agriculture, industry, and many different human activities, it can also have adverse impacts on public health and the environment. Countries should move away from dependence on fossil fuels toward alternative, sustainable sources of energy that do less damage to the environment and human health. However, because this transition cannot occur quickly without considerable disruption to the economy, fossil fuels sources should continue to be developed in the interim period. Because all forms of energy involve some risks to human health or the environment, a responsible energy policy is one that carefully balances benefits and risks while providing enough energy to sustain the human population.

POPULATION

Increases in the human population have widespread impacts on a variety of environmental and public health concerns, including pollution, deforestation, urban development, energy use, water shortages, agriculture, and climate change. Countries should use noncoercive measures, such as educational campaigns, economic incentives, provision of contraception,

and empowerment of women to promote sustainable population levels. International organizations should also assist countries in controlling population growth.

ENVIRONMENTAL JUSTICE

Many different environmental issues have implications for social justice. To promote distributive justice, environmental health policy decisions should take into account how
different choices impact the overall good of society, as well as equality of opportunity, property rights, and the welfare of the least advantaged members of society. Special protections
should be extended to vulnerable subpopulations, such as children and diseased individuals,
within practical limits.

To promote procedural justice, citizens should have an equal right to participate in
environmental policy choices that affect them. Social decision making should include
mechanisms for meaningful public deliberation on controversial issues and inclusion of
disenfranchised groups. International treaties related to the environment should promote
cooperation and a fair sharing of benefits and risks among nations.

HUMAN PARTICIPANT RESEARCH

Environmental health research with human participants raises a number of challenging
issues and dilemmas. Environmental health researchers should comply with relevant laws,
regulations, and ethical guidelines.

Research results should be returned to individuals participating in environmental studies only if 1) the testing methods used to obtain the results are accurate and reliable; 2) the
investigators are planning to provide counseling or referrals; and 3) the results have definite practical or clinical significance, or the results do not have definite practical or clinical
significance but the participants want to know the results and they are able to deal with
complexity and uncertainty.

Studies that intentionally expose human participants to environmental agents (such as
air pollution or pesticides) are morally acceptable if they are scientifically rigorous, likely to
yield important knowledge related to public health that cannot be obtained from animal
experiments or human observational studies, and meet other ethical requirements, such as
informed consent and risk minimization.

Studies of environmental interventions must be well designed and expected to yield
results that can benefit public health. Investigators must do their best to minimize risks to
participants and maximize benefits. They should inform participants about strategies they
may implement to reduce their exposures to potentially harmful environmental agents and
share research results with participants that are reliable, accurate, and useful.

Community-based participatory research (CBPR) is a useful strategy for benefiting
communities, enhancing recruitment and study design, and building public support for
research. For CBPR to be ethical and effective, investigators should reach agreements with

community representatives (such as advisory boards) on key issues, such as the purposes of the research, the study design, publication plans, and the use of biological samples/data. Investigators should hold regular meetings with community representatives to keep them updated about important developments. Informed consent documents should clearly indicate how samples and data will be used, stored, protected, and shared, and should provide research participants with instructions on how to withdraw their samples if they decide to stop participating in the study.

While this book has covered many different ethical and policy issues related to environmental health, it has only scratched the surface of this vast subject. Some important topics may have been omitted, and others may not have been discussed in sufficient depth. My goal in this book has not been to write a definitive treatise on environmental health ethics, but to call attention to important issues, problems, dilemmas, concepts, and frameworks, so that others may build upon my ideas, arguments, discussions, and conclusions. I acknowledge that much more work remains to be done, and I encourage others to expand upon what has been accomplished herein. A great deal has been written about ethical and policy issues pertaining to healthcare and the environment, but comparatively little has been written that focuses specifically on ethical and policy issues pertaining to environmental health. Hopefully, other scholars, scientists, and policy makers will use what I have written to help advance research and public debate about environmental health ethics.

REFERENCES

2point6billion.com. 2010. 2point6billion.com, August 23, 2010. India offering cash incentives to control birthrates. Available at: http://www.2point6billion.com/news/2010/08/23/ india-offering-cash-incentives-to-control-birthrates-6816.html. Accessed: August 31, 2010.

Abdel-Rahman A, Dechkovskaia AM, Goldstein LB, Bullman SH, Khan W, El-Masry EM, and Abou-Donia MB. 2004. Neurological deficits induced by malathion, DEET, and permethrin, alone or in combination in adult rats. Journal of Toxicology and Environmental Health A 67: 331–56.

Abee H. 2008. The black plague: revenge of the cats? Cats.com, April 8, 2008. Available at: http://www.cats.com/article/cattales/folklore/the-black-plague-revenge-of-the-cats/. Accessed: March 26, 2010.

Abou-Donia MB, Dechkovskaia AM, Goldstein LB, Abdel-Rahman A, Bullman SL, and Khan WA. 2004. Co-exposure to pyridostigmine bromide, DEET, and/or permethrin causes sensorimotor deficit and alterations in brain acetylcholinesterase activity. Pharmacology, Biochemistry, and Behavior 77: 253–62.

Achenbach J and Eilperin J. 2011. Climate change science makes for hot politics. Washington Post, August 19, 2011: A1.

Adler R. 2010. Global warming raising the risk of mega-drought in America's west. Suite 101, June 26, 2010. Available at: http://americanaffairs.suite101.com/article.cfm/global-warming-raising-the-risk-of-mega-drought-in-americas-west. Accessed: July 17, 2010.

Agency for Toxic Substances and Disease Registry. 2002. Toxicological profile for DDT, DDE, and DDD. Available at: http://www.atsdr.cdc.gov/toxprofiles/tp35.html. Accessed: March 22, 2010.

  2009. Priority list of toxic substances. Available at: http://www.atsdr.cdc.gov/cercla/07list. html. Accessed: December 14, 2010.

  2007. Lead toxicity: Who is at risk of lead exposure? Available at: http://www.atsdr.cdc. gov/csem/lead/pbwhoisat_risk2.html. Accessed: November 11, 2010.

Aiello AE, King NB, and Foxman B. 2006. Ethical conflicts in public health research and practice: antimicrobial resistance and the ethics of drug development. American Journal of Public Health 96: 1910–14.

Al Aqee A. 2007. Islamic ethical framework for research into and prevention of genetic diseases. Nature Genetics 39: 1293–98.

Alavanja MC, Hoppin JA, and Kamel F. 2004. Health effects of chronic pesticide exposure: cancer and neurotoxicity. Annual Review of Public Health 25: 155–97.

Alexis NE, Lay JC, Haczku A, Gong H, Linn W, Hazucha MJ, Harris B, Tal-Singer R, and Peden DB. 2008. Fluticasone propionate protects against ozone-induced airway inflammation and modified immune cell activation markers in healthy volunteers. Environmental Health Perspectives 116: 799–805.

Allen J. 2008. Vatican issues new document on biotechnology. National Catholic Reporter, December 12, 2008. Available at: http://ncronline.org/blogs/all-things-catholic/ vatican-issues-new-document-biotechnology. Accessed: March 1, 2011.

Allhoff F, Lin P, and Moore D. 2010. What Is Nanotechnology and Why Does It Matter? New York: Wiley-Blackwell.

Altman RG, Morello-Frosch R, Brody JG, Rudel R, Brown P, and Averick M. 2008. Pollution comes home and gets personal: women's experience of household chemical exposure. Journal of Health and Social Behavior 49: 417–35.

American Diabetes Association. 2010. Genetics of Diabetes. Available at: http://www. diabetes.org/diabetes-basics/genetics-of-diabetes.html. Accessed: March 26, 2010.

American Dietetic Association and Dieticians of Canada. 2003. Position of the American Dietetic Association and Dieticians of Canada: vegetarian diets. Journal of the American Dietetic Association 103: 748–65.

American Lung Association vs. EPA. 134 F.3d 388 (D.C. Cir. 1998).

Archibold RC. Cholera deaths up in Haiti, worse to come. The New York Times, November 14, 2010: A4.

Arias E. 2010. United States life tables by Hispanic origin. National Center for Health Statistics, Vital Health Statistics 2, 152. Available at: http://www.cdc.gov/nchs/data/ series/sr_02/sr02_152.pdf. Accessed: October 20, 2010.

Aristotle. 2003. Nichomachean Ethics. Tredennick H (ed.), Thomson JA (transl.). New York: Penguin Books.

Aruoma OI. 1998. Free radicals, oxidative stress, and antioxidants in human health and disease. Journal of the American Oil Chemists' Society 75: 199–212.

Asbestos.com. 2010. Asbestos exposure in jobsites & occupations. Available at: http://www. asbestos.com/exposure/. Accessed: April 6, 2010.

Attfield R. 2003. Environmental Ethics. Cambridge: Polity Press.

Audi R. 2004. The Good in the Right. Princeton, NJ: Princeton University Press.

Augustin L, Barbante C, Barnes PR, Barnola JM, Bigler M, Castellano E, Cattani O, Chappellaz J, Dahl-Jensen D, Delmonte B, Dreyfus G, Durand G, Falourd S, Fischer H, Flückiger J, Hansson ME, Huybrechts P, Jugie G, Johnsen SJ, Jouzel J, Kaufmann P, Kipfstuhl J, Lambert F, Lipenkov VY, Littot GC, Longinelli A, Lorrain R, Maggi V, Masson-Delmotte V, Miller H, Mulvaney R, Oerlemans J, Oerter H, Orombelli G, Parrenin F, Peel DA, Petit JR, Raynaud D, Ritz C, Ruth U, Schwander J, Siegenthaler

U, Souchez R, Stauffer B, Steffensen JP, Stenni B, Stocker TF, Tabacco IE, Udisti R, Van De Wal RS, Van Den Broeke M, Weiss J, Wilhelms F, Winther JG, Wolff EW, Zucchelli M, and EPICA community members. 2004. Eight glacial cycles from an Antarctic ice core. Nature 429: 623–28.

AVERT. 2009. History and science of HIV & AIDS. Available at: http://www.avert.org/history-science.htm. Accessed: April 7, 2010.

——. 2010. HIV and AIDS in Africa. Available at: http://www.avert.org/hiv-aids-africa.htm. Accessed: October 19, 2010.

Ayer AJ. 1946. Language, Truth, and Logic, 2nd ed. New York: Dover Books.

Baer P, Athanasiou T, Kartha S, and Kemp-Benedict E. 2008. The greenhouse development rights framework. Berlin: Heinrich Böll Foundation. Available at: http://www.ecoequity.org/docs/TheGDRsFramework.pdf. Accessed: November 15, 2010.

Baier A. 1984. For the sake of future generations. In: Regan T (ed.). Earthbound: New Introductory Essays in Environmental Ethics. New York: Random House: 214–46.

Bailar JC. 1997. The promise and problems of meta-analysis. N Engl J Med 337: 559–61.

Baker P. 2010. White House is lifting ban on deep-water drilling. New York Times, October 12, 2010: A1.

Bale JS, van Lenteren JC, and Bigler F. 2008. Biological control and sustainable food production. Philosophical Transactions of the Royal Society of London B: Biological Science 363: 761–76.

Ban Terminator. 2007. Ban terminator. Available at: http://www.banterminator.org/. Accessed: August 31, 2010.

Barboza D. 2000. Suburban genetics: scientists searching for the perfect lawn. The New York Times, July 8, 2000: A1.

Barcalow E. 1994. Moral Philosophy: Theory and Issues. Belmont, CA: Wadsworth.

Barinaga M. 2000. Asilomar revisited: lessons for today? Science 287: 1584–85.

Barr DA. 2008. Health Disparities in the United States. Baltimore, MD: Johns Hopkins University Press.

Barrionuevo A and Robbins L 2010. 1.5 million displaced after Chilean quake. The New York Times, February 28, 2010: A1.

Barry B. 1991. Theories of Justice, Volume One. Berkeley: University of California Press.

Barsky RB and Kilian L. 2004. Oil and the macroeconomy since the 1970s. Journal of Economic Perspective 18: 115–34.

Basel Convention. 2010. About the convention. Available at: http://www.basel.int/index.html. Accessed: July 23, 2010.

Batista R and Oliviera MM. 2009. Facts and fiction of genetically engineered food. Trends in Biotechnology 27: 277–86.

BBC News. 2006. The EU's baby blues. BBC News, March 27, 2006. Available at: http://news.bbc.co.uk/2/hi/europe/4768644.stm. Accessed: August 31, 2010.

Beauchamp T and Childress J. 2008. Principles of Biomedical Ethics, 6th ed. New York: Oxford University Press.

Beckoff M. 2002. Minding Animals: Awareness, Emotions, and Heart. New York: Oxford University Press.

Beecher HK. 1966. Ethics and clinical research. New England Journal of Medicine 274: 1354–60.

Beehler GP, Baker JA, Falkner K, Chegerova T, Pryshchepava A, Chegerov V, Zevon M, Bromet E, Havenaar J, Valdismarsdottir H, and Moysich KB. 2008. A multilevel analysis of long-term psychological distress among Belarusians affected by the Chernobyl disaster. Public Health 122: 1239–49.

Beitz C. 1999. Political Theory and International Relations, 2nd ed. Princeton, NJ: Princeton University Press.

Bell ML and Davis DL. 2001. Reassessment of the lethal London fog of 1952: novel indicators of acute and chronic consequences of acute exposures to air pollution. Environmental Health Perspectives 19, Suppl. 3: 389–94.

Bell ML and Samet JM. 2010. Air pollution. In: Frumkin H (ed.). Environmental Health: From Global to Local, 2nd ed. New York: John Wiley and Sons: 387–415.

Belluck P. 2010. Obesity rates hit plateau in U.S., data suggest. The New York Times, January 14, 2010: A20.

Benedict R. 1934. Patterns of Culture. Boston: Houghton-Mifflin.

Bentley WJ. 2009. The integrated control concept and its relevance to current integrated pest management in California fresh market grapes. Pest Management Science 12:1298–304.

Berenbaum, M. 2005. If malaria's the problem, DDT's not the only answer. Washington Post, June 5, 2005: B3.

Berg P, Baltimore D, Brenner S, Roblin III RO, and Singer MF. 1975. Summary statement of the Asilomar Conference on Recombinant DNA Molecules. Proceedings of the National Academy of Sciences 72: 1981–84.

Beyond Pesticides. 2010. What is beyond pesticides? Available at: http://www.beyondpesticides.org/about/mission.htm. Accessed: March 23, 2010.

Bill and Melinda Gates Foundation. 2010. Our approach: Malaria. Available at: http://www.gatesfoundation.org/topics/Pages/malaria.aspx. Accessed: May 21, 2010.

Biotechnology Industry Organization. Economic sustainability. Available at: http://www.valueofbiotech.com/employ/economic-sustainability. Accessed: March 9, 2011.

Black CG. 2005. Subsidizing disaster. National Center for Policy Analysis, Brief Analysis 525, September 7, 2005. Available at: http://www.ncpa.org/pdfs/ba525.pdf. Accessed: August 23, 2010.

Blackorby C, Bossert W, and Davidson D. 1995. Intertemporal population ethics: critical-level utilitarian principles. Econometrica 63: 1303–20.

Blaser M. 2011. Antibiotic overuse: stop killing the beneficial bacteria. Nature 476: 393–94.

Bloom DE and Canning D. 2000. The health and wealth of nations. Science 287: 1207–09.

Blumenthal I. 2001. Carbon monoxide poisoning. Journal of the Royal Society of Medicine 94: 270–72.

Bonan GB. 2008. Forest and climate change: forcings, feedbacks, and the climate benefits of forests. Science 320: 1444–49.

Boone CK. 1988. Bad axioms in genetic engineering. Hastings Center Report 18, 4: 9–13.

Boorse C. 1977. Health as a theoretical concept. Philosophy of Science 44: 542–73.

2004. On the distinction between disease and illness. In: Caplan AL, McCartney JJ, and Sisti DA (eds.). Health, Disease, and Illness. Washington, DC: Georgetown University Press: 77–90.

Borlaug N. 2002. Biotechnology and the green revolution. ActionBioscience interview. Available at: http://www.actionbioscience.org/biotech/borlaug.html. Accessed: May 23, 2010.

Borlaug NE. 2000. Ending world hunger. The promise of biotechnology and the threat of antiscience zealotry. Plant Physiology 124: 487–90.

Boschi-Pinto C, Velebit L, and Shibuya K. 2008. Estimating child mortality due to diarrhea in developing countries. Bulletin of the World Health Organization 86: 657–736.

Bouchard MF, Chevrier J, Harley KG, Kogut K, Vedar M, Calderon N, Trujillo C, Johnson C, Bradman A, Barr DB, and Eskenazi B. 2011. Prenatal exposure to organophosphate pesticides and IQ in 7-year old children. Environmental Health Perspectives 119: 1189–95.

Bourdés V, Boffetta P, and Pisani P. 2000. Environmental exposure to asbestos and risk of pleural mesothelioma: review and meta-analysis. European Journal of Epidemiology 16: 411–17.

Bovenkerk B, Brom FW, and van den Bergh BJ. 2002. Brave new birds: the use of 'animal integrity' in ethics. Hastings Center Report 32, 1: 16–22.

Braatne JH, Rood SB, Goater LA, Blair and CL. 2008. Analyzing the impacts of dams on riparian ecosystems: a review of research strategies and their relevance to the Snake River through Hells Canyon. Environmental Management 41: 267–81.

Brand S. 2009. Whole Earth Discipline: An Ecopragmatist Manifesto. New York: Viking.

Brandt R. 1998. A Theory of the Good and the Right, revised ed. New York: Prometheus Books.

Bread for the World. 2010. Global Hunger. Available at: http://www.bread.org/hunger/global/. Accessed: May 23, 2010.

Brennan A. 2008. Environmental ethics. Stanford Encyclopedia of Philosophy. Available at: http://plato.stanford.edu/entries/ethics-environmental/. Accessed: April 21, 2010.

Broder JM. 2009. E.P.A. clears way for greenhouse gas rules. New York Times, April 17, 2009: A1.

2010a. Obama to open offshore areas to oil drilling for the first time. New York Times, March 31, 2010: A1.

2010b. U.S. and China narrow differences at climate talks in Cancún. The New York Times, December 8, 2010: A1.

Broder JM and Krauss C. 2010a. Risk is clear in drilling; payoff isn't. New York Times, March 31, 2010: B1.

2010b. U.S halts plan to drill in Eastern Gulf. New York Times, December 1, 2010: A1.

Brody JG, Morello-Frosch R, Brown P, Rudel RA, Altman RG, Frye M, Osimo CA, Pérez C, and Seryak LM. 2007. "Is it safe?": new ethics for reporting personal exposures to environmental chemicals. American Journal of Public Health 97: 1547–54.

Bromenshenk JJ, Henderson CB, Wick CH, Stanford MF, and Zulich AW. 2010 Iridovirus and Microsporidian linked to honey bee colony decline. PLoS ONE 5, 10: e13181.

Brookes G. and Barfoot P. 2006. GM crops: The first ten years – global socio-economic and environmental impacts. International Service for the Acquisition of Agri-Biotech Applications, Brief No. 36. Ithaca, NY: International Service for the Acquisition of Agri-biotech Applications. Available at: http://www.isaaa.org/resources/publications/briefs/36/download/isaaa-brief-36–2006.pdf. Accessed: August 29, 2011.

Broughton E. 2005. The Bhopal disaster and its aftermath: a review. Environmental Health 4: 6.

Brown L. 2006. Starving for fuel: how ethanol production contributes to global hunger. The Globalist, August 2, 2006. Available at: http://www.theglobalist.com/storyid.aspx?StoryId=5518. Accessed: May 23, 2010.

Brown LP. 2008. Bakes sales fall victim to push for healthier foods. The New York Times, November 10, 2008: A1.

Buchanan D and Miller F. 2006. Justice and fairness in the Kennedy Krieger Institute lead paint study: the ethics of public health research on less expensive, less effective interventions. American Journal of Public Health 96: 781–87.

Buehr M and Hjorth JP. 2003. Genetically modified laboratory animals – what welfare problems do they face? Journal of Applied Animal Welfare Science 6: 319–38.

Bullard RD. 1994. Dumping in Dixie: Race, Class, and Environmental Quality, 2nd ed. Boulder, CO: Westview Press.

Burney JA, Davis SJ, and Lobell DB. 2010. Greenhouse gas mitigation by agricultural intensification. Proceedings of the National Academy of Science 107: 12052–57.

Buss D. 2004. Evolutionary Psychology: The New Science of the Mind. Boston: Pearson.

Butler D and Reichhardt T. 1999. Long-term effects of GM crops serves up food for thought. Nature 398: 651–56.

Butler RA. 2010. Deforestation in the Amazon. Mongabay.com. Available at: http://www.mongabay.com/brazil.html. Accessed: August 30, 2011.

Butti L. 2009. Hazardous waste management and the precautionary principle. Waste Management 29: 2415–16.

Buyx A and Tait J. 2011. Ethical framework for biofuels. Science 332: 540–41.

Bywater RJ. 2005. Identification and surveillance of antimicrobial resistance dissemination in animal production. Poultry Science 84: 644–48.

Caldwell LK and Shrader-Frechette KS. 1993. Policy for Land: Land and Ethics. Lanham, MD: Rowman and Littlefield.

Callahan D. 2000. Freedom, healthism, and health promotion: finding the right balance. In: Callahan D (ed.). Promoting Healthy Behavior. Washington, DC: Georgetown University Press: 138–52.

Callicott J. 1980. Animal liberation: a triangular affair. Environmental Ethics 2: 311–38.

   1989. In Defense of the Land Ethic. Albany, NY: State University of New York Press.

Campbell P. 2011. NSF clears Michael Mann of misconduct. Science 2.0, August 22, 2011. Available at: http://www.science20.com/cool-links/nsf_clears_michael_mann_misconduct-81904. Accessed: August 23, 2011.

Caplan AL. 1997. The concepts of health, disease, and illness. In: Veatch RM (ed.). Medical Ethics, 2nd ed. Boston: Jones and Bartlett: 57–74.

Carson R. 1962. Silent Spring. New York: Houghton Mifflin.

Catholic Answers. 2008. Birth Control. Available at: http://www.catholic.com/library/Birth_Control.asp. Accessed: August 30, 2010.

Cendrowicz L. 2010. Is Europe finally ready for genetically modified foods? Time/CNN, March 9, 2010. Available at: http://www.time.com/time/business/article/0,8599,1970471,00.html. Accessed: June 5, 2010.

Center for Food Safety. 2006a. Genetically Engineered Crops and Foods: Worldwide Regulation and Prohibition. Available at: http://www.centerforfoodsafety.org/pubs/World_Regs_Chart%20_6–2006.pdf. Accessed: June 6, 2010.

   2006b. Genetically engineered crops and foods: Regional regulation and prohibition. Available at: http://www.centerforfoodsafety.org/pubs/Regional_Regs_Chart_6–2006.pdf. Accessed: June 6, 2010.

Center for Science and the Public Interest. 2009. Banned food additives. Available at: http://www.cspinet.org/reports/chemcuisine.htm#banned_additives. Accessed: June 24, 2010.

Centers for Disease Control and Prevention. 2005. Campaign to prevent antimicrobial resistance. Available at: http://www.cdc.gov/drugresistance/healthcare/default.htm. Accessed: May 20, 2010.

   2007. Malaria. Available at: http://www.cdc.gov/malaria/ Accessed: March 23, 2010.

   2008a. Patient facts: Learn more about Legionnaire's Disease. Available at: http://www.cdc.gov/legionella/patient_facts.htm. Accessed: April 6, 2010.

   2008b. River blindness. Available at: http://www.cdc.gov/ncidod/dpd/parasites/onchocerciasis/factsht_onchocerciasis.htm. Accessed: July 17, 2010.

   2009a. Antibiotic/antimicrobial resistance. Available at: http://www.cdc.gov/drugresistance/index.htm. Accessed: May 18, 2010.

   2009b. Differences in prevalence of obesity among black, white, and Hispanic adults: United States, 2006–2008. Available at: http://www.cdc.gov/mmwr/preview/mmwrhtml/mm5827a2.htm. Accessed: October 20, 2010.

   2010. Tuberculosis. Available at: http://www.cdc.gov/tb/statistics/default.htm. Accessed: May 18, 2010.

2011. Dengue. Available at: http://www.cdc.gov/dengue/. Accessed: February 21, 2011.

Centers for Medicare and Medicaid Services. 2010. Clinical laboratory improvement amendments. Available at: https://www.cms.gov/clia/. Accessed: November 17, 2010.

Central Intelligence Agency. 2010. World Fact Book. Available at: https://www.cia.gov/library/publications/the-world-factbook/index.html. Accessed: October 20, 2010.

Chan AW and Yang SH. 2009. Generation of transgenic monkeys with human inherited genetic disease. Methods 49: 78–84.

Chapman HA, Kim DA, Susskind JM, and Anderson AK. 2009. In bad taste: evidence of the oral origins of moral disgust. Science 323: 1222–26.

Chaufan C, Hong GH, and Fox P. 2009. Taxing "sin foods" – obesity prevention and public health policy. New England Journal of Medicine 361: e113.

Childress JE, Faden RR, Gaare RD, Gostin LO, Kahn J, Bonnie RJ, Kass NE, Mastroianni AC, Moreno JD, and Nie P. 2002. Public health ethics: mapping the terrain. Journal of Law, Medicine, and Ethics 30: 170–78.

Chipman A. 2010. Fears over Europe's GM crop plan. Nature 466: 542–43.

Clapp JG. 1967. Locke, John. In: Edwards P (ed.). Encyclopedia of Philosophy, Volumes 3 and 4. New York: MacMillan: 487–503.

Clarke S and Simpson E (eds.). 1989. Anti-Theory in Ethics and Moral Conservatism. Albany, NY: State University of New York Press.

Clean Air Act. 1963 [1970, 1990]. 42 U.S.C. 7401.

Cochrane A. 2007. Environmental ethics. The Internet Encyclopedia of Philosophy. Available at: http://www.iep.utm.edu/e/envi-eth.htm. Accessed: April 21, 2010.

Cohen J. 1995. How Many People Can the Earth Support? New York: Norton.

2009. Philosophy, Politics and Democracy. Cambridge, MA: Harvard University Press.

Cole-Turner R. 1997. Genes, religion and society: the developing views of the churches. Science and Engineering Ethics 3: 273–88.

Committee on Defining Science-Based Concerns Associated with Products of Animal Biotechnology. 2002. Animal Biotechnology: Science Based Concerns. Washington, DC: National Academy Press.

Committee on the Future Role of Pesticides in U.S. Agriculture. 2000. The Future Role of Pesticides in US Agriculture. Washington, DC: National Academy Press.

Confucius. 1955. The Sayings of Confucius. Ware JR (transl.). New American Library: New York.

Congressional Budget Office. 2009. The economic effects of legislation to reduce greenhouse-gas emissions. Available at: http://www.cbo.gov/ftpdocs/105xx/doc10573/09-17--Greenhouse-Gas.pdf. Accessed: July 7, 2010.

Conner AJ, Glare TR, and Nap JP. 2003. The release of genetically modified crops into the environment. Part II. Overview of ecological risk assessment. Plant Journal 33: 19–46.

Conner AJ and Jacobs JM. 1999. Genetic engineering of crops as potential source of genetic hazard in the human diet. Mutation Research/Genetic Toxicology and Environmental Mutagenesis 443: 223–34.

Consumer Products Safety Commission. 2010. Carbon monoxide questions and answers. Available at: http://www.cpsc.gov/cpscpub/pubs/466.html. Accessed: April 8, 2010.

Cooper JM and Hutchinson DS (eds.). 1997. Plato: Complete Works. Indianapolis: Hackett.

Council for International Organizations of Medical Science. 2002. International ethical guidelines for biomedical research involving human subjects. Available at: http://www.cioms.ch/publications/layout_guide2002.pdf. Accessed: November 17, 2010.

Cranor C. 2008. (Almost) equal protection for genetically susceptible subpopulations: a hybrid regulatory compensation model. In: Sharp RR, Marchant GE, and Grodsky JA (eds.). Genomics and Environmental Regulation. Baltimore, MD: Johns Hopkins University Press: 267–89.

2011. Legally Poisoned: How the Law Puts Us at Risk from Toxicants. Cambridge, MA: Harvard University Press.

Crichton M. 2002. Prey. New York: Harper Collins.

Croplife America. 2010. Integrated pest management. Available at: http://www.croplife america.org/pesticide-issues/integrated-pest-management. Accessed: March 23, 2010.

Croplife America v. EPA (329 F.3d 876, U.S. Fed. Ct. App. Dist. Columbia, 2003).

Crutzen P. 2006. Albedo enhancement by stratospheric sulfur injections: a contribution to resolve a policy dilemma? Climate Change 77: 211–20.

Czech B. 2008. Prospects for reconciling the conflict between economic growth and biodiversity conservation with technological progress. Conservation Biology 22: 1389–98.

Czech B and Krausman PR. 2001. The Endangered Species Act: History, Conservation Biology, and Public Policy. Baltimore, MD: Johns Hopkins University Press.

Dale BJ, Clarke B, and Fontes EM. 2002. Potential for the environmental impact of transgenic crops. Nature Biotechnology 20: 567–74.

Daniels N. 1984. Just Health Care. Cambridge: Cambridge University Press.

2008. Just Health: Meeting Health Needs Fairly. Cambridge: Cambridge University Press.

Dare T. 2009. Parental rights and medical decisions. Paediatric Anaesthiology 10: 947–52.

Darwin C. 1859 [2003]. On the Origin of Species by Means of Natural Selection. New York: Signet Classics.

Davies JC. 2006. Managing the Effects of Nanotechnology. Washington, DC: Woodrow Wilson International Center.

Davila JC, Cezar GG, Thiede M, Strom S, Miki T, and Trosko J. 2004. Use and application of stem cells in toxicology. Toxicological Sciences 79: 214–23.

Davis JM. 1999. Inhalation health risks of manganese: an EPA perspective. Neurotoxicology. 20: 511–18.

Decaprio A. 1997. Biomarkers: coming of age in environmental health risk assessment. Environmental Science and Toxicology 31: 1837–48.

DeGeorge R. 2005. Business Ethics, 6th ed. Upper Saddle River, NJ: Prentice-Hall.

DeLeo F and Chambers H. 2009. Reemergence of antibiotic-resistant *Staphylococcus aureus* in the genomics era. Journal of Clinical Investigation 119: 2464–74.

de Melo-Martín I and Meghani Z. 2008. Beyond risk. A more realistic risk-benefit analysis of agricultural biotechnologies. EMBO Reports 9: 302–6.

Deng FD and Huang Y. 2004. Uneven land reform and urban sprawl in China: the case of Beijing. Progress in Planning 61: 211–36.

Department of Health and Human Services. 2009. Protection of Human Subjects. 45 CFR 46. Available at: http://www.hhs.gov/ohrp/humansubjects/guidance/45cfr46.htm. Accessed: November 16, 2010.

——— 2010. Health information privacy. Available at: http://www.hhs.gov/ocr/privacy/hipaa/administrative/privacyrule/index.html. Accessed: November 19, 2010.

Des Jardins J. 2005. Environmental Ethics, 5th ed. Belmont, CA: Wadsworth.

Dessler A and Parson E. 2006. The Science and Politics of Global Climate Change. Cambridge: Cambridge University Press.

de Waal F. 2009. Primates and Philosophers: How Morality Evolved. Princeton, NJ: Princeton University Press.

Diamanti-Kandarakis E, Bourguignon JP, Giudice LC, Hauser R, Prins GS, Soto AM, Zoeller RT, and Gore AC. 2009. Endocrine-disrupting chemicals: an Endocrine Society scientific statement. Endocrinology Review 30: 293–342.

Dibner JJ and Richards JD. 2005. Antibiotic growth promoters in agriculture: history and mode of action. Poultry Science 84: 634–43.

Dickert N and Sugarman J. 2005. Ethical goals of community consultation in research. American Journal of Public Health 95: 1123–27.

Diffey BL. 2009. Sunscreens as a preventative measure in melanoma: an evidence-based approach or the precautionary principle? British Journal of Dermatology 161, Supplement 3: 25–27.

Doney SC. 2010. The growing human footprint on coastal and open-ocean biogeochemistry. Science 328: 1512–16.

Dowling R. 2010. What social equity means. The Chapel Hill News, November 21, 2010: B1.

Dvir Y and Smallwood P. 2008. Serotonin syndrome: a complex but easily avoidable condition. General Hospital Psychiatry 30: 284–87.

Ehrlich AH and Ehrlich PR. 1990. The Population Explosion. New York: Simon and Schuster.

Eilperin J. 2011a. U.N. climate talks' real world outcome will be determined by Asia. The Washington Post, December 11, 2011: A1.

Eilperin J. 2011b. A great plains pipeline debate. Washington Post, January 24, 2011: A1.

Ekser B, Rigotti P, Gridelli B, and Cooper DK. 2009. Xenotransplantation of solid organs in the pig-to-primate model. Transplantation Immunology 21: 87–92.

Elbaz A, Clavel J, Rathouz PJ, Moisan F, Galanaud JP, Delemotte B, Alpérovitch A, and Tzourio C. 2009. Professional exposure to pesticides and Parkinson disease. Annals of Neurology 66: 494–504.

Elliott KC. 2010. Geoengineering and the precautionary principle. International Journal of Applied Philosophy 24: 237–53.

2011. Is A Little Pollution Good for You? Incorporating Societal Values in Environmental Research. New York: Oxford University Press.

Emanuel EJ, Grady C, Crouch RA, Lie R, Miller F, and Wendler D (eds.). 2008. The Oxford Textbook of Clinical Research Ethics. New York: Oxford University Press.

Emanuel EJ and Miller F. 2001. The ethics of placebo-controlled trials: a middle ground. New England Journal of Medicine 345: 915–19.

Energy Information Administration. 2010. Electric Power Monthly, September 2010. Available at: http://www.eia.doe.gov/cneaf/electricity/epm/epm_sum.html. Accessed: October 10, 2010.

Engberg J, Aarestrup FM, Taylor DE, Gerner-Smidt P, and Nachamkin I. 2001. Quinolone and macrolide resistance in Campylobacter jejuni and C. coli: resistance mechanisms and trends in human isolates. Emerging Infectious Disease 7: 24–34.

Engelder T. 2011. Fracking: too valuable. Nature 477: 274–75.

Enserink M. 2011. GM mosquito trial alarms opponents, strains ties in Gates-funded project. Science 330: 1030–31.

2011. Transgenic chickens could thwart bird flu, curb pandemic risk. Science 331: 131–32.

Environmental Defense Fund. 2011. How cap and trade works. Available at: http://www.edf.org/climate/how-cap-and-trade-works. Accessed: August 22, 2011.

Environmental Protection Agency. 1998. R.E.D. Facts – DEET. Available at: http://www.epa.gov/oppsrrd1/REDs/factsheets/0002fact.pdf. Accessed: May 13, 2010.

2002. Children are at greater risks for pesticide exposure. Available at: http://www.epa.gov/opp00001/factsheets/kidpesticide.htm. Accessed: November 11, 2010.

2006. Arsenic in drinking water. Available at: http://www.epa.gov/safewater/arsenic/index.html. Accessed: April 8, 2010.

2007. Air pollution and health risk. Available at: http://www.epa.gov/ttn/atw/3_90_022.html. Accessed: July 5, 2010.

2008. Recognition and management of pesticide poisonings. Available at: http://www.epa.gov/opp00001/safety/healthcare/handbook/handbook.htm. Accessed: May 13, 2010.

2009a. Pesticides: Health and safety. Available at: http://www.epa.gov/pesticides/health/index.htm. Accessed: March 23, 2010.

2009b. Importing and exporting hazardous waste. Available at: http://www.epa.gov/oecaerth/monitoring/programs/rcra/importexport.html. Accessed: July 23, 2010.

2009c. Nanotechnology: An EPA perspective factsheet. Available at: http://www.epa.gov/ncer/nano/factsheet/. Accessed: July 29, 2010.

2010a. What is a pesticide? Available at: http://www.epa.gov/pesticides/about/index.htm. Accessed: March 24, 2010.

2010b. Ozone depletion. Available at: http://www.epa.gov/ozone/strathome.html. Accessed: March 26, 2010.

2010c. Mandatory reporting of greenhouse gases rule. Available at: http://www.epa.gov/climatechange/emissions/ghgrulemaking.html. Accessed: March 27, 2010.

2010d. Federal Insecticide, Fungicide, and Rodenticide Act (FIFRA). Available at: http://www.epa.gov/oecaagct/lfra.html. Accessed: May 13, 2010.

2010e. Human-related sources and sinks of carbon dioxide. Available at: http://www.epa.gov/climatechange/emissions/co2_human.html. Accessed: August 23, 2010.

2010f. Clean Air Act. Available at: http://www.epa.gov/air/caa/. Accessed: July 7, 2010.

2010g. Safe Drinking Water Act. Available at: http://www.epa.gov/safewater/sdwa/. Accessed: July 17, 2010.

2010h. Environmental justice. Available at: http://www.epa.gov/compliance/environmentaljustice/. Accessed: October 11, 2010.

2010i. The Food Quality Protection Act (FQPA): Background. Available at: http://www.epa.gov/opp00001/regulating/laws/fqpa/backgrnd.htm. Accessed: November 11, 2010.

2010j. Pesticide issues in the works: Honeybee colony collapse disorder. Available at: http://www.epa.gov/pesticides/about/intheworks/honeybee.htm. Accessed: November 12, 2010.

2010k. About the national exposure research laboratory. Available at: http://www.epa.gov/aboutepa/nerl.html, Accessed: November 20, 2010.

2010l. Expanded Protections for Subjects in Human Studies Research. Available at: http://www.epa.gov/oppfead1/guidance/human-test.htm. Accessed: November 23, 2010.

2011a. About EPA. Available at: http://www.epa.gov/aboutepa/. Accessed: August 1, 2011.

2011b. Air quality trends. Available at: http://www.epa.gov/airtrends/aqtrends.html. Accessed: August 31, 2011.

Environmental Working Group. 1998. The English patients: Human experiments and pesticide policy. Available at: http://www.ewg.org/reports/english. Accessed: November 23, 2010.

Epstein R. 2001. Genetic engineering: a Buddhist assessment. Religion East and West, Issue 1, June 2001: 39–47. Available at: http://online.sfsu.edu/~rone/GEessays/GEBuddhism.html. Accessed: March 1, 2011.

European Environment Agency. 2006. Urban sprawl in Europe: The ignored challenge. Available at: http://www.eea.europa.eu/publications/eea_report_2006_10/eea_report_10_2006.pdf. Accessed: August 23, 2010.

Ewing R, Pendall R, Chen D. 2002. Measuring sprawl and its impact. Smart Growth America. Available at: http://www.smartgrowthamerica.org/sprawlindex/chart.pdf. Accessed: July 24, 2009.

Exxon Valdez Oil Spill Trustee Council. 2010. Oil spill facts. Available at: http://www.evostc.state.ak.us/facts/index.cfm. Accessed: September 7, 2010.

Falk MC, Chassy BM, Harlander SK, Hoban TJ 4th, McGloughlin MN, and Akhlaghi AR. 2002. Food biotechnology: benefits and concerns. Journal of Nutrition 132: 1384–90.

Federal Emergency Management Administration. 2010. Available at: http://www.fema.gov/index.shtm. Accessed: November 7, 2010.

Federal Mine Safety and Health Act. 1977. Public Law 91–173. Available at: http://www.msha.gov/REGS/ACT/ACTTC.HTM. Accessed: August 19, 2010.

Fent K, Weston AA, and Caminada D. 2006. Ecotoxicology of human pharmaceuticals. Aquatic Toxicology 76:122–59.

Ferguson LR. 2010. Meat and cancer. Meat Science 84: 308–13.

Ffrench-Constant RH. 2007. Which came first: insecticides or resistance? Trends in Genetics 23: 1–4.

Fiester A. 2005. Ethical issues in animal cloning. Perspectives in Biology and Medicine 48: 328–43.

Finkelman FD. 2010. Peanut allergy and anaphylaxis. Current Opinion in Immunology 22: 783–88.

Fiscella K and Williams DR. 2004. Health disparities based on socioeconomic inequities: implications for urban health care. Academic Medicine 79: 1139–47.

Fishkin J and Laslett P. 2003. Debating Deliberative Democracy. Somerset, NJ: Wiley-Blackwell.

Fitzpatrick L. 2009. A brief history of China's One-Child Policy. Time Magazine, July 27, 2009. Available at: http://www.time.com/time/world/article/0,8599,1912861,00.html. Accessed: August 31, 2010.

Food and Agriculture Organization of the United Nations. 2005. Major food and agricultural commodities producers. Available at: http://www.fao.org/es/ess/top/country.html?lang=en. Accessed: May 25, 2010.

2006. Livestock's long shadow. Available at: http://www.fao.org/docrep/010/a0701e/a0701e00.HTM. Accessed: June 20, 2010.

2007. Organic agriculture can contribute to fighting hunger. Available at: http://www.fao.org/newsroom/en/news/2007/1000726/index.html. Accessed: May 24, 2010.

2010. The Food Safety Risk Assessment of GM Animals. Available at: ftp://ftp.fao.org/es/esn/food/GMtopic4.pdf. Accessed: June 15, 2010.

Food and Drug Administration. 1999. Genetically engineered foods. Statement of James H. Maryanski before the Subcommittee on Basic Research, House Committee on Science, October 19, 1999. Available at: http://www.fda.gov/NewsEvents/Testimony/ucm115032.htm. Accessed: June 7, 2010.

2009. FDA releases final guidance on genetically engineered animals. Available at: http://www.fda.gov/ForConsumers/ConsumerUpdates/ucm092738.htm. Accessed: June 15, 2010.

2010a. Food ingredients and colors. Available at: http://www.fda.gov/Food/FoodIngredientsPackaging/ucm094211.htm. Accessed: June 25, 2010.

2010b. Information sheet: Guidance for Institutional Review Boards (IRBs), clinical investigators, and sponsors. Available at: http://www.fda.gov/ScienceResearch/

REFERENCES

SpecialTopics/RunningClinicalTrials/GuidancesInformationSheetsandNotices/ucm 113709.htm. Accessed: November 17, 2010.

Food First. 2000. Lessons from the green revolution. Available at: http://www.foodfirst.org/media/opeds/2000/4-greenrev.html. Accessed: May 23, 2010.

FoodSafety.gov. 2010. Food poisoning. Available at: http://www.foodsafety.gov/poisoning/index.html. Accessed: June 21, 2010.

Foot F. 1978. Virtues and Vice. Oxford: Blackwell.

Ford T. 2010. Water and health. In: Frumkin H (ed.). Environmental Health: From Global to Local, 2nd ed. New York: John Wiley and Sons: 487–555.

Fortin N. 2009. Food Regulation. New York: Wiley.

Fowler L. 2004. Complexity of factors involved in human population growth. Environmental Health Perspectives 112: A726-A727.

Fox M. 1986. The Case for Animal Experimentation. Berkeley: University of California Press.

Fox RM and DeMarco JP. 2000. Moral Reasoning: A Philosophical Approach to Applied Ethics, 2nd ed. New York: Harcourt Brace.

Framingham Heart Study. 2010. About the Framingham heart study. Available at: http://www.framinghamheartstudy.org/about/index.html. Accessed: April 4, 2010.

Frankena W. 1988. Ethics, 2nd ed. Upper Saddle River, NJ: Prentice Hall.

Freedman B. 1987 Equipoise and the ethics of clinical research. New England Journal of Medicine 317: 141–45.

Freudenberg WR, Gramling R, Laska S, and Erikson KT. 2009. Catastrophe in the Making: The Engineering of Katrina and the Disasters of Tomorrow. Washington, DC: Island Press.

Fried C. 1974. Medical Experimentation: Personal Integrity and Social Policy. New York: Elsevier Publishing.

Friedman L. 2009. The major players in the Copenhagen talks and their positions. The New York Times, December 8, 2009: A1.

Frey BS, Savage DA, and Torglerb B. 2010. Interaction of natural survival instincts and internalized social norms exploring the Titanic and Lusitania disasters. Proceedings of the National Academy of Sciences 107: 4862–65.

Frumkin H. 2002. Urban sprawl and public health. Public Health Reports 117: 201–17.
　2010a. Introduction. In: Frumkin H (ed.). Environmental Health: From Global to Local, 2nd ed. New York: John Wiley and Sons: xxix-lvii.
　2010b. Healthy Buildings. In: Frumkin H (ed.). Environmental Health: From Global to Local, 2nd ed. New York: John Wiley and Sons: 689–728.

Frumkin H, Frank L, and Jackson R. 2004. Urban Sprawl and Public Health. Washington, DC: Island Press.

Fuentes C and Sherman K. 2010. Science and Ethics Review of Protocol of Human Study of Mosquito Repellant Performance, Environmental Protection Agency, Office of

Pesticide Programs. Available at: www.epa.gov/hsrb/files/meeting…/oct-27…/1b-no-mas-003–10–1-10.pdf. Accessed: November 23, 2010.

Fukuyama F. 2003. Our Posthuman Future: Consequences of the Biotechnology Revolution. New York: Picador.

Furtaw EJ. 2001. An overview of human exposure modeling activities at the U.S. EPA's National Exposure Research Laboratory. Toxicology and Environmental Health 17: 302–24.

Gadsby P. 2004. The Inuit paradox. Discover Magazine, October 1, 2004. Available at: http://discovermagazine.com/2004/oct/inuit-paradox. Accessed: June 20, 2010.

Galbraith K. 2011. Gulf coast wind farms spring up, as do worries. The New York Times, February 10, 2011: A23.

Gardiner S. 2006. A perfect moral storm: climate change, intergenerational ethics, and the problem of moral corruption. Environmental Values 15: 397–413.

2010. Is "arming the future" with geoengineering really the lesser evil? Some doubts about the ethics of intentionally manipulating the climate system. In: Gardiner S, Caney S, Jamieson D, and Shue H (eds.). Climate Ethics: Essential Readings. New York: Oxford University Press: 284–312.

Gee GC and Payne-Sturges DC. 2004. Environmental health disparities: a framework integrating psychosocial and environmental concepts. Environmental Health Perspectives 112: 1645–53.

Gelt J. 1997. Sharing Colorado River water: history, public policy and the Colorado River Compact. Arroyo, August 1997, Volume 10, No. 1. Available at: http://ag.arizona.edu/azwater/arroyo/101comm.html. Accessed: July 19, 2010.

George JF. 2006. Xenotransplantation: an ethical dilemma. Current Opinion in Cardiology 21: 138–41.

Georgehiou GP. 1986. The magnitude of the resistance problem. In: Pesticide Resistance: Strategies for Tactics and Management. Washington, DC: National Academy Press: 14–44.

Gerde P. 2005. Animal models and their limitations: on the problem of high-to-low dose extrapolations following inhalation exposures. Experimental Toxicology and Pathology 57 (Supplement 1):143–46.

Gert B, Culver CM, and Clouser DK. 2006. Bioethics: A Systematic Approach, 2nd ed. New York: Oxford University Press.

Gewirth A. 2001. Human rights and future generations. In Boylan M (ed.). Environmental Ethics. Upper Saddle River, NJ: Prentice Hall: 207–11.

Gibbs W. 1997. Plantibodies: human antibodies produced by field crops enter clinical trials. Scientific American 277, 5: 44.

Gibson DG, Glass JI, Lartigue C, Noskov VN, Chuang RY, Algire MA, Benders GA, Montague MG, Ma L, Moodie MM, Merryman C, Vashee S, Krishnakumar R, Assad-Garcia N, Andrews-Pfannkoch C, Denisova EA, Young L, Qi ZQ, Segall-Shapiro TH,

Calvey CH, Parmar PP, Hutchison CA 3rd, Smith HO, and Venter JC. 2010. Creation of a bacterial cell controlled by a chemically synthesized genome. Science 329: 52–56.

Gilbert S. 2006. Supplementing the traditional institutional review board with an environmental health and community review board. Environmental Health Perspectives 114: 1626–29.

Gilligan C. 1993. In a Different Voice: Psychological Theory and Women's Development, 6th ed. Cambridge, MA: Harvard University Press.

Global Encasement. 2010. Lead based paint encapsulation/encasement and abatement information. Available at: http://encasement.com/site/encasement/lead-based-paint.html. Accessed: November 3, 2010.

Global Policy Forum. 2010. Water in conflict. Available at: http://globalpolicy.org/the-dark-side-of-natural-resources/water-in-conflict.html. Accessed: July 19, 2010.

Glover JD, Reganold JP, Bell LW, Borevitz J Brummer EC, Buckler ES, Cox CM, Cox TS, Crews TE, Culman SW, DeHaan LR, Eriksson D, Gill BS, Holland J, Hu F, Hulke BS, Ibrahim AM, Jackson W, Jones SS, Murray SC, Paterson AH, Ploschuk E, Sacks EJ, Snapp S, Tao D, Van Tassel DL, Wade LJ, Wyse DL, and Xu Y. 2010. Increased food and ecosystem security via perennial grains. Science 328: 1938–39.

Goklany IM. 2001. The Precautionary Principle: A Critical Appraisal of Environmental Risk Assessment. Washington, DC: Cato Institute.

Goldman KA. 2000. Bioengineered food – safety and labeling. Science 290: 457–59.

Goldner WS, Sandler DP, Yu F, Hoppin JA, Kamel F, and Levan TD. 2010. Pesticide use and thyroid disease among women in the Agricultural Health Study. American Journal of Epidemiology 171: 455–64.

Gómez-Galera S, Pelacho AM, Gené A, Capell T, and Christou P. 2007. The genetic manipulation of medicinal and aromatic plants. Plant Cell Reproduction 26: 1689–715.

Goodin R. 1990. No Smoking: The Ethical Issues. Chicago: University of Chicago Press.

Goodland R and Anhang J. 2009. Livestock and climate change. World Watch, November/December 2009. Available at: http://www.worldwatch.org/files/pdf/Livestock%20and%20Climate%20Change.pdf. Accessed: June 20, 2010.

Goodman B. 1997. Scientists exonerated by ORI report lingering wounds. The Scientist 11, 12: 1.

Goodpaster K. 1978. On being morally considerable. Journal of Philosophy 75: 308–25.

Gostin LO. 2007a. Law as a tool to facilitate healthier lifestyles and prevent obesity. Journal of the American Medical Association 297: 87–90.

    2007b. General justifications for public health regulation. Public Health 121: 829–34.

Goulson D, Lye GC, and Darvill B. 2008. Decline and conservation of bumble bees. Annu Rev Entomology 53: 191–208.

GoVeg.com. Cruelty to animals: Mechanized madness. 2010. Accessed: http://www.goveg.com/factoryFarming.asp. Accessed: June 19, 2010.

Govtrack.us. 2010. H.R. 5634: Offshore Drilling Safety Improvement Act. Available at: http://www.govtrack.us/congress/bill.xpd?bill=h111–5634. Accessed: October 10, 2010.

Greene JD, Sommerville RB, Nystrom LE, Darley JM, and Cohen JD. 2001. An fMRI investigation of emotional engagement in moral judgment. Science 293: 2105–08.

Greenpeace. 1996. Glyphosate fact sheet. Available at: http://archive.greenpeace.org/geneng/reports/gmo/gmo009.htm. Accessed: March 31, 2010.

____. 2010. Where does e-waste end up? Available at: http://www.greenpeace.org/international/en/campaigns/toxics/electronics/the-e-waste-problem/where-does-e-waste-end-up/. Accessed: July 23, 2010.

Gressel J. 2009. Evolving understanding of the evolution of herbicide resistance. Pest Management Science 65: 1164–73.

Griffith D. 2001. Animal Minds: Beyond Cognition to Consciousness. Chicago: University of Chicago Press.

Grimes v. Kennedy Krieger Institute, Inc. 782 A.2d 807 (Md 2001).

Grimes RW and Nuttall WJ. 2010. Generating the option of a two-stage nuclear renaissance. Science 329: 799–803.

Grossman M, Chaloupka FJ, and Shim K. 2002. Illegal drug use and public policy. Health Affairs 21: 134–45.

Grunwald M. 2008. Nuclear's comeback: still no energy panacea. Time Magazine, December 31, 2008. Available at: http://www.time.com/time/magazine/article/0,9171,1869203-1,00.html. Accessed: October 10, 2010.

Gulson B, McCall M, Korsch M, Gomez L, Casey P, Oytam Y, Taylor A, McCulloch M, Trotter J, Kinsley L, and Greenoak G. 2010. Small amounts of zinc from zinc oxide particles in sunscreens applied outdoors are absorbed through human skin. Toxicology Science 118: 140–49.

Gundacker C, Gencik M, and Hengstschläger M. 2010. The relevance of the individual genetic background for the toxicokinetics of two significant neurodevelopmental toxicants: mercury and lead. Mutation Research 705:130–40.

Gutmann A and Thompson D. 1998. Democracy and Disagreement. Cambridge, MA: Harvard University Press.

Haack S. 2003. Defending Science within Reason. New York: Prometheus Books.

Haidt J. 2007. The new synthesis in moral psychology. Science 316: 998–1002.

Hamlin HJ and Guillette LJ Jr. 2010. Birth defects in wildlife: the role of environmental contaminants as inducers of reproductive and developmental dysfunction. Systems Biology in Reproductive Medicine 56: 113–21.

Hasleberger AG. 2000. Monitoring and labeling for genetically modified products. Science 287: 431–32.

Hasler JF. 1992. Current status and potential of embryo transfer and reproductive technology in dairy cattle. Journal of Dairy Science 75: 2857–79.

Hauser M. 2006. Moral Minds: How Nature Designed our Universal Sense of Right and Wrong. New York: Harper Collins.

Health and Environment Alliance. 2010. Pesticides. Available at: http://www.env-health.org/r/68. Accessed: May 26, 2010.

Heaton SK, Balbus JM, Keck JW, and Dannenberg AL. 2010. Healthy communities. In: Frumkin H (ed.). Environmental Health: From Global to Local, 2nd ed. New York: John Wiley and Sons: 451–86.

Hecht MM. 2004. In Africa, DDT makes a comeback to saves lives. Executive Intelligence Review, June 18, 2004. Available at: http://www.larouchepub.com/other/2004/sci_techs/3124ddt_africa.html. Accessed: March 24, 2010.

Hegel GW. 1967 [1821]. The Philosophy of Right. Knox TM (trans.). Cambridge: Cambridge University Press.

Heinberg R and Fridley D. 2010. The end of cheap coal. Nature 468: 367–69.

Heinemann JA and Traavik T. 2004. Problems in monitoring horizontal gene transfer in field trials of transgenic plants. Nature Biotechnology 22: 1105–09.

Held V. 2007. The Ethics of Care: Personal, Political, Global. New York: Oxford University Press.

Hennessy-Fiske M and Zahniser D. 2008. Council bans new fast-food outlets in South L.A. Los Angeles Times, July 30, 2008: A1.

Hesketh T, Lu L, and Xing ZW. 2005. The effect of China's one-child family policy after 25 years. New England Journal of Medicine 353: 1171–76.

Hess JJ. 2010. Energy production. In: Frumkin H (ed.). Environmental Health: From Global to Local, 2nd ed. New York: John Wiley and Sons: 417–49.

Hill Jr. TH. 1983. Ideals of human excellence and preserving natural environments. Environmental Ethics 5: 211–24.

Hinrichsen D. 2010. Population pressure. In: Frumkin H (ed.). Environmental Health: From Global to Local, 2nd ed. New York: John Wiley and Sons: 259–78.

Hippocratic Oath. 2002 [4th century BCE]. North M (transl.). Available at: http://www.nlm.nih.gov/hmd/greek/greek_oath.html. Accessed: April 27, 2010.

Ho WC, Hartley WR, Myers L, Lin MH, Lin YS, Lien CH, and Lin RS. 2007. Air pollution, weather, and associated risk factors related to asthma prevalence and attack rate. Environmental Research 104: 402–09.

Hobbes T. 2006 [1651]. Leviathan. New York: Dover Books.

Hodge Jr. JG and Gostin LO. 2008. Confidentiality. In: Emanuel EJ, Grady C, Crouch RA, Lie R, Miller F, and Wendler D (eds.). The Oxford Textbook of Clinical Research Ethics. New York: Oxford University Press: 673–81.

Hoet P, Brüske-Hohlfield I, and Salata O. 2004. Nanoparticles – known and unknown health risks. Journal of Nanobiotechnology 2: 12–27.

Hogwarth R and Ingraffea A. 2011. Fracking: too high risk. Nature 477: 271–73.

Holtzman NA, Watson MS, and Task Force on Genetic Testing. 1997. Final Report of the Task Force on Genetic Testing. Available at: http://www.genome.gov/10001733. Accessed: November 17, 2010.

Holy Bible. 2004. King James Version. Peabody, MA: Hendrickson Publishers.

Hope D. 2003. Court rules laws on wetlands apply to family's farm. The Pittsburgh Post-Gazette, September 3, 2006: A1.

Hotopf M and Wessely S. 2005. Can epidemiology clear the fog of war? Lessons from the 1990–91 Gulf War. International Journal of Epidemiology 34: 791–800.

H.R. 5820. Toxic Chemical Safety Act of 2010. Available at: http://energycommerce.house. gov/documents/20100722/HR5820.pdf. Accessed: August 3, 2010.

Hrudey SE, Hrudey EJ, and Pollard SJ. 2006. Risk management for assuring safe drinking water. Environment International 32: 948–57.

Hsu SS. 2006. Katrina report spreads blame: Homeland Security, Chertoff singled out. The Washington Post, February 12, 2006: A1.

Hu FB and Malik VS. 2010. Sugar-sweetened beverages and risk of obesity and type 2 diabetes: epidemiologic evidence. Physiology and Behavior 100: 47–54.

Hughes JB, Daily GC, and Ehrlich PR. 1997. Population diversity: its extent and extinction. Science 278: 689–92.

Hughes MF. 2006. Biomarkers of exposure: a case study with inorganic arsenic. Environmental Health Perspectives 114: 1790–96.

Human Genome Project. 2009. Cloning fact sheet. Available at: http://www.ornl.gov/sci/ techresources/Human_Genome/elsi/cloning.shtml#whatis. Accessed: May 30, 2010.

Hume D. 1978 [1739–40]. Treatise of Human Nature. Nidditch PH (ed.). New York: Oxford University Press.

Hutchison WD, Burkness EC, Mitchell PD, Moon RD, Leslie TW, Fleischer SJ, Abrahamson M, Hamilton KL, Steffey KL, Gray ME, Hellmich RL, Kaster LV, Hunt TE, Wright RJ, Pecinovsky K, Rabaey TL, Flood BR, and Raun ES. 2010. Areawide suppression of European corn borer with BT maize reaps savings to non-BT maize growers. Science 330: 222–25.

Hvistendahl M. 2008. China's Three Gorges Dam: an environmental disaster? Scientific American, March 25, 2008. Available at: http://www.scientificamerican.com/article. cfm?id=chinas-three-gorges-dam-disaster. Accessed: July 18, 2010.

2010. Has China outgrown the one-child policy? Science 329: 1458–61.

Iltis AS. 2000. Bioethics as methodological case resolution: specification, specified principlism and casuistry. Journal of Medicine and Philosophy 25: 271–84.

Immerzeel WW, van Beek LP, and Bierkens MF. 2010. Climate change will affect the Asian water towers. Science 328: 1382–85.

Impact Project. 2009. Trade, health, and the environment. Available at: http://hydra.usc. edu/scehsc/web/Resources/Reports%20and%20Publications/THE%20Impact%20 Project%20Report%20-%20June%202009%20FINAL.pdf. Accessed: January 11, 2011.

Institute of Medicine. 2005. Ethical Considerations for Research on Housing-Related Health Hazards Involving Children. Washington, DC: National Academy Press.

2006. Gulf War and Health Volume 4: Health Effects of Serving in the Gulf War. Washington, DC: National Academy Press.

Interagency Working Group on Climate Change and Health. 2010. A human health perspective on climate change. Available at: http://ehp03.niehs.nih.gov/static/climatechange. action. Accessed: August 12, 2011.

International Conference on Harmonization. 2010. Good clinical practice guidelines. Available at: http://ichgcp.net/. Accessed: November 17, 2010.

International Energy Association. 2010. Key world energy statistics. Available at: http://iea.org/textbase/nppdf/free/2010/key_stats_2010.pdf. Accessed: September 20, 2010.

International Rivers. 2007. Environmental impacts of dams. Available at: http://www.internationalrivers.org/en/node/1545. Accessed: July 17, 2010.

Iraq Body Count. 2010. Available at: http://www.iraqbodycount.org/. Accessed: March 27, 2010.

Israel B, Schulz A, Parker E, and Becker A. 1998. Review of community-based research: assessing partnership approaches to improve public health. Annual Review Public Health 19: 173–94.

Jackson R and Kochtitzky C. 2009. Creating a healthy environment: The impact of the built environment and public health. Centers for Disease Control and Prevention. Available at: http://www.cdc.gov/healthyplaces/articles/Creating%20A%20Healthy%20Environment.pdf. Accessed: August 18, 2010.

Jacobson MF and Brownell KD. Small taxes on soft drinks and snack foods to promote health. American Journal of Public Health 90: 854–57.

Jameton A. 2010. Environmental health ethics. In: Frumkin H (ed.). Environmental Health: From Global to Local, 2nd ed. New York: John Wiley and Sons: 195–226.

Jamieson D. 1984. The city around us. In: Regan T (ed.). Earthbound: New Introductory Essays in Environmental Ethics. New York: Random House: 38–73.

1996. Intentional climate change. Climate Change 33: 323–36.

2002. Morality's Progress: Essays on Humans, Other Animals, and the Rest of Nature. Oxford: Clarendon Press.

2010. Can space reflectors save us? Why we shouldn't buy into geoengineering fantasies. Slate September 23, 2010. Available at: http://www.slate.com/id/2268034/. Accessed: July 25, 2011.

Jarvie JA and Malone RE. 2008. Children's secondhand smoke exposure in private homes and cars: an ethical analysis. American Journal of Public Health 98: 2140–45.

Jensen VF, Neimann J, Hammerum AM, Mølbak K, and Wegener HC. 2004. Does the use of antibiotics in food animals pose a risk to human health? An unbiased review? Journal of Antimicrobial Chemotherapy 54: 274–75.

Johnita M.D. v. David D.D., 740 N.Y.S.2d 811 (2002).

Johnson E. 1984. Treating the dirt: environmental ethics and moral theory. In: Regan T (ed.). Earthbound: New Introductory Essays in Environmental Ethics. New York: Random House: 336–65.

Johnson M. 2009. N.C. to impose 'fat tax'. Raleigh News and Observer, October 7, 2009: A1.

Jones JH. 1981. Bad Blood. London: Free Press.

Jones M. 2010. Food: a taste of things to come? Nature 468: 752–53.

Jones R. 2007. What have we learned from public engagement? Nature Nanotechnology 2: 262–63.

Jonsen A, Siegler M, and Winslade W. 2006. Clinical Ethics, 6th ed. New York; McGraw-Hill.

Jonsen A and Toulmin S. 1988. The Abuse of Casuistry: A History of Moral Reasoning. Berkeley: University of California Press.

Kamel F and Hoppin JA. 2004. Association of pesticide exposure with neurologic dysfunction and disease. Environmental Health Perspectives 112: 950–58.

Kamel F, Tanner C, Umbach D, Hoppin J, Alavanja M, Blair A, Comyns K, Goldman S, Korell M, Langston J, Ross G, and Sandler D. 2007. Pesticide exposure and self-reported Parkinson's disease in the agricultural health study. American Journal of Epidemiology 165: 364–74.

Kant I. 1964 [1785]. Groundwork of the Metaphysics of Morals. Paton HD (transl.). New York: Harper and Rowe.

Kapp C. 2004. Help or hazard? Lancet 364: 1113–14.

Kass L. 2008. Toward a More Natural Science. New York: Free Press.

Katz E and Light A (eds.). 1996. Environmental Pragmatism. New York: Routledge.

Katz TM, Miller JH, and Hebert AA. 2008. Insect repellents: historical perspectives and new developments. Journal of the American Academy of Dermatology 58: 865–71.

Kawachi I and Kennedy BP. 2006. The Health of Nations: Why Inequality Is Harmful to Your Health. New York: New Press.

Keasling JD. 2010. Manufacturing molecules through metabolic engineering. Science 330:1355–58.

Keegan J. 2005. The Second World War. New York: Penguin Books.

Keese P. 2008. Risks from GMOs due to horizontal gene transfer. Environmental Biosafety Research 7: 123–49.

Keesing F, Brunner J, Duerr S, Killilea M, Logiudice K, Schmidt K, Vuong H, and Ostfeld RS. 2009. Hosts as ecological traps for the vector of Lyme disease. Proceedings of the Royal Society: Biological Sciences 276: 3911–19.

Keith DW. 2010. Photophoretic levitation of engineered aerosols for geoengineering. Proceedings of the National Academy of Sciences 107: 16428–31.

Keith DW, Parson E, and Morgan EG. 2010. Research on global sun block needed now. Nature 463: 426–27.

Kercsmar C, Dearborn D, Schluchter M, Xue L, Kirchner H, Sobolewski J, Greenberg S, Vesper S, and Allan T. 2006. Reduction in asthma morbidity in children as a result of home remediation aimed at moisture sources. Environmental Health Perspectives 114: 1574–80.

Kerr RA. 2010. Do we have the energy for the next generation? Science 329: 780–81.

———. 2011. Light at the end of the radwaste disposal tunnel could be real. Science 333: 150–52.

Kessler R. 2011. Engineered nanoparticles in consumer products: understanding a new ingredient. Environmental Health Perspectives 119: A120–25.

Kimmelman J. 2009. Gene Transfer and the Ethics of First-in-Human Research: Lost in Translation. Cambridge: Cambridge University Press.

King R. 2000. Environmental ethics and the built environment. Environmental Ethics 22: 115–31.

Kintisch E. 2007. Power generation: making dirty coal plants cleaner. Science 317: 184–86.
  2010a. Asilomar 2 takes small steps toward rules for geoengineering. Science 328: 22–23.
  2010b. Out of site. Science 329: 788–89.

Kleeberger SR, Reddy S, Zhang LY, and Jedlicka AE. 2000. Genetic susceptibility to ozone-induced lung hyperpermeability. American Journal of Respiratory Cell and Molecular Biology 22: 620–27.

Klevens RM, Morrison MA, Nadle J, Petit S, Gershman K, Ray S, Harrison LH, Lynfield R, Dumyati G, Townes JM, Craig AS, Zell ER, Fosheim GE, McDougal LK, Carey RB, Fridkin SK; and Active Bacterial Core surveillance (ABCs) MRSA Investigators. 2007. Invasive methicillin-resistant Staphylococcus aureus infections in the United States. Journal of the American Medical Association 298: 1763–71.

Kohlberg L. 1981. The Philosophy of Moral Development: Moral Stages and the Idea of Justice. New York: Harper and Row.

Kohler BA, Ward E, McCarthy BJ, Schymura MJ, Ries LA, Eheman C, Jemal A, Anderson RN, Ajani AU and Edwards BK. 2011. Annual report to the nation on the status of cancer, 1975–2007, featuring tumors of the brain and other nervous system, Journal of the National Cancer Institute 103: 1–23.

Körner S. 1955. Kant. New York: Pelican Books.

Kovács J. 1998. The concept of health and disease. Medicine, Health Care, and Philosophy 1: 31–39.

Krebs JR, Wilson JB, Bradbury RB, and Siriwardena GM. 1999. The second silent spring? Nature 400: 611–12.

LaFollette H and Shanks N. 1997. Brute Science: Ethical Dilemmas of Animals Experimentation. New York: Routledge.

La Tzu. 1984. Tao Te Ching. Lau DC (ed.). New York: Penguin Books.

Laumbach RJ. 2010. Outdoor air pollutants and patient health. American Family Physician 81: 175–80.

Lear LJ. 2009. Rachel Carson: Witness for Nature. New York: Mariner Books.

Lederer SE. 1995. Subjects to Science: Human Experimentation in America before the Second World War. Baltimore, MD: Johns Hopkins University Press.

Le CT and Boen JR. 1995. Health and Numbers: Basic Biostatistical Methods. New York: John Wiley.

Lee C. 2002. Environmental justice: building a unified vision of health and the environment. Environmental Health Perspectives 110, supplement: 2141–44.
  2010. Environmental justice. In: Frumkin H (ed.). Environmental Health: From Global to Local, 2nd ed. New York: John Wiley and Sons: 227–56.

Lee JA. 1976. Recent trends of large bowel cancer in Japan compared to the United States and Wales. International Journal of Epidemiology 6: 187–94.

Lemaux PG. 2008. Genetically engineered plants and foods: a scientist's analysis of the issues (part I). Annual Review of Plant Biology 59: 771–812.

Leonhardt D. 2009. Fat tax. The New York Times, August 16, 2009: MM9.

Leopold A. 1949. A Sand County Almanac and Sketches Here and There. Oxford: Oxford University Press.

Leopold A. 1989. A Sand County Almanac: And Sketches Here and There, Commemorative edition. Oxford: Oxford University Press.

Levin RJ. 2008. Incidence of thyroid cancer in residents surrounding the Three Mile Island nuclear facility. Laryngoscope 118: 618–28.

Levy D. 1992. The Antibiotic Paradox. New York: Plenum Press.

Lewin T. 2001. U.S. investigating Johns Hopkins study of lead paint hazard. The New York Times, August 24, 2001: A1.

Lewis AS. 2007. Organic versus inorganic arsenic in herbal kelp supplements. Environmental Health Perspectives 115: A575.

Lewis CS. 1952. Mere Christianity. New York: Harper.

Lieberman B. 2010. The economics of global warming policy. Heritage Foundation Lecture 1156, June 16, 2010. Available at: http://www.heritage.org/Research/Lecture/The-Economics-of-Global-Warming-Policy. Accessed: September 30, 2010.

Lifton RJ. 2000. The Nazi Doctors. New York: Basic Books.

Lillico SG, McGrew MJ, Sherman A, and Sang HM. 2005. Transgenic chickens as bioreactors for protein-based drugs. Drug Discovery Today 10: 191–96.

Lizzio v. Lizzio, 618 N.Y.S.2d 934, 936 (N.Y. Fam. Ct. 1994).

Locke J. 1980 [1689]. Second Treatise of Civil Government. Indianapolis: Hackett.

Lockwood A. 2004. Human testing of pesticides: scientific and ethical considerations American Journal of Public Health 94: 1908–16.

Logan JG, Stanczyk NM, Hassanali A, Kemei J, Santana AE, Ribeiro KA, Pickett JA, and JA Mordue. 2010. Arm-in-cage testing of natural human-derived mosquito repellents. Malaria Journal 9: 239.

LoGiudice K, Ostfeld RS, Schmidt KA, and Keesing F. 2003. The ecology of infectious disease: effects of host diversity and community composition on Lyme disease risk. Proceedings of the National Academy of Sciences 100: 567–71.

Longley M and Sotherton NW. 1997. Factors determining the effects of pesticides upon butterflies inhabiting arable farmland. Agriculture, Ecosystems & Environment 61: 1–12.

Longnecker MP, Rogan WJ, and Lucier G. 1997. The human health effects of DDT (dichlorodiphenyltrichloroethane) and PCBs (polychlorinated biphenyls) and an overview of organochlorines in public health. Annual Review of Public Health 18: 211–44.

Lorenz K. 2002. On Aggression, 2nd ed. New York: Routledge.

Losey JE, Rayor LS, and Carter ME. 1999. Transgenic pollen harms monarch larvae. Nature 399: 214.

Lovett GM, Tear TH, Evers DC, Findlay SE, Cosby BJ, Dunscomb JK, Driscoll CT, and Weathers KC. 2009. Effects of air pollution on ecosystems and biological diversity in the eastern United States. Annals of the New York Academy of Science 1162: 99–135.

Lubick N. 2010. Drugs in the environment: do pharmaceutical take-back programs make a difference? Environmental Health Perspectives 118: A211–14.

Lubin JH and Caporaso NE. 2006. Cigarette smoking and lung cancer: modeling total exposure and intensity. Cancer Epidemiology, Biomarkers & Prevention 15: 517–23.

Luster MI and Rosenthal GJ. 1993. Chemical agents and the immune response. Environmental Health Perspectives 100: 219–26.

Lynch T and Price A. 2007. The effect of cytochrome P450 metabolism on drug response, interactions, and adverse effects. American Family Physician 76: 391–96.

Lynd L, Laser M, Bransby D, Dale B, Davison B, Hamilton R, Himmel M, Keller M, McMillan J, Sheehan J, and Wyman C. 2008. How biotech can transform biofuels. Nature Biotechnology 26: 169–72.

Lytle MH. 2007. The Gentle Subversive: Rachel Carson, Silent Spring, and the Rise of the Environmental Movement. New York: Oxford University Press.

MacIntyre A. 1984. After Virtue. South Bend, IN: University of Notre Dame Press.

2006. A Short History of Ethics, revised ed. New York: Routledge.

MacDorman MF and Mathews TJ. 2008. Recent trends in infant mortality in the United States. National Center for Health Statistics, Data Brief, Number 9, October 2008. Available at: http://www.cdc.gov/nchs/data/databriefs/db09.htm. Accessed: October 20, 2010.

Malakoff D. 2011. Landmark study reveals oil quagmire. Science 333: 809.

Malthus T. 1798 [2008]. Essay on the Principle of Population. New York: Oxford University Press.

Maquire DC. 2003. Sacred Rights: The Case for Contraception and Abortion in World Religions. New York: Oxford University Press.

Mann CC and Plummer ML. 2002. Forest biotech edges out of the lab. Science 295: 1626–29.

Marchant GE. 2008a. Toxicogenomics and environmental regulation. In: Sharp RR, Marchant GE, and Grodsky JA (eds.). Genomics and Environmental Regulation. Baltimore, MD: Johns Hopkins University Press: 11–24.

2008b. Setting air quality standards in the postgenomic era. In: Sharp RR, Marchant GE, and Grodsky JA (eds.). Genomics and Environmental Regulation. Baltimore, MD: Johns Hopkins University Press: 116–38.

Marchant GE and Grodsky JA. 2008. Genomics and environmental justice: some preliminary thoughts. In: Sharp RR, Marchant GE, and Grodsky JA (eds.). Genomics and Environmental Regulation. Baltimore, MD: Johns Hopkins University Press: 98–115.

Margawati ET. 2003. Transgenic animals: their benefits to human welfare. Acitonbioscience, January 3, 2003. Available at: http://www.actionbioscience.org/biotech/margawati. html. Accessed: June 14, 2010.

Marlow HJ, Hayes WK, Soret S, Carter RL, Schwab ER, and Sabaté J. 2009. Diet and the environment: does what you eat matter? American Journal of Clinical Nutrition 89: 1699S-1703S.

Marshall E. 2004. Public enemy number one: tobacco or obesity? Science 304: 804.

 2005. Nuclear power: is the friendly atom poised for a comeback? Science 309: 1168–69.

Martin A and Severson K. 2008. Sticker shock in the organic aisles. The New York Times, April 18, 2008: B1.

Martmot M and Wilkinson RG (eds.). 2005. Social Determinants of Health, 2nd ed. New York: Oxford University Press.

Marx K. 1992 [1867]. Capital, vol. 1. Fowkes B (transl.). New York: Penguin Classics.

Maslin M and Scott J. 2011. Carbon trading needs a multi-level approach. Nature 475: 445–47.

Masood S. 2010. 800,000 in Pakistan reachable only by air. The New York Times, August 25, 2010: A1.

Master Z and Crozier GK. 2011. The ethics of moral compromise for stem cell research policy. Health Care Analysis April 12, 2011. [Epub ahead of print].

Mastroianni AC and Kahn JP. 2002. Risk and responsibility: ethics, Grimes v Kennedy Krieger, and public health research involving children. American Journal of Public Health 92: 1073–76.

Mathew AG, Cissell R, and Liamthong S. 2007. Antibiotic resistance in bacteria associated with food animals: a United States perspective of livestock production. Foodborne Pathogen Discovery 4:115–33.

Mayr E. 2001. Evolution. New York: Basic Books.

McDonnell G and Russell AD. 1998. Antiseptics and disinfectants: activity, action, and resistance. Clinical Microbiology Reviews 12, 1: 147–79.

McDowell N. 2002. Africa hungry for conventional foods as biotech row drags on. Nature 418: 571–72.

McKelvey W, Brody JG, Aschengrau A, and Swartz CH. 2003. Association between residence on Cape Cod, Massachusetts and breast cancer. Annals of Epidemiology 14: 89–94.

McMichael AJ, Powles JW, Butler CD, and Uauy R. 2007. Food, livestock production, energy, climate change, and health. Lancet 370: 1253–63.

McSwane D. 2010. Food safety. In: Frumkin H (ed.). Environmental Health: From Global to Local, 2nd ed. New York: John Wiley and Sons: 635–88.

Mead M. 2001. Sex and Temperament in Three Primitive Societies, 4th ed. New York: Harper Perennial.

Medical News Today. 2006. France's high birth rate partly due to government incentives. Medical News Today, September 27, 2006. Available at: http://www.medicalnewstoday. com/articles/52654.php. Accessed: August 31, 2010.

Medline Plus. 2009a. Acetaminophen overdose. Available at: http://www.nlm.nih.gov/medlineplus/ency/article/002598.htm. Accessed: March 31, 2010.

2009b. Alcoholism. Available at: http://www.nlm.nih.gov/medlineplus/ency/article/000944.htm. Accessed: April 1, 2010.

Mello MM and Wolf LE. 2010. The Havasupai Indian tribe case – lessons for research involving stored biologic samples. New England Journal of Medicine 363: 204–07.

Melnick RL and Huff J. 2004. Testing toxic pesticides in humans: health risks with no health benefits. Environmental Health Perspectives 112: A459–61.

Mendelsohn M, Kough J, Vaituzis Z, and Matthews K. 2003. Are BT crops safe? Nature Biotechnology 21: 1002–09.

Metcalf S. 1997. Water rights law for municipal lawyers: the basics, ruthlessly simplified. Proceedings of the Washington State Association of Municipal Attorneys' Annual Fall Conference, October 8–10, 1997. MRSC Information Bulletin No. 499, October 1997. Available at: http://www.mrsc.org/Subjects/Environment/water/IB499–8a.aspx. Accessed: July 19, 2010.

Metz B, Davidson OR, Bosch PR, Dave R, and Meyer LA (eds.). 2007. Contribution of Working Group III to the Fourth Assessment Report of the Intergovernmental Panel on Climate Change, 2007. Cambridge: Cambridge University Press.

Meyer O. 2003. Testing and assessment strategies, including alternatives and new approaches. Toxicology Letters 140–141: 21–30.

Micha R, Wallace SK, and Mozaffarian D. 2010. Red and processed meat consumption and risk of incident coronary heart disease, stroke, and diabetes mellitus: a systematic review and meta-analysis. Circulation 121: 2271–83.

Mikhail J. 2007. Universal moral grammar: theory, evidence, and the future. Trends in Cognitive Sciences 11: 143–52.

Mill JS. 2003 [1859, 1863]. Utilitarianism and On Liberty. New York: Wiley-Blackwell.

Miller F and Brody H. 2002. What makes placebo-controlled trials unethical? American Journal of Bioethics 2, 2: 3–9.

Miller FG and Rosenstein DL. 2008. Challenge experiments. In: Emanuel EJ, Grady C, Crouch RA, Lie R, Miller F, and Wendler D (eds.). The Oxford Textbook of Clinical Research Ethics. New York: Oxford University Press: 273–79.

Miller G. 2008. The roots of morality. Science 320: 734–37.

Miller P and Weijer C. 2003. Rehabilitating equipoise. Kennedy Institute of Ethics Journal 13: 93–118.

Mills JN, Gage KL, and Khan AS. 2010. Potential influence of climate change on vector-borne and zoonotic disease: a review and proposed research plan. Environmental Health Perspectives 118: 1507–14.

Minkler M. 2004. Ethical challenges for the "outside" researcher in community-based participatory research. Health Education and Behavior 31: 684–97.

Mohan S and Campbell NR. 2009. Salt and high blood pressure. Clinical Science 117: 1–11.

Mohr SH and Evans GM. 2009. Forecasting coal production until 2100. Fuel 88: 2059–67.

Monheit AC. 2008. Ideology, politics, and health care reform. Inquiry 44: 377–80.

Monsanto. 2009. Is Monsanto going to develop or sell "terminator" seeds? Available at: http://www.monsanto.com/monsanto_today/for_the_record/monsanto_terminator_seeds.asp. Accessed: June 1, 2010.

Mooney C. 2005. The Republican War on Science. New York: Basic Books.

Moore GE. 1903. Principia Ethica. Cambridge: Cambridge University Press.

Morello-Frosch R and Lopez R. 2006. The riskcape and the colorline: examining the role of segregation in environmental health disparities. Environmental Research 102: 181–96.

Moreno JD. 2005. In the wake of Katrina: has "bioethics" failed? American Journal of Bioethics 5, 5: W18–19.

Morgan SP. 2003. Is low fertility a twenty-first century demographic crisis? Demography 40: 589–603.

Morgan WJ, Crain EF, Gruchalla RS, O'Connor GT, Kattan M, Evans R 3rd, Stout J, Malindzak G, Smartt E, Plaut M, Walter M, Vaughn B, Mitchell H, and Inner-City Asthma Study Group. 2004. Results of a home-based environmental intervention among urban children with asthma. New England Journal of Medicine 351: 1068–80.

Moss M. 2010. The hard sell on salt. The New York Times, May 29, 2010: A1.

Munthe C. 2011. The Price of Precaution and the Ethics of Risk. Dordrecht: Springer.

Murray I. 2007. Silent alarmism: a centennial we could do without. National Review Online, May 31, 2007. Available at: http://article.nationalreview.com/317031/isilenti-alarmism/iain-murray. Accessed: March 22, 2010.

Mutter J. 2010. Disasters widen the rich-poor gap. Nature 466: 1042.

Naess A. 1973. The shallow and the deep, long-range ecology movement. Inquiry 16, 97–107.
   1986. The deep ecological movement: Some philosophical aspects. Philosophical Inquiry 8: 10–31.

Naranjoa SE and Ellsworth PC. 2009. Fifty years of the integrated control concept: moving the model and implementation forward in Arizona. Pest Management Science 65: 1267–86.

National Aeronautics and Space Administration. 2010a. Global Climate Change. Available at: http://climate.nasa.gov/. Accessed: September 27, 2010.
   2010b. GISS Surface Temperature Analysis. Available at: http://data.giss.nasa.gov/gistemp/graphs/. Accessed: September 27, 2010.
   2011. Climate change: how do we know? Available at: http://climate.nasa.gov/evidence/. Accessed: September 20, 2011.

National Cancer Institute. 2010. Cancer health disparities. Available at: http://www.cancer.gov/cancertopics/types/disparities. Accessed: October 19, 2010.

National Commission for the Protection of Human Subjects of Biomedical and Behavioral Research. 1979. The Belmont Report. Washington, DC: Department of Health, Education, and Welfare.

National Institute on Aging. 2010. Alzheimer's disease fact sheet. Available at: http://www. nia.nih.gov/Alzheimers/Publications/adfact.htm. Accessed: April 1, 2010.

National Institute for Environmental Health Sciences. 2006. Strategic plan. Available at: http://www.niehs.nih.gov/about/od/strategicplan/strategicplan2006/strategicplan06. pdf. Accessed: August 25, 2011.

National Institute of Environmental Health Sciences. 2010a. Endocrine disruptors. Available at: http://www.niehs.nih.gov/health/topics/agents/endocrine/index.cfm. Accessed: April 8, 2010.

2010b. Environmental justice and community-based participatory research. Available at: http://www.niehs.nih.gov/research/supported/programs/justice/. Accessed: October 12, 2010.

2010c. Environmental justice and community-based participatory research: Grantees. Available at: http://www.niehs.nih.gov/research/supported/programs/justice/grantees/ index.cfm. Accessed: October 12, 2010.

2011. NIH launches largest oil spill study. Available at: http://www.niehs.nih.gov/news/ releases/2011/gulfstudyfinal/. Accessed: July 26, 2011.

National Institutes of Health. 2009. About Recombinant DNA Advisory Committee (RAC). Available at: http://oba.od.nih.gov/rdna_rac/rac_about.html. Accessed: May 31, 2010.

National Nanotechnology Initiative. 2010a. Nanotechnology: Big things from a small world. Available at: http://www.nano.gov/Nanotechnology_BigThingsfromaTiny Worldspread.pdf. Accessed: July 27, 2010.

2010b. Funding. Available at: http://www.nano.gov/html/about/funding.html. Accessed: July 28, 2010.

National Oceanic and Atmospheric Administration. 2010. Endangered Species Act. Available at: http://www.nmfs.noaa.gov/pr/laws/esa/. Accessed: August 11, 2010.

National Park Service. 2010. About us. Available at: http://www.nps.gov/aboutus. Accessed: August 20, 2010.

National Partnership for Action. 2010. Health Disparities. Available at: http://minority-health.hhs.gov/npa/templates/browse.aspx?lvl=1&lvlid=13. Accessed: October 19, 2010.

National Research Council 2004. Intentional Human Dosing Studies for EPA Regulatory Purposes: Scientific and Ethical Issues. Washington, DC:National Academy Press.

National Toxicology Program. 2009. 11th Report on Carcinogens. Available at: http:// ntp.niehs.nih.gov/index.cfm?objectid=32BA9724-F1F6–975E-7FCE50709CB4C932. Accessed: October 10, 2010.

NationMaster.com. 2010. Health statistics by country. Available at: http://www.nationmaster. com/cat/hea-health. Accessed: October 19, 2010.

Nature. 2003. Don't believe the hype. Nature 424: 237.

2010. How to feed a hungry world. Nature 466: 531–32.

Nature Conservancy. 2010. About us. Available at: http://www.nature.org/aboutus/?src=t5. Accessed: August 23, 2010.

Needleman HL, Reigart JR, Landrigan P, Sass J, and Bearer C. 2005. Benefits and risks of pesticide testing on humans. Environmental Health Perspectives 113: A804–05.

Neuman W and Pollack A. 2010. Farmers cope with roundup-resistant weeds. The New York Times, May 3, 2010: A1.

Newberry B. 2010. Katrina: macro-ethical issues for engineers. Science and Engineering Ethics 16: 535–71.

Nguyen DM and El-Serag HB. 2010. The epidemiology of obesity. Gastroenterology Clinics of North America 39: 1–7.

Nicholl DS. 2008. An Introduction to Genetic Engineering. Cambridge: Cambridge University Press.

Nobelprize.org. 2010. Paul Müller. Available at: http://nobelprize.org/nobel_prizes/medicine/laureates/1948/muller-bio.html. Accessed: April 3, 2010.

Nohynek GJ, Lademann J, Ribaud C, and Roberts MS. 2007. Grey goo on the skin? nanotechnology, cosmetic and sunscreen safety. Critical Reviews in Toxicology 37: 251–77.

Nordlee JA, Taylor SL, Townsend JA, Thomas LA, and Bush RK. Identification of a Brazilnut allergen in transgenic soybeans. 1996. New England Journal of Medicine 334: 688–92.

North Carolina Wind Energy. 2010. North Carolina wind energy. Available at: http://www.wind.appstate.edu/. Accessed: October 11, 2010.

Norton B. 1987. Why Preserve Natural Variety? Princeton, NJ: Princeton University Press.
   1991. Toward Unity Among Environmentalists, New York: Oxford University Press.
   2005. Sustainability: A Philosophy of Adaptive Ecosystem Management. Chicago: University of Chicago Press.

Nozick R. 1974. Anarchy, State, and Utopia. New York: Basic Books.

Nuclear Regulatory Commission. 2010. About NRC. http://www.nrc.gov/about-nrc.html. Accessed: September 17, 2010.

Nuffield Council. 1999. Genetically modified crops: The ethical and social issues. London: Nuffield Council. Available at: http://www.nuffieldbioethics.org/sites/default/files/GM%20crops%20-%20full%20report.pdf. Accessed: February 25, 2011.

Nuremberg Code. 1947. Directives for human experimentation. Available at: http://ohsr.od.nih.gov/guidelines/nuremberg.html. Accessed: November 16, 2010.

Oberdörster G, Oberdörster E, Oberdörster J. 2005. Nanotoxicity: an emerging discipline evolving from studies of ultrafine particles. Environmental Health Perspectives 113: 823–39.

O'Fallon LR and Dearry A. 2002. Community-based participatory research as a tool to advance environmental health science. Environmental Health Perspectives 110 (suppl. 2): 155–59.

Office of Human Research Protections. 2010. Policy guidance. Available at: http://www.hhs.gov/ohrp/policy/index.html. Accessed: November 17, 2010.

Olden K. 2006. Toxicogenomics – a new systems toxicology approach to understanding of gene–environment interactions. Annals of the New York Academy of Sciences 1076: 703–06.

O'Mathuna DP. 2009. Nanoethics: Big Ethical Issues With Small Technology. London: Continuum.

O'Neill I. 2010. Is a devastating solar flare coming to a city near you? Discovery News, June 16, 2010. Available at: http://news.discovery.com/space/is-a-devastating-solar-flare-coming-to-a-city-near-you.html. Accessed: July 13, 2010.

O'Neill O. 1990. Constructions of Reason: Explorations of Kant's Practical Philosophy. Cambridge: Cambridge University Press.

    1997. Environmental values, anthropocentrism and speciesism. Environmental Values 6: 127–42.

Onishi N, Sanger DE, and Wald ML. 2011. High radiation severely hinders emergency work to cool Japanese plant. The New York Times, March 17, 2011: A1.

Orlik DK. 2007. Ethics for the Legal Professional, 7th ed. Upper Saddle River, NJ: Prentice-Hall.

Osotimehin B. 2011. Population and development. Science 333: 499.

Owen MD. 2008. Weed species shifts in glyphosate-resistant crops. Pest Management Science 64: 377–87.

Owen MD and Zelaya IA. 2005. Herbicide-resistant crops and weed resistance to herbicides. Pest Management Science 61: 301–11.

Pafit D. 1986. Reasons and Persons. New York: Oxford University Press.

Pansare M and Kamat D. 2010. Peanut allergy. Current Opinion in Pediatrics 22: 642–46.

Passmore J. 1980. Man's Responsibility for Nature, 2nd ed. London: Duckworth.

Paterson J. 2007. Sustainable development, sustainable decisions and the precautionary principle. Natural Hazards 42: 515–28.

Patz JA. 2010. Climate change. In: Frumkin H (ed.). Environmental Health: From Global to Local, 2nd ed. New York: John Wiley and Sons: 279–328.

Pence G. 2007. Medical Ethics: Accounts of the Cases that Shaped and Defined Medical Ethics, 7th ed. New York: McGraw-Hill.

Perrett RW. 1998. Hindu Ethics: A Philosophical Study. Honolulu: University of Hawaii Press.

Perry M and Hu H. 2010. Workplace health and safety. In: Frumkin H (ed.). Environmental Health: From Global to Local, 2nd ed. New York: John Wiley and Sons: 729–67.

Personal Dividends. 2010. 7 Income tax breaks – thanks to your children. Available at: http://personaldividends.com/money/miranda/income-tax-breaks-children. Accessed: August 31, 2010.

Pesticide Action Network International. 2010. About PAN. Available at: http://www.pan-international.org/panint/?q=node/33. Accessed: May 22, 2010.

Pesticide Action Network of North America. 2007. Safe malaria solutions – beyond DDT. Available at: http://www.panna.org/ddt. Accessed: March 23, 2010.

Peters T. 2002. Playing God? Genetic Determinism and Human Freedom, 2nd ed. New York: Routledge.

Phillips I, Casewell M, Cox T, De Groot B, Friis C, Jones R, Nightingale C, Preston R, and Waddell J. 2004. Does the use of antibiotics in food animals pose a risk to human health? A critical review of published data. Journal of Antimicrobial Chemotherapy 53: 28–52.

Phillips L. 2010. EU commission approves first cultivation of GM crop in 12 years. EU Observer, March 3, 2010. Available at: http://euobserver.com/885/29598. Accessed: June 5, 2010.

Physicians' Desk Reference. 2010. Williston, VT: PDR Network.

Piaget J. 1997. The Moral Judgment of the Child. New York: Free Press.

Pierce J and Jameton A. 2001. Environmentally Responsible Healthcare. New York: Oxford University Press.

Pimental D. 1996. Green revolution agriculture and chemical hazards. Science of the Total Environment 188, Supplement 1: S86–98.

Pinstrup-Andersen P and Schiøler E. 2000. Seeds of Contention: World Hunger and the Controversy over GM Crops. Washington, DC: International Food Policy Research Institute.

Pojman LP. 2005. Ethics: Discovering Right and Wrong, 5th ed. Belmont, CA: Wadsworth.

Pollack A. 2010a. Genetically altered salmon get close to the table. The New York Times, June 27, 2010: A1.

2010b. Antibiotic research subsidies weighed by U.S. The New York Times, November 5, 2010: B1.

PollingReport.com. 2011. Abortion and birth control. Available at: http://www.pollingreport.com/abortion.htm. Accessed: July 14, 2011.

Pope CA 3rd, Burnett RT, Krewski D, Jerrett M, Shi Y, Calle EE, and Thun MJ. 2009. Cardiovascular mortality and exposure to airborne fine particulate matter and cigarette smoke: shape of the exposure-response relationship. Circulation 120: 941–48.

Population Reference Bureau. 2009. 2009 World population data sheet. Available at: http://www.prb.org/Publications/Datasheets/2009/2009wpds.aspx. Accessed: March 30, 2010.

Posner GA and Weisbach D. 2010. Climate Change Justice. Princeton, NJ: Princeton University Press.

Potera C. 2011. Can transgenic plants root out pollutants? Environmental Health Perspectives 119: A206–07.

Potrykus I. 2010. Regulation must be revolutionized. Nature 466: 561.

Powles SB. Evolved glyphosate-resistant weeds around the world: lessons to be learnt. Pest Management Science 2008; 64: 360–65.

Preservation of Antibiotics for Medical Treatment Act, H.R. 1549. 2009. Available at: http://www.govtrack.us/congress/bill.xpd?bill=h111–1549. Accessed: May 28, 2010.

Radakovits R, Jinkerson Re, Darzins A, and Posewitz MC. 2010. Genetic engineering of algae for enhanced biofuel production. Eukaryotic Cell 9: 486–501.

Rahmstorf S. 2007. A semi-empirical approach to projecting future sea-level rise. Science 315: 368–70.

Rain-tree.com. 2010. Rainforest Facts. Available at: http://www.rain-tree.com/facts.htm. Accessed: August 9, 2010.

Ramessar K, Capell T, Twyman RM, and Christou P. 2010. Going to ridiculous lengths – European coexistence regulations for GM crops. Nature Biotechnology 28: 133–36.

Ramsey P. 1980. Fabricated Man: The Ethics of Genetic Control. New Haven: Yale University Press.

Ranson H, Abdallah H, Badolo A, Guelbeogo WM, Kerah-Hinzoumbé C, Yangalbé-Kalnoné E, Sagnon N, Simard F, and Coetzee M. 2009. Insecticide resistance in Anopheles gambiae: data from the first year of a multi-country study highlight the extent of the problem. Malaria Journal 8: 299.

Rasko J, O'Sullivan G, and Ankeny R (eds.). 2006. The Ethics of Inheritable Genetic Modification: A Dividing Line? Cambridge: Cambridge University Press.

Rawls J. 1971. A Theory of Justice. Cambridge, MA: Harvard University Press.

1999. The Law of Peoples. Cambridge, MA: Harvard University Press.

2005. Political Liberalism, 2nd ed. New York: Columbia University Press.

Rawls J and Herman B. 2000. Lectures on the History of Moral Philosophy. Cambridge, MA: Harvard University Press.

Regan T. 2004. The Case for Animal Rights, 2nd ed. Berkeley, CA: University of California Press.

Reinecke SA and Reinecke AJ. 2007. The impact of organophosphate pesticides in orchards on earthworms in the Western Cape, South Africa. Ecotoxicology and Environmental Safety 66: 244–51.

Reiss MJ and Straughan R. 1996. Improving Nature? The Science and Ethics of Genetic Engineering. Cambridge: Cambridge University Press.

Renegar G, Webster CJ, Stuerzebecher S, Harty L, Ide SE, Balkite B, Rogalski-Salter TA, Cohen N, Spear BB, Barnes DM, and Brazell C. 2006. Returning genetic research results to individuals: points-to-consider. Bioethics 20: 24–36.

Resnik, DB. 2003a. Is the precautionary principle unscientific? Studies in the History and Philosophy of Biology and the Biomedical Sciences 34: 329–44.

2003b. A pluralistic account of intellectual property. The Journal of Business Ethics 46: 319–35.

2004. The precautionary principle and medical decision making. Journal of Medicine and Philosophy 29: 281–99.

2006. Intentional exposure studies of environmental agents on human subjects: assessing benefits and risks. Accountability in Research 14: 35–55.

2007a. The Price of Truth. New York: Oxford University Press.

2007b. The new EPA regulations for protecting human subjects: haste makes waste. Hastings Center Report 37, 1: 17–21.

2007c. Are the new EPA regulations concerning intentional exposure studies with children overprotective? IRB 29, 5: 5–7.

2008a. Environmental health research involving human subjects: ethical issues. Environmental Health Insights 2: 27–34.

2008b. Randomized controlled trials in environmental health research: ethical issues. Journal of Environmental Health 70, 6: 28–31.

2009a. Human health and the environment: in harmony or conflict? Health Care Analysis 17: 261–76.

2009b. Playing Politics with Science. New York: Oxford University Press.

2009c. The investigator-subject relationship: A contextual approach. Journal of Philosophy, Ethics, Humanities in Medicine 4: 16.

2009d. Environmental health research and the observer's dilemma. Environmental Health Perspectives 117: 1191–94.

2010a. Trans fat bans and human freedom. American Journal of Bioethics 10, 3: 27–32.

2010b. Urban sprawl, smart growth, and democratic deliberation. American Journal of Public Health 100: 1852–56.

Resnik DB and Kennedy CE. 2010. Balancing scientific and community interests in community-based participatory research. Accountability in Research 17:198–210.

Resnik DB and Portier C. 2005. Pesticide testing on human subjects: Weighing benefits and risks. Environmental Health Perspectives 113: 813–17.

Resnik DB and Roman G. 2007. Health, justice, and the environment. Bioethics 21: 230–41.

Resnik DB and Sharp R. 2006. Protecting third parties in human subjects research. IRB 28, 4: 1–7.

Resnik DB, Steinkraus H, Langer P. 1999. Human Germ-line Gene Therapy: Scientific, Moral and Political Issues. Georgetown, TX: RG Landes.

Resnik DB and Tinkle SS. 2007. Ethical issues in clinical trials involving nanomedicine. Contemporary Clinical Trials 28: 433–41.

Resnik DB and Wing S. 2007. Lessons learned from the Children's Environmental Exposure Research Study. American Journal of Public Health 97: 414–18.

Resnik DB and Zeldin D. 2008. Environmental health research on hazards in the home and the duty to warn. Bioethics 22: 209–17.

Reston M. 2011. Rick Perry calls global warming an unproven, costly theory. Los Angeles Times, August 17, 2011: A1.

Revkin AC. 2006. Climate change expert says NASA tried to silence him. The New York Times, January 29, 2009: A1.

2009. Hacked e-mail is new fodder for climate dispute. The New York Times, November 20, 2009: A1.

Richardson H. 2000. Specifying, balancing, and interpreting bioethical principles. Journal of Medicine and Philosophy 25: 285–307.

Richardson JR and Miller GW. 2010. Toxicology. In: Frumkin H (ed.). Environmental Health: From Global to Local, 2nd ed. New York: John Wiley and Sons: 49–78.

Richman KA. 2004. Ethics and the Metaphysics of Medicine. Cambridge, MA: M.I.T. Press.

Rifkin J. 1984. Algeny. New York: Penguin.

1985. Declaration of a Heretic. Boston: Routledge and Kegan Paul.

Ritter JM, Harding I, and Warren JB. 2009. Precaution, cyclooxygenase inhibition, and cardiovascular risk. Trends Pharmacological Science 30: 503–08.

Roberts DR, Manguin S, and Mouchet J. 2000. DDT house spraying and re-emerging malaria. Lancet 356: 330–32.

Robertson GP, Dale VH, Doering OC, Hamburg SP, Melillo JM, Wander MM, Parton WJ, Adler PR, Barney JN, Cruse RM, Duke CS, Fearnside PM, Follett RF, Gibbs HK, Goldemberg J, Mladenoff DJ, Ojima D, Palmer MW, Sharpley A, Wallace L, Weathers KC, Wiens JA, and Wilhelm WW. 2008. Agriculture: sustainable biofuels redux. Science 322: 49–50.

Robertson JA. 1994. Children of Choice: Freedom and the New Reproductive Technologies. Princeton, NJ: Princeton University Press.

Roberts M. 2009. The non-identity problem. Stanford Encyclopedia of Philosophy. http:// plato.stanford.edu/entries/nonidentity-problem/. Accessed: May 6, 2010.

Robinson AS, Knols BG, Voigt G, and Hendrichs J. 2009. Conceptual framework and rationale. Malaria Journal 8, Supplement 2: S1.

Robles F. 2010. Haiti not the first stop for cholera strain that's killed 2,000. Miami Herald, December 12, 2010: A1.

Robson MG, Hamilton GC, and Siriwong W. 2010. Pest control and pesticides. In: Frumkin H (ed.). Environmental Health: From Global to Local, 2nd ed. New York: John Wiley and Sons: 592–634.

Rockström J, Steffen W, Noone K, Persson A, Chapin FS 3rd, Lambin EF, Lenton TM, Scheffer M, Folke C, Schellnhuber HJ, Nykvist B, de Wit CA, Hughes T, van der Leeuw S, Rodhe H, Sörlin S, Snyder PK, Costanza R, Svedin U, Falkenmark M, Karlberg L, Corell RW, Fabry VJ, Hansen J, Walker B, Liverman D, Richardson K, Crutzen P, and Foley JA. 2009. A safe operating space for humanity. Nature 461: 472–75.

Rodenbeck S, Orloff K, and Falk H. 2010. Solid and hazardous waste. In: Frumkin H (ed.). Environmental Health: From Global to Local, 2nd ed. New York: John Wiley and Sons: 559–90.

Roemer JE. 1998. Theories of Justice. Cambridge, MA: Harvard University Press.

Roll Back Malaria. 2010. About RBM. Available at: http://www.rollbackmalaria.org/index. html. Accessed: May 21, 2010.

Rollin B. 1995. The Frankenstein Syndrome: Ethical and Social Issues in the Genetic Engineering of Animals. Cambridge: Cambridge University Press.

2006. Animal Rights and Human Morality, 3rd ed. New York: Prometheus Books.

Rolston III H. 1994. Environmental ethics: values in and duties toward the natural world. In Gruen L and Jamieson D (eds.). Reflecting on Nature. New York: Oxford University Press: 65–84.

Romeis J, Meissle M, and Bigler F. 2006. Transgenic crops expressing Bacillus thuringiensis toxins and biological control. Nature Biotechnology 24: 63–71.

Romero S. 2010. Haiti lies in ruins; grim search for untold dead. The New York Times, January 14, 2010: A1.

Rosenberg A. 2000. Darwinism in Philosophy, Social Science and Policy. Cambridge: Cambridge University Press.

Rosenthal E. 2008. As more eat meat, a bid to cut emissions. The New York Times, December 8, 2008: A1.

2009. Climate change treaty, to go beyond the Kyoto Protocol, is expected by the year's end. The New York Times, June 12, 2009: A5.

2010. Skeptics find fault with U.N. climate panel. The New York Times, February 9, 2010: A1.

2011. For many species, no escape as temperature rises. The New York Times, January 21, 2011: A1.

Rosner H. 2004. Turning genetically engineered trees into toxic avengers. The New York Times, August 3, 2004: A1.

Ross WD. 1930. The Right and the Good. Oxford: Oxford University Press.

Rowland FS. 2006. Stratospheric ozone depletion. Philosophical Transactions of the Royal Society of London B: Biological Science 361: 769–90.

Rudant J, Menegaux F, Leverger G, Baruchel A, Nelken B, Bertrand Y, Patte C, Pacquement H, Vérité C, Robert A, Michel G, Margueritte G, Gandemer V, Hémon D, and Clavel J. 2007. Household exposure to pesticides and risk of childhood hematopoietic malignancies: The ESCALE study (SFCE). Environmental Health Perspectives 115: 1787–93.

Ryan PB. 2010. Exposure assessment, industrial hygiene, and environmental management. In: Frumkin H (ed.). Environmental Health: From Global to Local, 2nd ed. New York: John Wiley and Sons: 109–36.

Sagoff M. 1984. Ethics and economics in environmental law. In: Regan T (ed.). Earthbound: New Introductory Essays on Environmental Ethics. New York: Random House: 147–78.

Sailor WC, Bodansky D, Braun C, Fetter S, and van der Zwaan B. 2000. Nuclear power: a nuclear solution to climate change? Science 288: 1177–78.

Saletan W. 2008. Food apartheid: banning fast food in poor neighborhoods. Slate, July 31, 2008. Available at: http://www.slate.com/id/2196397. Accessed: June 24, 2010.

Samet JM, Avila-Tang E, Boffetta P, Hannan LM, Olivo-Marston S, Thun MJ, and Rudin CM. 2009. Lung cancer in never smokers: clinical epidemiology and environmental risk factors. Clinical Cancer Research 15: 5626–45.

Samuelson P and Nordhaus W. 2009. Economics, 19th ed. New York: McGraw-Hill.

Sandel M. 1981. Liberalism and the Limits of Justice. Cambridge: Cambridge University Press.

Sandin P. 2004. Better Safe than Sorry: Applying Philosophical Methods to the Debate on Risk and the Precautionary Principle. Stockholm: Theses in Philosophy from the Royal Institute of Technology.

Sanger DE and Broad WJ. 2010. Inspectors say Iran worked on warhead. The New York Times, February 18, 2010: A1.

Sattar N, Preiss D, Murray HM, Welsh P, Buckley BM, de Craen AJ, Seshasai SR, McMurray JJ, Freeman DJ, Jukema JW, Macfarlane PW, Packard CJ, Stott DJ, Westendorp RG, Shepherd J, Davis BR, Pressel SL, Marchioli R, Marfisi RM, Maggioni AP, Tavazzi L, Tognoni G, Kjekshus J, Pedersen TR, Cook TJ, Gotto AM, Clearfield MB, Downs JR, Nakamura H, Ohashi Y, Mizuno K, Ray KK, and Ford I. 2010. Statins and risk of incident diabetes: a collaborative meta-analysis of randomised statin trials. Lancet 375: 735–42.

Savolainen K, Alenius H, Norppa H, Pylkkänen L, Tuomi T, and Kasper G. 2010. Risk assessment of engineered nanomaterials and nanotechnologies – a review. Toxicology 269: 92–104.

Scheirmeier Q. 2011. Increased flood risk linked to global warming. Nature 470: 316.

Schulze WD, Brookshire DS, Hageman RK, and Tschirhart J. 1987. Benefits and costs of earthquake resistant buildings. Southern Economics Journal 53: 934–51.

Schwarzman MR and Wilson MP. 2010. New science for chemicals policy. Science 326: 1065–66.

Schweitzer A. 1959. The Philosophy of Civilization. New York: MacMillan.

Science Daily. 2009. How to deflect asteroids and save the Earth. Science Daily, April 20, 2009. Available at: http://www.sciencedaily.com/releases/2009/04/090416125212.htm. Accessed: March 27, 2010.

Scientific American. 2010. Reservations about toxic waste: Native American tribes encouraged to turn down lucrative hazardous disposal deals. March 31, 2010. Available at: http://www.scientificamerican.com/article.cfm?id=earth-talk-reservations-about-toxic-waste. Accessed: July 24, 2010.

Seabloom EW, Dobson AP, and Stoms DM. 2002. Extinction rates under nonrandom patterns of habitat loss. Proceedings of the National Academy of Sciences 99: 11229–34.

Sears MK, Hellmich RL, Stanley-Horn DE, Oberhauser KS, Pleasants JM, Mattila HR, Siegfried BD, and Dively GP. 2001. Impact of BT corn pollen on monarch butterfly populations: a risk assessment. Proceedings of the National Academy of Sciences 98: 11937–42.

Selgelid M. 2007. Ethics and drug resistance. Bioethics 21: 218–29.

Sen A. 2000. Development as Freedom. New York: Anchor Books.

Service R. 2008. Eyeing oil, synthetic biologists mine microbes for black gold. Science 322: 522–23.

  2010. Is there a road ahead for cellulosic ethanol? Science 329: 784–85.

Severance CA. 2009. Business risks to utilities as nuclear power costs escalate. The Electricity Journal 22: 112–20.

Shamoo A and Resnik DB. 2006. Strategies to minimize risks and exploitation in Phase One trials on healthy subjects. American Journal of Bioethics 6, 3: W1–13.

2009. Responsible Conduct of Research, 2nd ed. New York: Oxford University Press.

Shannon MA, Bohn PW, Elimelech M, Georgiadis JG, Mariñas BJ, and Mayes AM. 2008. Science and technology for water purification in the coming decades. Nature 452: 301–10.

Shelton D. 2005. Encyclopedia of Genocide and Crimes Against Humanity. Detroit, MI: Macmillan Reference.

Shrader-Frechette KS. 1988. Agriculture, ethics, and restrictions on property rights. Agricultural and Environmental Ethics 1: 21–40.

1991. Risk and Rationality. Berkeley: University of California Press.

1994. Ethics of Scientific Research. Lanham, MD: Rowman and Littlefield.

2002. Environmental Justice: Creating Equity, Reclaiming Democracy. New York: Oxford University Press.

2007a. Taking Action, Saving Lives. New York: Oxford University Press.

2007b. EPA's 2006 human-subjects rule for pesticide experiments. Accountability in Research 14: 211–54.

Sierra Club. 2010. Toxics: Pesticides and Global Warming. Available at: http://www.sierraclub.org/toxics/pesticides/default.aspx. Accessed: May 26, 2010.

Simon RL. 2003. Fair Play: The Ethics of Sport, 2nd ed. Boulder, CO: Westview Press.

Singer P. 1993. Practical Ethics, 2nd ed. Cambridge: Cambridge University Press.

Singer P and Mason J. 2007. The Ethics of What We Eat: Why Our Food Choices Matter. New York: Rodale Books.

Sister Study. 2010. Frequently asked questions. Available at: http://www.sisterstudy.org/English/faq2.htm#1. Accessed: April 6, 2010.

Sly PD, Eskenazi B, Pronczuk J, Srám R, Diaz-Barriga F, Machin DG, Carpenter DO, Surdu S, and Meslin EM. 2009. Ethical issues in measuring biomarkers in children's environmental health. Environmental Health Perspectives 117: 1185–90.

Small-Farm-Permaculture-And-Sustainable-Living.com. 2010. Advantages and disadvantages of organic farming. Available at: http://www.small-farm-permaculture-and-sustainable-living.com/advantages_and_disadvantages_organic_farming.html. Accessed: May 23, 2010.

Smart JJC and Williams B. 1973. Utilitarianism: For and Against. Cambridge: Cambridge University Press.

Smith G. 2011. Southern Illinois flood: appeals court oks levee blast. Chicago Tribune, May 1, 2011: A1.

Smith J. 2011. A long shadow over Fukushima. Nature 472: 7.

Smith MD, Asche F, Guttormsen AG, and Wiener JB. 2010. Genetically modified salmon and full impact assessment. Science 330: 1052–53.

Snyder B. 2008. How to reach a compromise on drilling in ANWR. Energy Policy 36: 937–39.

Soberón M, Pardo-López L, López I, Gómez I, Tabashnik BE, and Bravo A. 2007. Engineering modified BT toxins to counter insect resistance. Science 318: 1640–42.

Solomon S, Qin D, Manning M, Marquis M, Averyt K, Tignor M, Miller Jr. HL, and Chen Z. 2007. Climate Change 2007: The Physical Basis. Working Group I Contribution to the Fourth Assessment Report of the Intergovernmental Panel on Climate Change. Cambridge: Cambridge University Press.

Sorrell S, Speirs J, Bentley R, Brandt A, and Miller R. 2010. Global oil depletion: a review of the evidence. Energy Policy 38: 5290–95.

Spencer RW. 2010. Climate Confusion. New York: Encounter Books.

Spriggs M. 2004. Canaries in the mines: children, risk, non-therapeutic research, and justice. Journal of Medical Ethics 30: 176–81.

Stebbins GL. 1982. Darwin to DNA, Molecules to Humanity. New York: WH Freeman.

Steenland K and Moe C. 2010. Environmental and occupational epidemiology. In: Frumkin H (ed.). Environmental Health: From Global to Local, 2nd ed. New York: John Wiley and Sons: 79–108.

Stenfors N, Bosson J, Helleday R, Behndig AF, Pourazar J, Törnqvist H, Kelly FJ, Frew AJ, Sandström T, Mudway IS, and Blomber A. 2010. Ozone exposure enhances mast-cell inflammation in asthmatic airways despite inhaled corticosteroid therapy. Inhalation Toxicology 22: 133–39.

Stern VM, Smith RF, van den Bosch R, and Hagen KS. 1959. The integrated control concept. Hilgardia 29: 81–101.

Stokstad E. 2002. Engineered fish: friend or foe of the environment? Science 297: 1797–99.

2008. Spotted owl recovery plan flaws, review panel finds. Science 320: 594–95.

2011. Can biotech and organic farmers get along? Science 322: 166–69.

Stone R. 2010. Climate talks still at impasse, China buffs its green reputation. Science 330: 305.

2011. The legacy of Three Gorges Dam. Science 333: 817.

Strong, C. 2000. Specified principlism: what is it, and does it really resolve cases better than casuistry? Journal of Medicine and Philosophy 25: 323–41.

Sudhira HS, Ramachandra TV, and Jagadish KS. 2004. Urban sprawl: metrics, dynamics and modelling using GIS. International Journal of Applied Earth Observation and Geoinformation 5: 29–39.

Sunstein CR. 2005. Laws of Fear: Beyond the Precautionary Principle. Cambridge: Cambridge University Press.

Taylor P. 1986. Respect for Nature: A Theory of Environmental Ethics. Princeton NJ: Princeton University Press.

Taubenberger JK and Morens DM. 2006. 1918 Influenza: the mother of all pandemics. Emerging Infectious Diseases 12: 15–22.

Teitel M. 2001. Genetically engineered food: not ready for prime time. Nutrition 17: 61–62.

Thompson DF. 2004. Restoring Responsibility: Ethics in Government, Business, and Healthcare. Cambridge: Cambridge University Press.

Thompson PB. 2010. Food Biotechnology in Ethical Perspective, 2nd ed. Dordrect, Netherlands: Springer.

Thompson PB and Hannah W. 2008. Food and agricultural biotechnology: a summary and analysis of ethical concerns. Advances in Biochemical Engineering and Biotechnology 111: 229–64.

Thomson JJ. 1976. Killing, letting die, and the trolley problem. The Monist 59: 204–27.

1992. The Realm of Rights. Cambridge, MA: Harvard University Press.

Thorton M. 1991. Alcohol prohibition was a failure. Policy Analysis 157, July 17, 1991. Available at: http://www.cato.org/pub_display.php?pub_id=1017. Accessed: June 21, 2010.

Tollefson J. 2010. Geoengineering faces ban. Nature 468: 13–14.

2011. The sceptic meets his match. Nature 475: 440–41.

Travis J. 2005. Hurricane Katrina: scientists' fears come true as hurricane floods New Orleans. Science 309: 1656–59.

UNAIDS. 2010. A global view of HIV infection. Available at: http://data.unaids.org/pub/GlobalReport/2008/GR08_2007_HIVPrevWallMap_GR08_en.jpg. Accessed: October 20, 2010.

Unger P. 1996. Living High and Letting Die. Oxford: Oxford University Press.

Union of Concerned Scientists. 2006. European Union bans antibiotics for growth promotion. Available at: http://www.ucsusa.org/food_and_agriculture/solutions/wise_antibiotics/european-union-bans.html. Accessed: May 27, 2010.

2009. Clean energy 101. Available at: http://www.ucsusa.org/clean_energy/clean_energy_101/. Accessed: September 18, 2010.

2010a. Roundup ready soybeans. Available at: http://www.ucsusa.org/food_and_agriculture/science_and_impacts/impacts_genetic_engineering/roundup-ready-soybeans.html. Accessed: June 1, 2010.

2010b. Got water? Nuclear power plant cooling needs. Available at: http://www.ucsusa.org/assets/documents/nuclear_power/20071204-ucs-brief-got-water.pdf. Accessed: September 17, 2010.

2011. Scientific consensus on global warming. Available at: http://www.ucsusa.org/ssi/climate-change/scientific-consensus-on.html. Accessed: August 18, 2011.

United Nations. 1992. Rio Declaration on Environment and Development. Available at: http://www.un-documents.net/rio-dec.htm. Accessed: May 7, 2010.

2005a. World urbanization prospects: 2005 revision. Available at: http://www.un.org/esa/population/publications/WUP2005/2005wup.htm. Accessed: August 5, 2010.

2005b. Population challenges and development goals. Available at: http://www.un.org/esa/population/publications/pop_challenges/Population_Challenges.pdf. Accessed: August 29, 2010.

2009. World population prospects: the 2008 revision. Population Newsletter, June 2009, 87: 1. Available at: http://www.un.org/esa/population/publications/popnews/Newsltr_87.pdf. Accessed: May 25, 2010.

United Nations Framework Convention on Climate Change. 2010. Kyoto Protocol. Available at: http://unfccc.int/kyoto_protocol/items/2830.php. Accessed: July 8, 2010.

U.S. Census Bureau. 2010a. International database. Available at: 2010 http://www.census.gov/cgi-bin/broker. Accessed: August 28, 2010.

2010b. Expectation of life at birth and projections. Available at: http://www.census.gov/compendia/statab/2010/tables/10s0102.xls. Accessed: October 19, 2010.

U.S. Constitution. 1787. Available at: http://www.archives.gov/exhibits/charters/constitution.html. Accessed: October 27, 2010.

U.S. Department of Agriculture. 2009. Organic agriculture: Organic market overview. Available at: http://www.ers.usda.gov/Briefing/Organic/Demand.htm. Accessed: May 24, 2010.

2010. Organic production. Available at: http://www.ers.usda.gov/Data/Organic/. Accessed: May 24, 2010.

2011a. Invasive species – plants. Available at: http://www.invasivespeciesinfo.gov/plants/main.shtml. Accessed: March 21, 2011.

2011b. Adoption of genetically engineered crops in the U.S. Available at: http://www.ers.usda.gov/Data/BiotechCrops/. Accessed: August 29, 2011.

U.S. Department of Veterans Affairs. 2010. Agent Orange: Diseases associated with Agent Orange exposure. Available at: http://www.publichealth.va.gov/exposures/agentorange/diseases.asp. Accessed: November 12, 2010.

U.S. Fish and Wildlife Service. 2010a. Environmental contaminants program. Available at: http://www.fws.gov/contaminants/issues/pesticides.cfm. Accessed: May 22, 2010.

2010b. Extinct species. Available at: http://www.fws.gov/midwest/endangered/lists/extinct.html. Accessed: August 20, 2010.

2010c. Endangered species program. Available at: http://www.fws.gov/endangered/species/us-species.html. Accessed: August 20, 2010.

Van Bortel W, Trung HD, Thuan le K, Sochantha T, Socheat D, Sumrandee C, Baimai V, Keokenchanh K, Samlane P, Roelants P, Denis L, Verhaeghen K, Obsomer V, and Coosemans M. 2008. The insecticide resistance status of malaria vectors in the Mekong region. Malaria Journal 5: 102.

van den Berg H. 2009. Global status of DDT and its alternatives for use in vector control to prevent disease. Environmental Health Perspectives 117: 1656–63.

Vanengelsdorp D, Evans JD, Saegerman C, Mullin C, Haubruge E, Nguyen BK, Frazier M, Frazier J, Cox-Foster D, Chen Y, Underwood R, Tarpy DR, and Pettis JS. 2009. Colony collapse disorder: a descriptive study. PLoS One 4: e6481.

van Luijn HE, Aaronson NK, Keus RB, and Musschenga AW. 2006. The evaluation of the risks and benefits of phase II cancer clinical trials by institutional review board (IRB) members: a case study. Journal of Medical Ethics 32:170–76.

Varner G. 1998. In Nature's Interests? Interests, Animal Rights, and Environmental Ethics. Oxford: Oxford University Press.

Varner GE. 1995. Can animal rights activists be environmentalists?. In: Pierce C and Van de Veer D (eds.). Basic Issues in Environmental Ethics, 2nd ed. Belmont, CA: Wadsworth: 254–73.

Vetrica. 2004. Chocolate poisoning in the dog. Available at: http://www.vetrica.com/care/dog/chocolate.shtml. Accessed: March 31, 2010.

Viscusi WK. 1983. Risk by Choice: Regulating Health and Safety in the Workplace. Cambridge, Harvard University Press.

    1992. Fatal Tradeoffs: Public and Private Responsibility for Risk. New York: Oxford University Press.

vom Saal FS and Hughes C. 2005. An extensive new literature concerning low-dose effects of Bisphenol-A shows the need for new risk assessment. Environmental Health Perspectives 113: 926–33.

von Braum J. 2010. Strategic body needed to beat food crises. Nature 465: 548–49.

Wakabayashi D and Inada D. 2009. Baby bundle: Japan's cash incentive for parenthood. The Wall Street Journal, October 9, 2009. Available at: http://personaldividends.com/money/miranda/income-tax-breaks-children. Accessed: August 31, 2010.

Walker K. 2000. Cost-comparison of DDT and alternative insecticides for malaria control. Medical and Veterinary Entomology 14: 345–54.

Wall S. 2010. Wind energy in North Carolina. North Carolina Bar Association, June 29, 2010. Available at: http://environmentenergyandnaturalresourceslaw.ncbar.org/newsletters/environmentalnewsjune2010/windenergy.aspx. Accessed: October 3, 2010.

Wallace SS. 2005. ANWR: the great divide. Smithsonian, 36, 7: 48–56.

Waltz E. 2011. GM grass eludes outmoded USDA oversight. Nature Biotechnology 29: 772–73.

Walzer M. 1983. Spheres of Justice. Oxford: Blackwell.

Warren MA. 2000. The moral difference between infanticide and abortion: a response to Robert Card. Bioethics 14: 352–59.

Water.org. 2011. Water facts. Available at: http://water.org/learn-about-the-water-crisis/facts/. Accessed: August 30, 2011.

Watkins B, Shepard P, and Corbin-Mark C. 2009. Completing the circle: a model for effective community review of environmental health research. American Journal of Public Health 99: S567–77.

Weale A. 2010. Ethical arguments relevant to the use of GM crops. Nature Biotechnology 27: 582–87.

Weckert J and Moore J. 2006. The precautionary principle in nanotechnology. International Journal of Applied Philosophy 2: 191–204.

Weeks JL. 1991. Occupational health and safety regulation in the coal mining industry: public health at the workplace. Annual Review of Public Health 12: 195–207.

Wegener HC. 2003. Antibiotics in animal feed and their role in resistance development. Current Opinion in Microbiology 6: 439–45.

Weijer C and Emanuel EJ. 2000. Protecting communities in biomedical research. Science 289: 1142–44.

Weiss R. 2008. USDA recommends that foods from clones stay off the market. The Washington Post, January 16, 2008: A3.

Wendler D and Miller FG. 2008. In: Emanuel EJ, Grady C, Crouch RA, Lie R, Miller F, and Wendler D (eds.). The Oxford Textbook of Clinical Research Ethics. New York: Oxford University Press: 503–12.

Wertheimer A. 1999. Exploitation. Princeton, NJ: Princeton University Press.

White Jr. L. 1967. The historical roots of our ecological crisis. Science 55: 1203–07.

Whitman DB. 2000. Genetically modified foods: harmful or helpful? ProQuest, April 2000. Available at: http://www.csa.com/discoveryguides/gmfood/overview.php. Accessed: June 1, 2010.

Wigle DT, Turner MC, and Krewski D. 2009. A systematic review and meta-analysis of childhood leukemia and parental occupational pesticide exposure. Environmental Health Perspectives 117: 1505–13.

Wijffels RH and Barbosa MJ. An outlook on microalgal biofuels. Science 329: 796–99.

Wilcox B and Jessop H. 2010. Ecology and environmental health. In: Frumkin H (ed.). Environmental Health: From Global to Local, 2nd ed. New York: John Wiley and Sons: 3–47.

Wiley LF and Gostin LO. 2009. The international response to climate change: an agenda for global health. Journal of the American Medical Association 302: 1218–20.

Williams D. 2009. Radiation carcinogenesis: lesson from Chernobyl. Oncogene 27: S9–18.

Wilson AM, Wake CP, Kelly T, and Salloway JC. 2005. Air pollution, weather, and respiratory emergency room visits in two northern New England cities: an ecological time-series study. Environmental Research 97: 312–21.

Wilson EO. 1984. Biophilia. Cambridge, MA: Harvard University Press.

Wing S and Wolf S. 2000. Intensive livestock operations, health, and quality of life among eastern North Carolina residents. Environmental Health Perspectives 108: 233–238.

Winn WC. 1988. Legionnaire's Disease: historical perspective. Clinical Microbiology Reviews 1: 60–81.

Winograd IJ and Roseboom EH Jr. 2008. Nuclear waste. Yucca Mountain revisited. Science 320: 1426–27.

Wolf SM, Lawrenz FP, Nelson CA, Kahn JP, Cho MK, Clayton EW, Fletcher JG, Georgieff MK, Hammerschmidt D, Hudson K, Illes J, Kapur V, Keane MA, Koenig BA, Leroy BS, McFarland EG, Paradise J, Parker LS, Terry SF, Van Ness B, and Wilfond BS. 2008. Managing incidental findings in human subjects research: analysis and recommendations. Journal of Law, Medicine and Ethics 36: 219–48.

Wolff A. 2001. Jewish perspectives genetic engineering. Tishrei 5762, 2, October 2001. Available at: http://www.jcpa.org/art/jep2.htm. Accessed: March 1, 2011.

Wolfenbarger LL and Phifer PR. 2000. The ecological risks and benefits of genetically engineered plants. Science 290: 2088–92.

Woodside J, McKinley M, and Young I. 2008. Saturated and trans fatty acids and coronary heart disease. Current Atherosclerosis Reports 10: 460–66.

World Bank. 2010a. What is poverty? Available at: http://web.worldbank.org/WBSITE/ EXTERNAL/TOPICS/EXTPOVERTY/EXTPA/0,,contentMDK:20153855~menuP K:435040~pagePK:148956~piPK:216618~theSitePK:430367,00.html. Accessed: May 23, 2010.

2010b. World development indicators database, revised July 9, 2010. Available at: http:// siteresources.worldbank.org/DATASTATISTICS/Resources/GNIPC.pdf. Accessed: August 25, 2010.

World Commission on Environment and Development. 1987. Our Common Future. New York: Oxford University Press.

World Food Programme. 2010. What causes hunger? Available at: http://www.wfp.org/ hunger/causes. Accessed: May 23, 2010.

World Health Organization. 2002. Antimicrobial resistance. Available at: http://www.who. int/mediacentre/factsheets/fs194/en/. Accessed: May 28, 2010.

2006. Malaria vector control and personal protection. Available at: http://whqlibdoc. who.int/trs/WHO_TRS_936_eng.pdf. Accessed: March 23, 2010.

2007. Iraq. Available at: http://www.who.int/countryfocus/cooperation_strategy/ccs-brief_irq_en.pdf. Accessed: March 27, 2010.

2010a. WHO global malaria programme. Available at: http://www.who.int/malaria/ about_us/en/index.html. Accessed: March 23, 2010.

2010b. Environmental health. Available at: http://www.who.int/topics/environmental_ health/en/. Accessed: March 26, 2010.

2010c. Frequently asked questions. Available at: http://www.who.int/suggestions/faq/en/ index.html. Accessed: April 1, 2010.

2010d. Food security. Available at: http://www.who.int/trade/glossary/story028/en/. Accessed: May 25, 2010.

2010e. 20 questions on genetically modified foods. Available at: http://www.who.int/ foodsafety/publications/biotech/20questions/en/. Accessed: June 11, 2010.

2010f. Obesity and overweight. Available at: http://www.who.int/dietphysicalactivity/ publications/facts/obesity/en/. Accessed: June 24, 2010.

2010g. Water sanitation and health. Available at: http://www.who.int/water_sanitation_ health/mdg1/en/index.html. Accessed: July 13, 2010.

2010h. Global health observatory. Available at: http://www.who.int/gho/en/. Accessed: October 20, 2010.

2010i. Progress and prospects for the use of genetically modified mosquitoes to inhibit disease transmission. Available at: http://apps.who.int/tdr/publications/training-guideline-publications/gmm-report/pdf/gmm-report.pdf. Accessed: February 21, 2011.

World Hunger Education Service. World hunger facts 2010. Available at: http://www.worldhunger.org/articles/Learn/world%20hunger%20facts%202002.htm. Accessed: May 23, 2010.

World Medical Association. 2008. Declaration of Helsinki. Available at: http://www.wma.net/en/30publications/10policies/b3/index.html. Accessed: November 16, 2010.

World Resources Institute. 2008. June 2008 monthly update: Genetically modified crops and the future of world agriculture. Available at: http://earthtrends.wri.org/updates/node/313. Accessed: June 1, 2010.

    2010. Energy consumption: Total energy consumption per capita. Available at: http://earthtrends.wri.org/searchable_db/index.php?theme=6&variable_ID=351&action=select_countries. Accessed: October 11, 2010.

    2011. Deforestation: The assault continues. Available at: http://www.wri.org/publication/content/8368. Accessed: August 30, 2011.

Worldwatch Institute. 2009. Water scarcity looms as population, temperature rise. Available at: http://www.worldwatch.org/node/6217. Accessed: July 18, 2010.

Xu J, Kochanek KD, Murphy SL, and Tejada-Vera B. 2010. Deaths: final data for 2007. National Vital Statistics Report 58, 19. Available at: http://www.cdc.gov/nchs/data/nvsr/nvsr58/nvsr58_19.pdf. Accessed: October 20, 2010.

York G and Mick H. 2008. 'Last ghost' of the Vietnam War. The Globe and Mail, July 12, 2008. Available at: http://www.theglobeandmail.com/archives/article697346.ece. Accessed: May 13, 2010.

Young MC, Muñoz-Furlong A, and Sicherer SH. 2009. Management of food allergies in schools: a perspective for allergists. Journal of Allergy and Clinical Immunology 124:175–82.

Zehnder G, Gurr GM, Kühne S, Wade MR, Wratten SD, and Wyss E. 2007. Arthropod pest management in organic crops. Annual Review Entomology 52: 57–80.

Zeller Jr. T. 2010. E.P.A. considers risks of gas extraction. New York Times, July 23, 2010: B1.

Zhang J, Mauzerall DL, Zhu T, Liang S, Ezzati M, and Remais JV. 2010. Environmental health in China: progress towards clean air and safe water. Lancet 375: 1110–19.

INDEX